SERS-Based Advanced Diagnostics for Infectious Diseases

Online at: https://doi.org/10.1088/978-0-7503-5920-7

IOP Series in Global Health and Radiation Oncology

Series editor
Wilfred Ngwa
Dana-Farber/Harvard Cancer Center, University of Massachusetts Lowell, Johns Hopkins University, USA

Editor biography
Wilfred Ngwa is the Director of the Global Health Catalyst, a cross-institutional collaboration initiative launched at Harvard to catalyze high impact collaborations in global health. He currently serves as Adjunct Professor at the University of Massachusetts, as Associate Professor of Radiation Oncology at Johns Hopkins University and as ICTU Distinguished Professor of Public Health. He is a chair of the Lancet Oncology Commission for Sub-Saharan Africa, has published three books on global health and serves on the editorial board of a number journals, including ASCO's *Journal of Global Oncology, Ecancermedicalsciences*, and *Frontiers in Oncology*. He has won many awards from Harvard, the USA National Institutes of Health, and International professional organizations for his innovations and leading work in global health to address disparities in the USA and globally.

Aims and scope
This series includes books in the emerging area of global radiation oncology and its applications in global health. Building on the published book by the series editor entitled *Emerging Models for Global Health in Radiation Oncology*, it will further detail the work being done globally to promote cancer research and awareness, particularly in lower-income countries.

SERS-Based Advanced Diagnostics for Infectious Diseases

Edited by

Raju Khan, Shalu Yadav and Mohd Abubakar Sadique

CSIR-Advanced Materials & Processes Research Institute (AMPRI), India

IOP Publishing, Bristol, UK

Permission to make use of IOP Publishing content other than as set out above may be sought at permissions@ioppublishing.org.

Raju Khan, Shalu Yadav and Mohd Abubakar Sadique have asserted their right to be identified as the editors of this work in accordance with sections 77 and 78 of the Copyright, Designs and Patents Act 1988.

ISBN   978-0-7503-5920-7 (ebook)
ISBN   978-0-7503-5917-7 (print)
ISBN   978-0-7503-5918-4 (myPrint)
ISBN   978-0-7503-5919-1 (mobi)

DOI   10.1088/978-0-7503-5920-7

Version: 20230501

IOP ebooks

British Library Cataloguing-in-Publication Data: A catalogue record for this book is available from the British Library.

Published by IOP Publishing, wholly owned by The Institute of Physics, London

IOP Publishing, No.2 The Distillery, Glassfields, Avon Street, Bristol, BS2 0GR, UK

US Office: IOP Publishing, Inc., 190 North Independence Mall West, Suite 601, Philadelphia, PA 19106, USA

*All knowledge that the world has ever received comes from the mind;
the infinite library of the universe is in our mind.*
—Swami Vivekananda

Contents

3 Historical review of SERS in biomedical applications: infectious diseases

Muhammad Usman, Jia-Wei Tang, Zheng-Kang Li, Jin-Xin Lai, Kai-Xuan Yuan, Qing-Hua Liu, Xiao Zhang and Liang Wang

Preface

Raman spectroscopy enables the identification of molecular vibrations giving characteristic specific signals of each molecule. However, it has some limitations of its own such as that low-density scattering signals are very weak and they get capped with other noise signals. Surface enhanced Raman spectroscopy (SERS) is a powerful technique which has gained much attention in the research community due to its several advantages. Among emerging novel detection techniques, SERS has come out as a robust analytical tool for analysis of single-molecule-level sensitivity and capacity of quantitative detection. In the SERS sensing technique, amplified inelastic light scatters from the molecules after being absorbed on the surface of metals. The frequency modulation of excitation light and localized surface plasmonic resonance (LSPR) of the metallic nanomaterial could enhance the scattering signal by a thousand times. The potential of SERS significantly increased after the discovery of its detection of microorganisms. The future clinical applications paved the way in healthcare for the rapid detection of pathogens, especially viruses. Infectious diseases, which are caused by pathogens such as bacteria and viruses, are responsible for millions of deaths worldwide. Respiratory infectious diseases, such as influenza, tuberculosis, and pneumonia, lead to 5 million deaths every year. Recently, the advent of coronavirus disease has resulted in an ongoing global COVID-19 pandemic. Driven by the growing demand for healthcare and point-of-care test applications, next-generation diagnostic tools of diseases require sensing platforms that enable rapid, quantitative readout of analytes with excellent specificity and sensitivity. SERS-based detection methods have shown promise in overcoming the low sensitivity and multiplex detection problems inherent to conventional detection methods like RT-PCR, ELISA, LFIA, CRISPR, LAMP, etc. SERS technology has appeared as one of the most reliable emerging technologies among the various other biosensors and gained much attention due to its extraordinary properties like ultra-sensitivity and specificity, and its utilization in different fields of science like biomedical, energy conversion, physics, chemical sensing, biosensing, material science, photocatalysis,etc.

The book mainly deals with the integration of SERS with other conventional diagnostic tools to overcome the inaccuracy, time-consuming and expensive nature of conventional methods like ELISA, RT-PCR, LFIA. It also highlights the investigation of the current status and future opportunities associated with other SERS-based devices for the point-of-care (POC) diagnosis of infectious diseases. The miniaturization ability of SERS-based devices makes them promising in biosensor applications and gives them the potential to make a better alternative to conventional diagnostic methods.

A brief description of the chapters of the book is given below.

At the outset, the first chapter 'Fundamentals of Raman and surface-enhanced Raman spectroscopy in diagnostics' includes the basic applications of Raman characterization technique and the need of SERS technique with its working principle for disease diagnosis. This Chapter briefly introduces the book and importance of SERS and its application in the healthcare industry.

The subsequent chapter 'Overview of infectious diseases and their diagnostic techniques' includes the various infectious diseases like influenza, tuberculosis, coronavirus diseases, Zika, HIV, Ebola etc, and the action of mechanism and their detection techniques are discussed in detail.

The third chapter 'Historical preview of SERS in biomedical applications: infectious diseases' includes the use of SERS as a diagnostic tool in medical industry with its previous developments and applications. It includes the early age development of the technique, its primary uses and how SERS gradually came into the medical industry.

The next chapter 'Use of nanotechnology in SERS-based diagnostics', includes the utility of nanomaterials to build the SERS setup, process optimization and performance enhancement with the use of nanotechnology.

The chapter entitled 'Significance, design, and synthesis method of SERS tags/probes', includes fabrication and advancements in the SERS tags or nanotags that play an important role in signal enhancement. The use of different types of nanostructures for fabrication of SERS tags properties responsible for the SERS effect and its practical use in biomedical application is explored.

The chapter 'SERS integrated detection techniques for clinical samples, overcoming the challenges', includes the integration of SERS with other available diagnostic techniques for the application of SERS in real samples and the challenges associated with it.

The chapter 'SERS-based point-of-care biosensors for rapid detection of viral infections: SARS-CoV-2 study', comprises currently developed point-of-care-based biosensors for the rapid detection of the viral infections such as lateral flow immunoassay, optical, microfluidics electrochemical etc, and their integration with SERS to enhance and give more accurate, sensitive results.

The chapter 'SERS-based lateral flow immunoassay for viral infections', includes the use of integrated SERS and lateral flow immunoassay platform to diagnose disease more effectively, with better performance parameters. It will also discuss the probable futuristic advancements as per demand and to overcome present bottlenecks.

The chapter 'SERS-based microfluidics for real sample detection' discusses the combined use of SERS along with microfluidics-based detection setup in order to achieve high sensitivity, throughput and enhanced results for viral infections, specifically the SARS-CoV-2 virus.

The chapter 'IoMT-based SERS detection as advanced diagnostics' includes the use of computational techniques such as artificial intelligence and internet of medical things to solve the limitations of current diagnostics. The integration of digital technology in SERS-based devices would aid the characteristics of detection as a futuristic approach for viral infections, even significant help in COVID-19 pandemic management.

The penultimate chapter 'Optimization of SERS setup for high efficiency, rapid detection of infectious diseases', includes the optimization, improvement and analysis of various parameters responsible for giving gold standard results. High demand, accurate results, sensitivity, portability, ease and rapid testing are needs which can only be fulfilled after proper analysis and optimization of each and every component of the SERS technique and the device design.

The last chapter 'Future potential of SERS-based advanced diagnosis in real-life conditions', includes the conclusion of the book, the ideas gathered from the in-depth literature, practical challenges and their solutions. Theree is discussion about feasible advancements in the SERS technique and its better utilization in real-life conditions such as pandemics, outbreaks, other microbiological infections. SERS has the potential to be a helping hand in current pandemic management and for any future need as well.

The overall aim of this book is intended to collect, organize, aware, establish a link between researchers and manufacturers for the successful end-user commercialization of technology with effective approach to control and manage the infectious diseases. The use of SERS-based techniques and their utilization in diagnostic applications is a great breakthrough in medical, material science and bio-nano-technology as an effective tool to fight against infectious diseases. This will be a multidisciplinary book with the interface between nano-biotechnology, material science, chemistry, physics and healthcare industry.

Raju Khan
Shalu Yadav
Mohd Abubakar Sadique

Acknowledgements

The editors are sincerely thankful to every contributor to the book. Their heartfelt efforts, hard work, and rational approach are greatly acknowledged. At the same time, the editors would like to acknowledge the publisher and the associated team for their constant support, guidance, and inspiration which regularly thrust us to the fore to complete this book.

The beneficial suggestion and support given by Dr Avanish Kumar Srivastava, Director, CSIR-Advanced Materials and Processes Research Institute, Bhopal, MP, India, is duly acknowledged.

Raju Khan expresses his special thanks to his parents, wife Shazia M Siddiqui, daughter Sara Khan and son Aayan Khan for their everlasting love, enthusiasm for science, and encouragement to pursue every task successfully.

Shalu Yadav would like to acknowledge with gratitude, the support and love of her family—her parents, Usha and Sudhir; her brother Ashish and sister Bhavna. They all kept her going, and the work done by her would have not been possible without the continual support of them.

Mohd Abubakar Sadique expresses particular gratitude to his parents, family members, colleagues and friends for their continual care and encouragement.

Additionally, the editors are sincerely appreciative of all who have directly or indirectly offered important input to this book.

Raju Khan
Shalu Yadav
Mohd Abubakar Sadique

Editor biographies

Raju Khan

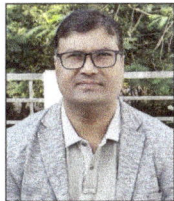

Raju Khan is currently a Senior Principal Scientist and Professor in the Industrial Waste Utilization, Nano and Biomaterials division at the CSIR-Advanced Materials and Processes Research Institute. He received his PhD in Physical Chemistry from Jamia Millia Islamia, Central University, New Delhi, India and was a Postdoctoral Fellow at the Sensor Research Laboratory in the Department of Chemistry at the University of the Western Cape in Cape Town, South Africa. He has more than 15 years of R&D experience at CSIR and other academic R&D Institutes. He has published more than 80 articles SCI journals, which have attracted more than 2500 citations, published more than 25 book chapters in the reputed books of Elsevier and Taylor Francis, and edited 15 books published by Elsevier, Institute of Physics Publishing and CRC Press. His current research is on electrochemical biosensor for clinical applications.

Shalu Yadav

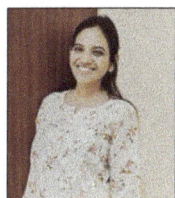

Shalu Yadav is currently working as PhD (research scholar) under supervision of Dr Raju Khan in CSIR-AMPRI, Bhopal. She has completed her BSc and MSc degree from Dr Bhimrao Ambedkar University, Agra, Uttar Pradesh, India. Her research interest is electrochemistry, nanotechnology and material sciences, synthesis of 2D nanomaterials, fabrication of biosensors, and applications concerning Infectious diseases. She has several research and review articles and book chapters under her profile.

Mohd Abubakar Sadique

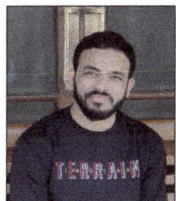

Mohd Abubakar Sadique is currently a Junior Research Fellow at CSIR-AMPRI in Bhopal, India. He is working on a DST-SERB project entitled 'Development of Rapid Electrochemical based Diagnostics for Detection of SARS-CoV-2 Infection'. Mr Sadique was a Gold Medalist in MTech and received his post-graduate degree in Nanotechnology from Aligarh Muslim University. Mr Sadique's particular research interest involves carbon-based nano-structures and their effectiveness in the purview of biosensing, diagnostics, therapeutics, and healthcare applications.

List of contributors

Sarbari Acharya
Department of Biology, School of Applied Sciences, KIIT, India

Puja Adhikari
Department of Biotechnology, Maharishi Markandeshwar University, Mullana, Ambala, India

Lal Singh Banjara
Government Indira Gandhi Home Science Girls PG College, Shahdol, India

Soumyadeep Basu
Amity University, Kolkata, India

Ioana Brezeştean
National Institute of R&D of Isotopic and Molecular Technologies, Cluj-Napoca, Romania

Santhosh Chidangil
Centre of Excellence for Biophotonics, Department of Atomic and Molecular Physics, Manipal Academy of Higher Education, Manipal, India

Nicoleta Elena Dina
National Institute of R&D of Isotopic and Molecular Technologies, Cluj-Napoca, Romania

Kritika Gaur
NIMS Institute of Allied Medical Science and Technology, NIMS University, Jaipur, Rajasthan, India

Sajan D George
Centre of Excellence for Biophotonics, Department of Atomic and Molecular Physics, Manipal Academy of Higher Education, Manipal, India

Ana Maria Raluca Gherman
National Institute of R&D of Isotopic and Molecular Technologies, Cluj-Napoca, Romania
Faculty of Physics, Babe-Bolyai University, Cluj-Napoca, Romania

Samar Ghopry
Jazan University, Jazan, Saudi Arabia

Shagun Gupta
Department of Biotechnology, Maharishi Markandeshwar University, Mullana, Ambala, India

Anwesha Kanungo
Department of Biology, School of Applied Sciences, KIIT, India

Ankur Kaushal
Department of Biotechnology, Maharishi Markandeshwar University, Mullana, Ambala, India

Raju Khan
Academy of Scientific and Innovative Research (AcSIR), Ghaziabad, UP, India
Industrial Waste Utilization, Nano and Biomaterials, CSIR-Advanced Materials and Processes Research Institute (AMPRI), Bhopal, MP, India

Vedika Khare
School of Nanotechnology, UTD, RGPV Campus, Gandhi Nagar, Bhopal, India

Neeraj Kumar
CSIR-Advanced Materials and Processes Research Institute (AMPRI), Bhopal, India
Academy of Scientific and Innovative Research (AcSIR), Ghaziabad, India

Jin-Xin Lai
Guangdong Provincial People's Hospital, Guangzhou, Guangdong, China

Zheng-Kang Li
Guangdong Provincial People's Hospital, Guangzhou, Guangdong, China

Qing-Hua Liu
Macau University of Science and Technology, Taipa, Macau, China

Jijo Lukose
Centre of Excellence for Biophotonics, Department of Atomic and Molecular Physics, Manipal Academy of Higher Education, Manipal, India

Arpana Parihar
Industrial Waste Utilization, Nano and Biomaterials, CSIR-Advanced Materials and Processes Research Institute (AMPRI), Hoshangabad Road, Bhopal, MP, India

Shadhan Raja
Department of Biotechnology, Maharishi Markandeshwar University, Mullana, Ambala, India

Pushpesh Ranjan
CSIR-Advanced Materials and Processes Research Institute (AMPRI), Bhopal, India
Academy of Scientific and Innovative Research (AcSIR), Ghaziabad, India

Mohd Abubakar Sadique
CSIR-Advanced Materials and Processes Research Institute (AMPRI), Bhopal, India
Academy of Scientific and Innovative Research (AcSIR), Ghaziabad, India

Apoorva Shrivastava
Dr D Y Patil Biotechnology and Bioinformatics Institute, Dr D Y Patil Vidyapeeth, Tathawade, Pune, Maharashtra, India

Ayushi Singhal
Academy of Scientific and Innovative Research (AcSIR), Ghaziabad, UP, India
Industrial Waste Utilization, Nano and Biomaterials, CSIR-Advanced Materials and Processes Research Institute (AMPRI), Bhopal, MP, India

Sumit
Department of Biotechnology, Maharishi Markandeshwar University, Mullana, Ambala, India

Jia-Wei Tang
Xuzhou Medical University, Xuzhou, Jiangsu Province, China

Garima Tripathi
VIT University, Vellore, India

Shweta Tripathi
Amity University, Kolkata, India

Muhammad Usman
Xuzhou Medical University, Xuzhou, Jiangsu Province, China

Liang Wang
Guangdong Provincial People's Hospital, Guangzhou, Guangdong, China

Judy Wu
University of Kansas, Lawrence, Kansas, USA

Shalu Yadav
CSIR-Advanced Materials and Processes Research Institute (AMPRI), Bhopal, India
Academy of Scientific and Innovative Research (AcSIR), Ghaziabad, India

Kai-Xuan Yuan
Guangdong Provincial People's Hospital, Guangzhou, Guangdong, China

Xiao Zhang
Xuzhou Medical University, Xuzhou, Jiangsu Province, China

Chapter 1

Fundamentals of surface-enhanced Raman spectroscopy in diagnostics

Soumyadeep Basu, Garima Tripathi and Shweta Tripathi

Raman spectroscopy is a vibrational technique in the field of spectroscopic analysis that deals with the quantification of inelastic light scattering processes. Moreover, the potential applicability of the Raman spectroscopic technique in a diverse range of fields, such as chemical sensing, biological imaging, and material characterization, has helped it gain increasing interest from varied scientific disciplines. In inelastic scattering, monochromatic light experiences an alteration in its frequency at the interface with any sort of vibrational mode of molecules. The rapid increase in the advancement of science and technology has resulted in the availability of improved laser sources, compact spectrometers, and efficient detectors, thereby leading to the development of Raman spectroscopy as a highly sensitive spectrometric technique that can probe the structural details of complex molecular configurations. The inherent characteristic of this technique of exhibiting a low scattering cross-section has restricted the implementation of traditional Raman spectroscopy. With the inception of surface-enhanced Raman spectroscopy (SERS), an approach based on the intensified amplification of Raman scattering by metallic nanostructures, Raman spectroscopy has established its place as a diagnostic method in the research community. This phenomenon has inspired a multitude of highly discerning diagnostic technologies in analytical chemistry, medical biotechnology, nanomedical engineering, drug delivery, and life sciences. In this chapter we highlight the fundamental characterization of Raman spectroscopy as a balanced and cogent method that will provide promising directions for future research and growth in the repertoire of diagnostics.

1.1 Introduction

The human body is always experiencing broad exposure to a diverse range of infectious pathogenic activities, such as viral, bacterial, fungal, protozoan, and helminthic, which lead to the degeneration of tissue through varied mechanisms. These microbes have an immense ability to manipulate the host-cell organization in many ways and continuously evolve to preserve their survival and thrive in all species.

Since the emergence of COVID-19, the novel coronavirus disease, in December 2019, the virus has become a global pandemic that has raised significant concern in terms of public health. The advent of this unusual coronavirus has emphasized the importance of speed, sensitivity, and specificity in the diagnostic machinery for the detection and prevention of infectious diseases [1]. Nucleotide identification strategies, such as the polymerase chain reaction (PCR), which comprises the amplification of DNA, RNA, and miRNA and their detection with the use of fluorescence, are the current standard. Although it is such a sensitive technique, PCR requires certain specific strains, advanced devices (such as thermocyclers), and expensive reagents such as primers, aptamers, buffers, and so on [2–4]. The procedure for PCR is, moreover, a time-consuming process, running repetitive cycles. Many antigen detection immunoassays such as the enzyme-linked immunosorbent assay (ELISA) have greatly complemented PCR protocols. These techniques also pose challenges, as special attention has to be given to the target antigen or antibody for binding with the pathogen, and the inadequate sensitivity levels and the long assay times in ELISA have raised questions around ease-of-use and effectiveness [5].

In contrast to these ultra-modern methodologies, Raman spectroscopy is a promising approach that helps in delivering the requirements of specificity, sensitivity, and rapidity of action without the involvement of various expression sequence tags (EST), primers, or antibodies/antigens. The inelastic scattering of photons, the exchange of energy between the photon particles, accompanied by the vibrational motion of the photonic components with low energy, denoting Raman's Stoke shift, or with increased energy interaction, denoting anti-Stokes Raman shift, in Raman spectroscopy, has initiated a favorable application in the field of biomedical science, depicted in the figure 1.1. Principally, its implementation as a label-free method which is based on internal signals from the specimens of interest can help in the direct diagnosis of microorganisms, diseased cells, or molecules in the absence of a marker. An impressive attribute of Raman reporters is their resistance to photobleaching. The sharp spectral peaks in Raman spectroscopy aid in superior multiplexing to specifically designed biomarkers at effective rates. The procedure is more resistant to water absorption than infrared spectroscopy, which is a crucial aspect of probing biological samples [6].

Although Raman spectroscopy has a good level of portability, the possibility of being used in personalized medication with careful application can be attributed by the property of one of the photons undergoing inelastic scattering, Raman signals can be improved with the use of controlled interactivity of light and matter, thereby leading to a specialized approach—surface-enhanced Raman spectroscopy (SERS) [7]. SERS is dependent on the plasmonic resonance of metallic substrates and their chemical charge transfer efficiency, which favors simultaneously the localized electric field from the incident light along with the light that is dispersed from the target specimen [8, 9]. The detection of clinically relevant biomarkers such as

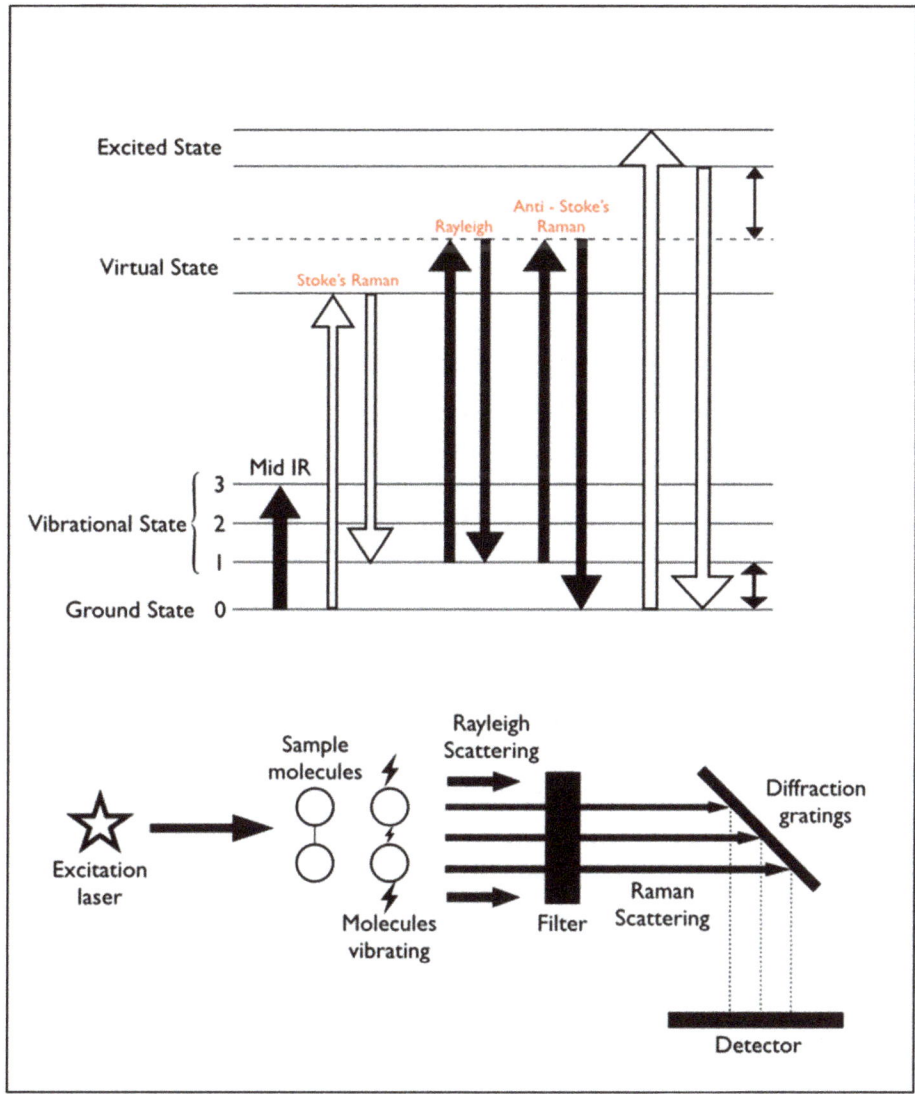

Figure 1.1. Schematic representation of the architecture of Raman spectroscopy and the principles of Raman effects.

antibodies, nucleic acids [10, 11], and peptides at a molecular level [12–14] is possible using Raman spectroscopy, hence it is a potential tool for the diagnosis of tumor markers, and for managing conditions such as chronic diabetes and hypertension.

SERS has been used in practice as a diagnostic tool for infectious diseases by targeting viral and bacterial microbes, e.g. rhinovirus, influenza, and parainfluenza, with 90% specificity, which stands in contrast to the current quantitative reverse transcription PCR (RT-qPCR). It has been highly valuable in determining antibiotic susceptibility, the identification of bacterial elements, analysing colonial growths in microbes, examining intracellular signaling pathways, and the detection and monitoring of the p24 antigen in blood plasma for HIV, as the robust SERS signaling mechanism does not require sample amplification, allowing its efficacy in intracellular mutation detection and antiviral resistance testing. In this chapter we intend to highlight the fundamentals of Raman spectroscopy and SERS as promising techniques in the arena of diagnostics that will efficiently help in accelerating the tracking and testing of virulent diseases, personalized medicative strategies, and precision health.

1.2 The fundamental principle behind Raman spectroscopy and surface-enhanced Raman spectroscopy (SERS)

The idea behind Raman spectroscopy is that as radiation can be reflected, absorbed, or scattered, monochromatic radiation can be passed through a sample in such a manner that the above inference can be obtained. The frequency of scattered photons is different from the incident photons as the rotational and vibrational properties vary. This causes a change in the wavelength, which is examined in the infra-red (IR) spectra [15].

The variance between a scattered photon and the incident photon is called the Raman shift. When the energy related to the dispersed photons is lower than the energy of an incident photon, the scattering is called Stokes's scattering. When the energy of the dispersed photons is higher than that of the incident photon, the scattering is called anti-Stokes's scattering.

1.2.1 Quantum theory of the Raman effect

The polarizability of molecules is the basis of the classical theory of the Raman effect, which considers how easily the electron cloud of a molecule is deformed by an electric field. The method is based on molecular distortion in an electric field E detected by molecular polarizability. The dispersed light has a significant equivalent to the incident light (Rayleigh), equivalent to the incident light plus the vibrational frequency (anti-Stokes), and equivalent to the incident light minus the vibrational frequency (Stokes) [16].

Upon interaction of light with matter, the photons that comprise the light may be absorbed or dispersed or may not interact with the material and in some instances pass directly through it [17]. When there is an interaction between monochromatic light and molecules, the majority of the photons are dispersed without significant alteration in their energy. This process is termed elastic or Rayleigh scattering, and it occurs when the electrons in a molecule vibrate (oscillate) in resonance with the administered electric field of the incident light. However, a minute number of photons (1 out of 10^6–10^9) are inelastically dispersed and experience a change in energy. The correlations between frequency, wavenumber, wavelength, and energy are as follows:

- $E = h\nu$ (ν is the frequency in s^{-1} and h is Planck's constant).
- $E = hc\nu'$ (ν' is the wavenumber in cm^{-1} and c is the speed of light in cm s^{-1}).
- $N = 1/\lambda$ (wavelength is represented in nm by λ).

The inelastic dispersing process is called the Raman effect (Raman scattering). The change in photon energy occurs because a molecule may vibrate during that time and an electric field is applied which causes the electrons to oscillate in resonance. A vibrational mode that alters the dipole moment induced by an electric field (molecular polarizability) causes a change in incident photon energy. The variance in energy between the inelastically scattered photons and the incident photons is called the Raman shift. The representation of the intensity of the inelastically dispersed light as an outcome of the energy change is called the Raman spectrum [18].

1.2.2 Stoke's shift

The Stokes shift term can also be used in Raman spectroscopy, where it explains whether the Raman dispersed radiation is at higher energy (anti-Stokes shifted) or lower energy (Stokes shifted) than the Rayleigh dispersed radiation [15]. The majority of photons scatter molecules elastically with no change in the vibrational energy of molecules during the scattering process (Rayleigh scattering) when radiation is scattered from a molecule. In Stokes Raman scattering the molecule attains a quantum of vibrational energy from the photon during the dispersing process and the Stokes radiation, hence it has a longer wavelength than the incident radiation [18]. In anti-Stokes Raman scattering the opposite happens, with the molecule ejecting a quantum of vibrational energy in the dispersing process, and the anti-Stokes radiation hence has a shorter wavelength than the incident radiation.

1.2.3 Efficacy of SERS compared to conventional Raman spectroscopy

Surface-enhanced Raman spectroscopy has the ability to manipulate the ability of metallic nanoscale structures to concentrate upon the electromagnetic energy through optical nodes that are referred to as surface plasmons. In contrast to conventional Raman spectroscopy, the major advantage of SERS is the enhanced level and improvement of the Raman intensity for varied orders of magnitude, which is established widely to arise from the congruence of electromagnetic and chemical mechanisms. Raman scattering deals with the interactivity between the molecule and the incoming radiation. At the same time, for the occurrence of SERS, the presence of metallic nanostructures is imperative. SERS deals with the interaction between the light radiation, the molecule, and the metallic structure. When irradiation of a metallic nanostructure occurs within the course of incident light exposure, delocalization of the electrons into collective oscillatory pathways take place, which leads to the emergence of an electromagnetic field at the interface of the metal nanostructure and the dielectric surrounding (figure 1.2(A)).

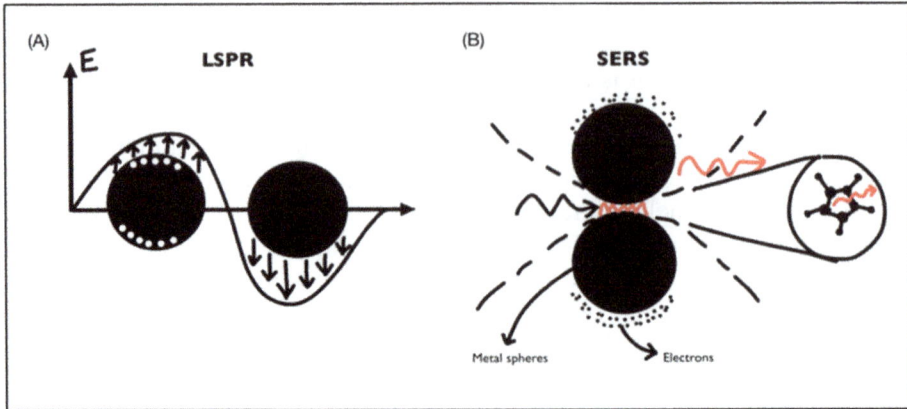

Figure 1.2. (A) Localized surface plasmon resonance (LSPR) effect—the electrons are undergoing excitation within the oscillation which results in an electromagnetic field that is localized at the interface where light is irradiated. (B) Interactivity between the nanoparticle and the molecule causing the Raman polarizability (red arrow) and the localized field (black arrow) inducing enhanced Raman signaling through SERS.

Factors that affect the frequency of such oscillations are the electron density, the mass of the electrons, and the shape and size of the distributive charge. In general, the local electromagnetic field that is produced within the localized surface plasmon resonance is higher in correspondence to the magnitude of the field, which helps in the improved levels of the electromagnetic field in SERS. Moreover, the interaction of molecules with the adjoining metallic nanostructures creates a resultant excitation phase, which denotes the Raman polarizability by the localized field. This, in turn, increases the SERS scale four-fold, due to the overall enhancement of the localized electromagnetic field (figure 1.2(B)) [19].

Raman spectroscopy has the following disadvantages that reduce its level of effectiveness in the field of diagnostics. They are as follows:

- The equipment required is quite costly.
- Metallic structures or alloys are not supported.
- There is difficulty in the measurement of lower concentrations of samples.
- The process of heating of samples from using the laser radiation mechanism can lead to the destruction of samples.

Enhancement in the Raman signal by 10–15-fold, using SERS, can lead to the quantification of a single molecule. SERS includes enhancement at both the electromagnetic and chemical level, of which the electromagnetic enhancement exhibits greater significance. Electromagnetic enhancement contributes significantly as it increases the improvement level up to ten-fold. The effect is visible after the absorption of an analyte onto a rough surface that causes an excitation phase triggering the formation of plasmons. The energy is traversed back into the plasmon and the scattering of the radiation can be easily recorded by the use of a spectrometer. When two nanostructures are in close proximity to each other it generates a coupling action, and this is denoted as hotspots. The resident molecules of the hotspots experience increased levels of localized electromagnetic field, resulting in a further enhancing effect. This enhancement leads to lower magnitudes of laser power, thereby protecting the samples from any sort of radiation destruction, reducing the time for integration and speeding up the process of acquisition.

1.3 Label-free Raman and SERS improving spectral analysis

A spectroscopic fingerprint of biological agents is obtained specifically through the use of label-free SERS. Hence, this technique can be incorporated easily into screening a wide spectrum of patient samples. This is very effective for the detection of bacterial inflammations such as infections of the bloodstream and urinary tract, or the sites where we can detect an overexpression of more than 30–35 bacterial species, each having different complexities in their susceptibility towards antibiotic interaction in the least masking concentrations [20]. Label-free SERS is a promising approach for segregating various viral agents and the expressivity of their species.

Through label-free SERS, data analysis has taken an advanced trajectory and provided prediction algorithms that enable proper elucidation and characterization of the spectra. Knowledge engineering-based methodologies that include principal component analysis (PCA) clustering can detect certain undetermined Raman or SERS spectral information sets and can lead to the visualization of different spectral variations obtained without having any previous knowledge of the characterized categories. Moreover, Raman signatures have remained advantageous with the emergence of advanced data analysis methods such as neural network (NN) techniques and support vector machines (SVMs), which have become critical approaches in Raman spectral analysis. Raman spectral interpretation can be achieved directly by NNs without the involvement of pre-processing, i.e. artifact elimination and background de-rectification, thereby avoiding of all the possible misinterpretations that might be a result of signal pre-processing.

Taking this further, beyond the general prospects of spectral analysis, computer-based mechanistic algorithms can cater to the next generation of SERS substrate design. One major characteristic feature of SERS diagnostics is that it requires crucially an increased electromagnetic enriched field that imparts a specific level of uniformity across the desired biomarkers. In the case of viral and bacterial pathogens, the signal enhancements are fixed at a determined range between several tens of nanometers to micrometers. The localized electromagnetic characteristics can be modified easily with the use of metasurfaces that act upon the nanoscale architectural framework, whose composition can be of gold or silver microfilms. The most striking feature is that they provide an increased efficacy of uniform signal enhancement distributed over a large surface area, giving rise to standardized enhancements [21] (figure 1.3).

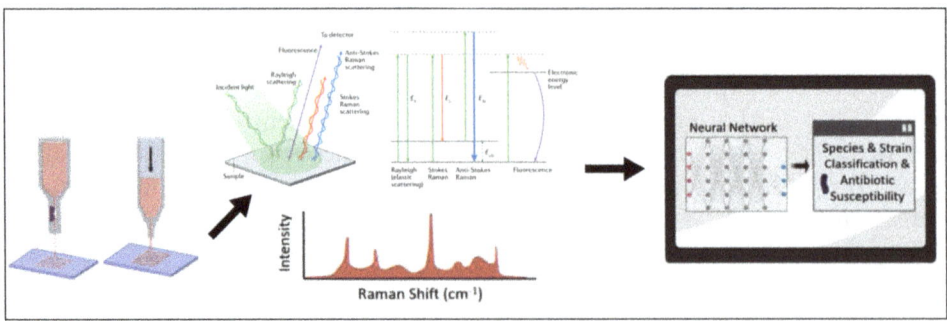

Figure 1.3. Schematic depiction of the utilization of Raman spectroscopy from the process of sample preparation to spectral interpretation.

1.4 Rapid, sensitive, and analyte-dependent diagnosis using SERS affinity agents and nanotags

Label-free SERS has been accepted categorically for providing an increased magnitude of sensitivity and specificity for quantifying analytical samples. Various infectious disease conditions require different approaches for loading the pathogen of the sample obtained from the patient, based on the stage to which the infection has progressed, and the sample source, which can be obtained, for example, through nasopharyngeal swabs or broncho tracheal lavage. Then finally comes the type of disease. Label-free SERS, with help of its novel approach, can investigate, at a much more rapid pace, complex entities such as blood, not involving any sort of amplification in the process.

As a result, this increases the sensitivity and specificity levels, thereby helping in the proper diagnosis of several multiplexed biomarkers. The unique nature of label-free SERS has led to its use for a plethora of affinity agents, comprising antibodies, aptamers, and so on. Along with this strategy, where SERS can successfully deliver in targeting analytes on affinity agents, the use of Raman reporters, such as resonant fluorescent dyes or aromatic thiols, has helped in increasing the signaling spectrum of the technique. The mechanism involved in this technique shows how these Raman reporters can be effectively administered into the SERS substrate or directly into the affinity agent and favor the quantification and interpretation of less concentrated sample specimens. Recombinant antibody fragments are incorporated very well to address the major drawbacks that arise in for monoclonal antibodies, as they are small in shape and size and are immobilized rapidly on the SERS substrate [22].

In addition to antibodies, versatility, specificity, and compact target binding capabilities along with an increased density for packing have been exhibited on SERS substrates. From a different viewpoint, polymers, such as polyethylene glycol, are highly volatile biocompatible polymers with intense flexibility, resulting in correct stabilization of SERS metal particles for a controlled level of synthesizing prowess with a properly defined administration of thiol groups. N-isopropyl

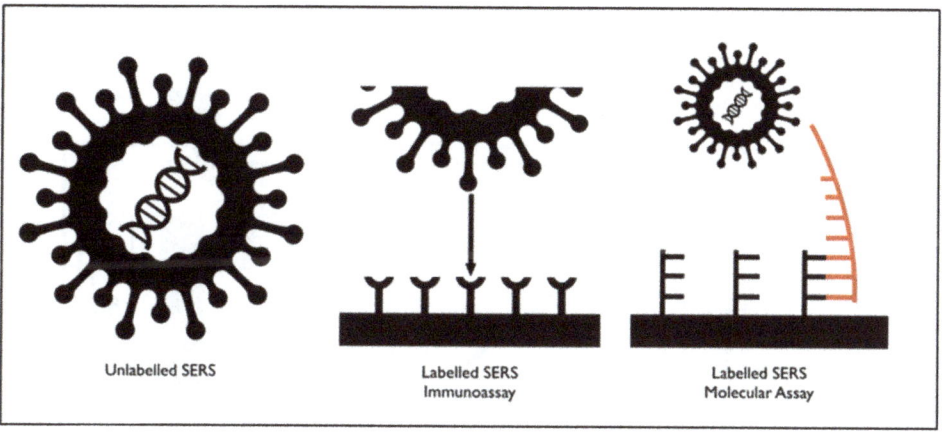

Figure 1.4. Modes of performance for SERS-based influenza testing.

acrylamide (PNIAM), fashioned to be a porous structure, allows the insertion of a Raman reporter with a potential mechanism of diffusion and entrapment without the requirement for any specific affinity for any metal [22, 23]. Thanks to its extremely cost-effective nature, versatile attributes in chemical moiety targeting, binding sites, and close distance from the SERS substrate, this technology has the potential to be confirmed as a sophisticated and powerful weapon in the diagnostics of pathogens (figure 1.4).

1.5 SERS enables sample processing in the field of microfluidics and bioprinting

Sample preparation plays a critical role in the application of SERS. The current clinical standards, such as ELISA, PCR processing, mass spectrometry, etc, require an incubation period for a sample, amplification of smaller quantities of desired compound components, and purification to limit any background signals from contemporaneous components of samples [24]. Advanced technical methodologies and developments in the sphere of microfluidics and bioprinting can increase the aptitude for SERS sample creation. In the sector of point-of-care diagnosis and for clinical applicability these methods can prove advantageous for both labeled and unlabeled SERS.

Microfluidics is defined as the manipulative power of fluid flows that remain functional at very low Reynolds numbers. Microfluidics in sub-millimeter channels undergo some type of diffusion-based mixing, giving rise to considerably predictable fluid behavior. Many elements combine to form lab-on-chip (LOC) designs for the integration of the preparation of the sample and site specific [25]. Microfluidic integration and optical spectrometric approaches have been able to achieve certain effective results for robust and reproducible SERS measurements. The integration of systems facilitates the reproducible nature of SERS and imparts it with a sensitive applicable feature in detecting minute analyte concentrations.

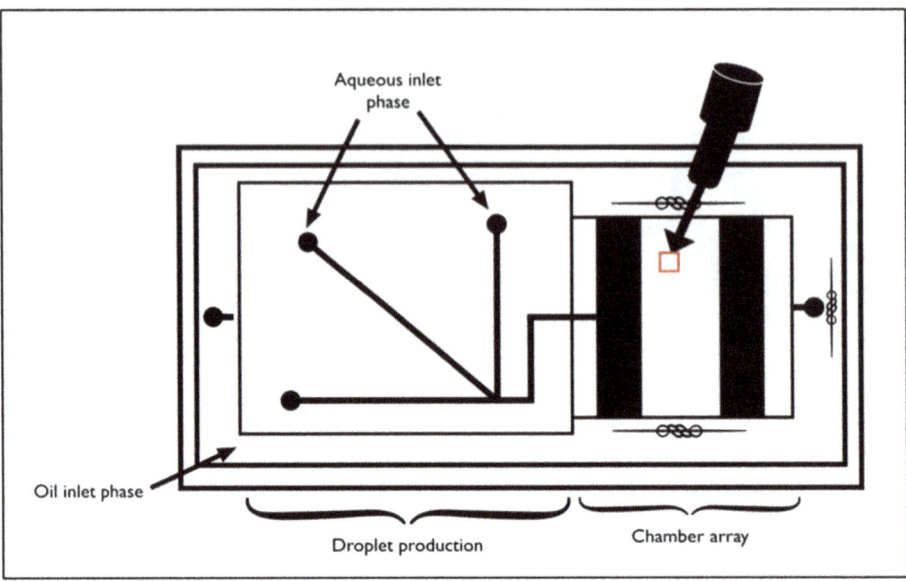

Figure 1.5. Representation of an integrated SERS–microfluidic platform.

The integration of bioprinting platforms in association with Raman spectroscopy is nascent, wherein inkjet printing has gradually achieve the precision to be used in conjunction with SERS, making way for future single-cell SERS interrogation. In this approach, an inkjet dispensed SERS that is commercially available as the HP D300e or D100 thermal inkjet digital dispenser and its associated HP bio-patterning are utilized for patterning microdroplets of 1,2-bis(4-pyridyl) ethylene (BPE) onto the substrate for SERS that contains a concentration at various levels. The droplet production technique using the bioprinting principle can help in designing of several assays for diagnostic purposes leading to a useful clinical adaptation of SERS [26, 27] (figure 1.5).

1.6 Applications of surface-enhanced Raman scattering spectroscopy (SERS) in diagnostics

SERS is used for different diagnostic processes in the medical field. The advantage of using SERS is that it can be used for marking organelles, non-invasive tagging of tissues, and ultra-detection of relevant biomolecules [28]. Among the available techniques of ELISA, fluorescence immunoassay (FIA), and radio immunoassay (RIA), SERS has risen to be a versatile technique with remarkable sensitivity and specificity for structural information of biological processes and media. It helps us to provide deeper knowledge about molecular systems and the different vibrational modes in the Raman spectrum. The technique works on the effect at nanoscale levels and, hence, this provides an electromagnetic field at the nano-metal surface. As the bio-analytes are highly sensitive to changes in the environment, such as pH, temperature, and ionic strength, they can be better detected in the SERS spectrum than in mass spectroscopy which requires prior processing of two biomolecules. Thus, the biomolecule under consideration can be diagnosed better using SERS [29].

1.6.1 Biomolecular sensing

In this type of diagnostic technique, SERS fingerprinting is used, detecting the target analyte directly. This is achieved by the sensitive binding of nanostructures and their consequent detection through SERS. Standard SERS is the technique that facilitates the formation of well-defined SERS spectra with a sufficient reproducible intensity as the signal acquired is from a dynamic system and not from discrete particles [30]. The limitation of this sensing technique lies in the fact that it is carried out on a dilute analyte, which is present in a colloidal state. Hence, the interaction of the particles is inhibited. Hence, the probability of obtaining the Raman spectrum and signals decreases [31].

Nanostructured films of gold and silver are used as direct sensing elements for SERS. This can be used for the ultra-detection and *in vivo* monitoring of biomolecules, pathogens, and metabolites. Statistics are also used along with the Raman spectrum, resolving and characterizing the complex patterns [32, 33]. This can help us in the further in-depth diagnosis of the molecules involved in various biological pathways and systems. With the help of a diagnostics test such as PCA the components can be analysed and can be used for the detection of drug design and components [34].

1.6.2 Point-of-care diagnostics

Flexible biosensors working on the principle of Raman spectroscopy and SERS are capable of fingerprinting and label-free detection of particles and their consequent development in low concentrations and non-invasive sample [35, 36]. In particular, SERS technology built from flexible materials offers superior advantages over traditional SERS detection instruments based on rigid substrates [37]. For example, a common approach to rigid-substrate-based traditional SERS detection in environmental monitoring applications is the complex extraction of analytes from outdoor objects and their application on SERS substrates for analysis. This means a long sample preparation step in a laboratory environment before adsorption of the analyte.

Based on the variety of purposes that flexible SERS aims to achieve, there are three main categories of current flexible SERS platforms: (i) actively tunable SERS; (ii) the swab-sampling SERS strategy; and (iii) the *in situ* SERS detection approach.

The SERS platform allows point-of-care diagnostics, a very detailed area of study and research. These different subfields are explored via macromolecular identification and efficient extraction. SERS works on plasmonic nanostructures and substrates which are even functional for lower analytes and the analytes which show little adhesion with the particles [38].

1.6.3 Bioprinting

Diffusion-based mixing occurs in microflows in sub-millimeter channels, resulting in consistent fluid behavior. Although depending exclusively on diffusion results in extensive mixing durations, a variety of active and passive mixing and separation techniques are available to meet the challenges of sample preparation, speed, and signal homogeneity in clinical samples [39, 40]. Many parts can be merged on a single device, resulting in an LOC that combines bioreactions, sample preparation, and detection.

For reliable and repeatable SERS experiments, integrated microfluidic and optical spectroscopic devices have lately gained attention [41]. The development of high temporal resolution spectroscopy devices that fit the kilohertz range enabled the integration of Raman spectroscopy.

1.6.4 Single-molecule detection

Single-molecule detection is one of the most relevant and useful applications of SERS. The SERS tests use excitation wavelengths located close to the resonance effect and the transition observed on the target molecule. In an experiment, Nie and Emory acquired an enhancement factor for a single molecule of rhodamine used in silver nanoparticle synthesis [42]. The hot aggregates produced can be detected by SERS which help in the development of the drug and its consequent action and effect on the target molecules.

Because SERS enhancement is primarily based on the electromagnetic (EM) enhancement process, which is caused by plasmon excitation in the substrate metal, SERS spectra with metals in the UV are not as common as in the visible spectral region. As a result, the UV–SERS activity of alternative substrate metals must be studied. Until now, UV–SERS investigations have used a 325 nm excitation wavelength. Ren *et al* reported the first UV–SERS enhancement in 2003 [43], using roughened rhodium and ruthenium electrodes as SERS substrates and demonstrating an enhancement for pyridine as a model molecule.

1.6.5 Tissue imaging and detection

The SERS-based detection system has made the detection of molecules and biomarkers involved directly and indirectly in the initiation and growth of disease an accessible mode of diagnosis [44]. In one study, gold nanoparticles coupled with SERS-based analysis were used in the detection of a specific prostate-specific antigen, associated with prostate cancer. This helps in the non-invasive and high-end diagnosis of the related disease and determining the localization of other components in the same [45]. SERS can also help to overcome the limitations posed by immune histopathological techniques. As SERS imaging is not bound to the tissue region and receptors, it can also be used in drug-delivery systems. Functionalized nanotags with antibodies can be used in clinical tissue samples and have been characterized by higher sensitivity and detection compatibility for the growth and development of various cancers and their biomarkers [46, 47].

1.6.6 SERS biosensors

These biosensors are highly sensitive and not only help in the enumeration of the disease-causing pathogens but also help in understanding the type of interaction involved with biomolecules and vital information to check the viability of the cells [48]. These sensors can also be used for breath analysis, which can detect the smallest amount of ethanol or acetone in the breath [49, 50]. *In situ* SERS-based nanosensors can be used for the detection of gastric cancer and its diagnostic sensitivity can be further assessed by gas chromatography-mass spectrometry (GC-MS) and quantitative characterization [51]. A SERS biosensor made by Qiao *et al* contains gold nanoparticles coated with ZIF-8 which can be used for the clinical analysis of lung cancer and can be used for the real-time understanding of its development [52].

Gold nanoparticles are used in sensors for SERS imaging purposes. They can be used in different biological systems for different applications. The characteristics of AuNPs after uptake and processing through the endocytic circulation pathways of the body, was investigated with diffusion rates and tracking down of the particle [53]. The Brain Research through Advancing Innovative Neurotechnology (BRAIN) Initiative in 2013 led to an over-all increase in the development of neurological studies and consequently helped in the development of nanoparticle use in SERS applications. Silver nanoparticles were used in the detection of GABA accumulation in the case of neurodegenerative diseases such as epilepsy.

In the case of diabetes, SERS is used in biosensor technology for quantifying the amount of glucose in urine samples. Kong *et al* performed an extensive study of the peaks obtained during the quantification of a glucose content sample and formed a new sensor that helped them to identify the amount more accurately and efficiently [54].

1.6.7 SERS use in the treatment of diseases

The use of nanostructures in the SERS analytical technique helps in the theranostics of disease [55]. Gold nanostars associated with the detection of SERS signals were used in the treatment of breast cancer. SERS functionalization with the TAT peptide was observed to be critical in the successful treatment of cancerous cells [56]. Several cases of drug-delivery-facilitating treatment using SERS analysis have been reported in the case of lung cancer and related disorders [57]. A SERS-based immunoassay is being used for the detection of several interleukins and cytokines. These are the biomarkers of several autoimmune disorders and hence help in the detection of their development and severity [58, 59].

The diagnosis of numerous viral and tropical diseases has been made possible by using the technology of SERS. Multilayered combinatorial Au/Ag nanorods were used to formulate a SERS substrate to be implemented on an array for effective fusion with rhodamine. This served as a probe that exhibited an incredible magnification factor and helped in detecting viral strains of influenza A (e.g. H2N2, H3N2, and H1N1). Nanospheres made of Au were linked with multi-branched gold nanostars to effectively integrate antibodies. The desired analytes present in the sample were rendered into lateral flow immunoassay (LFIA) strips, thereby inhibiting the migration of nucleoprotein complexes. The spectral data were recorded at the very point of accumulation on the strip. Further analysis of the allantoic fluid comprising the viral strain H1N1 of influenza A was conducted to consolidate the technique as an effective diagnostic for viral elements in the matrix [60, 61].

Gold nanoparticles in commercial diagnostic lateral flow assay (LFA) kit were exchanged with AuNPs linked with Raman reporter malachite green isothiocyanate (MGITC). The technique was able to determine the severity of influenza A with increased sensitivity [62, 63]. Hepatitis is a major source of liver diseases, which include liver cancer, ensuring the need for proper diagnosis. The maximum detection of hepatitis sample can often lead to complicated sample synthesis and is expensive, while surface-enhanced techniques for the diagnosis of hepatitis B virus (HBV) can be achieved with little to no sample synthesis and in a cost-efficient fashion.

There is a requirement for sensitive analysis for the detection of human immunodeficiency virus (HIV), which would permit the earlier detection of HIV infection. This initial diagnosis would permit the commencement of antiretroviral treatment earlier to avoid severe immuno-compromised repercussions, and diagnosis via SERS has developed as a unique technique due to the sensitivity provided by the method. A SERS-based HIV-1 DNA LFA biosensor, consisting of gold nano-particles labeled with Raman reporter MGITC, was integrated to thiolated ssDNA complementary to HIV-1 [64]. This SERS-based perspective also indicated three orders of magnitude lower LOD than color intensity and fluorescent diagnosis techniques. Mosquito-borne viruses such as West Nile (WNV), dengue (DENV), and Zika (ZIKV) have been the subject of research in recent years due to recent outbreaks of the diseases.

Similar symptomatic effects, pathogenicity, and prevalance over geographic regions have made it very difficult to segregate the vector borne tropical viral pathogens ZIKV and DENV. SERS-based nanostars made of gold can be used to create SERS-based immunoassays for proper integration into the antibodies that are specific for the respective viruses, wherein the Raman reporter molecules help in screening the non-structural protein 1 (NS1) biomarkers. Nanoparticle Au based SERS probes conjugated with anti-flavivirus antibodies can help in visualizing the two viral elements. The vector borne pathogen Chikungunya virus served as the negative control producing no Raman signals. The spectral variations helped in deducing the differences between two viruses [65, 66].

Difficulty in the clinical detection of dengue is hastening the implementation of point-of-care therapeutic support for febrile patients. In this chapter we intend to establish SERS applied diagnosis of dengue virus using blood samples clinically procured from a lot of patients. Standard NS1 antigen and IgM antibody ELISA kits were administered for all the samples collected. A glancing angle deposition technique was utilized to design the silver nanorods to be used as the SERS substrate. Appropriate quantities of blood serum from the patients were collected, examined, and reviewed [66]. Spectral readings of pure NS1 protein along with the spike protein in the serum were noted individually. For distinguishing dengue positives or healthy negatives statistically, PCA was carried out. Therefore, SERS

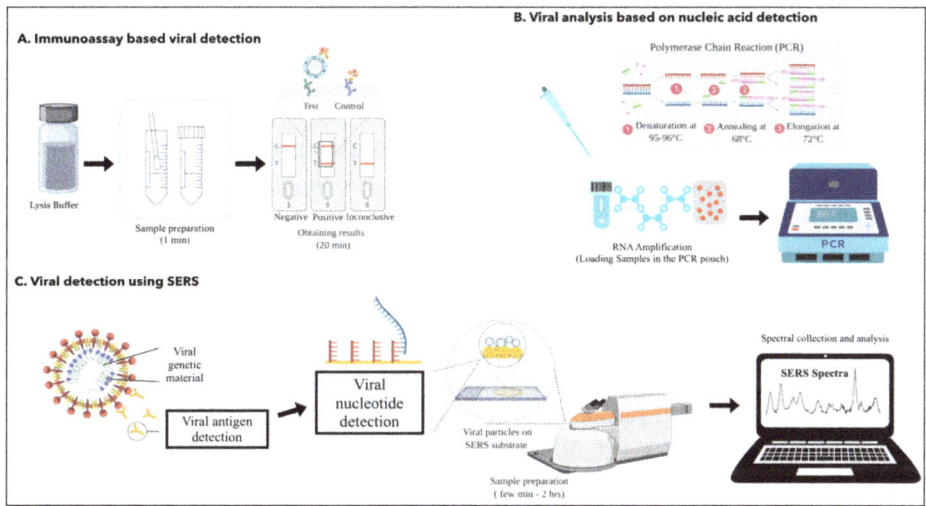

Figure 1.6. Schematic representation of clinical standard approaches and viral diagnostic procedures based on SERS.

technology is applicable for delivering a rapid and sensitive diagnostic confirmation of dengue during the presymptomatic phase [63] (figure 1.6).

1.7 Conclusion and future outlook

Raman spectroscopy has undoubtedly taken a significant position as a diagnostic tool in the field of biomedicine. The high specificity and sensitivity from the bioprinting approach for biomarkers, provides faster and multifaceted analytic support in an easily transportable and cost-effective medium. In the past, Raman spectroscopy experienced fewer coherent interfaces, an abundance of complexity in the spectral interpretation, and an absence of structured work efficacy from the collection of the sample specimens to spectral addition, making clinical interpretations challenging. Recent times have seen the modernization of nanophotonic SERS substrates, computational learning, microfluidity, and bioprinting that are potentially establishing some effective strategies to overcome these difficulties.

Label-free SERS, moreover, has been able to revolutionize the diagnostic disciplines based on Raman spectroscopy. This has led to advancements in enhancing the spectral interpretation of Raman signatures, which results in increased levels of accuracy and identification of microbial targets. Upon comparison of the different types of spectral analysis in protein level, macromolecular, nucleic acid, carbohydrates, and so on, Raman spectroscopy is used for better understating of cell–drug interactions, clinical trials including phase I in mouse models, phase II in secondary animals such as chimpanzees, and finally human trials along with the production of new antibiotics and antivirals. Advances in the computational approaches that are dependent on optical design methodologies have aided in enhancing the Raman specificity levels and clinical applicability.

Raman reporters have gained recognition in the detection of particular pathogens and their affinity agents in diagnostic assays. The versatile nature of the aptamers and polymers, with their smaller sizes, have enabled obtaining a larger packaging density, a minimum level of interference on the SERS signature, and a very cost-effective fabrication technique. These principles make it possible for SERS to target a particular pathogenic activity and identify pathogenic agents with a rapid processing time.

The approaches that have been extended into the areas of microfluidics and bioprinting have helped SERS to acquire proper validation to serve as an enabling and effective clinical interpretation tool that is based on the principles and mechanisms of Raman spectroscopy. Proper mixing, separation, and multiplexing strategies have favored the microfluidic media. This in turn has caused improved homogeneity and throughput. The bioprinting mechanism has created a wealth of suitable output procedures for infectious pathogen detection and diagnosis. SERS can be utilized as a sophisticated diagnostic tool that might be envisioned as having an advancing nanophotonic SERS substrate, computer-based learning approach, and bioprinting objectives for clinical diagnosis. The emergence of a pressing need for a rapid mode of infectious disease detection and susceptibility of drug examination has induced accelerated implementation of SERS for designing personalized patient care and accurate treatments.

Acknowledgments

We would like to thank Amity University Kolkata for giving us this opportunity to write this book chapter

References

[1] World Health Organization 2022 Laboratory testing for coronavirus disease 2019 (COVID-19) in suspected human cases: interim guidance, 2 March 2020 *Technical document* World Health Organization, Geneva https://apps.who.int/iris/handle/10665/331329

[2] Yeh Y *et al* 2019 A rapid and label-free platform for virus capture and identification from clinical samples *Proc. Natl Acad. Sci.* **117** 895–901

[3] Shanmukh S, Jones L, Driskell J, Zhao Y, Dluhy R and Tripp R 2006 Rapid and sensitive detection of respiratory virus molecular signatures using a silver nanorod array SERS substrate *Nano Lett.* **6** 2630–6

[4] Park H, Yang S and Choo J 2016 Early diagnosis of influenza virus A using surface-enhanced Raman scattering-based lateral flow assay *Bull. Korean Chem. Soc.* **37** 2019–24

[5] Schloter M, Aßmus B and Hartmann A 1995 The use of immunological methods to detect and identify bacteria in the environment *Biotechnol. Adv.* **13** 75–90

[6] Holly J B *et al* 2016 Using Raman spectroscopy to characterize biological materials *Nat. Protoc.* **11** 664–87

[7] Xiaoyu Z, Matthew A Y, Olga L and Richard P V D 2005 Rapid detection of an anthrax biomarker by surface-enhanced Raman spectroscopy *J. Am. Chem. Soc.* **127** 4484–9

[8] Kneipp K and Kneipp H 2006 Surface-enhanced Raman scattering on silver nanoparticles in different aggregation stages *Isr. J. Chem.* **46** 299–305

[9] Latorre F *et al* 2016 Spatial resolution of tip-enhanced Raman spectroscopy—DFT assessment of the chemical effect *Nanoscale* **8** 10229–39

[10] Kim W, Lee J, Song S, Kim S, Choi Y and Sim S 2019 A label-free, ultra-highly sensitive and multiplexed SERS nanoplasmonic biosensor for miRNA detection using a head-flocked gold nanopillar *Analyst* **144** 1768–76

[11] Hamm L, Gee A and Indrasekara A 2019 Recent advancement in the surface-enhanced Raman spectroscopy-based biosensors for infectious disease diagnosis *Appl. Sci.* **9** 1448

[12] Sharma B, Frontiera R, Henry A, Ringe E and Van Duyne R 2012 SERS: materials, applications, and the future *Mater. Today* **15** 16–25

[13] Le R E and Etchegoin P 2012 Single-molecule surface-enhanced Raman spectroscopy *Annu. Rev. Phys. Chem.* **63** 65–87

[14] Crozier K, Zhu W, Wang D, Lin S, Best M and Camden J 2014 Plasmonics for surface enhanced Raman scattering: nanoantennas for single molecules *IEEE J. Sel. Top. Quantum Electron.* **20** 152–62

[15] Butler H *et al* 2016 Using Raman spectroscopy to characterize biological materials *Nat. Protoc.* **11** 664–87

[16] Ball D W 2004 *Modern Spectroscopy* ed J Michael Hollas (New York: Wiley)

[17] Smith E and Dent G 2005 *Modern Raman Spectroscopy—a Practical Approach* (Chichester: Wiley)

[18] Schmitt M and Popp J 2006 Raman spectroscopy at the beginning of the twenty-first century *J. Raman Spectrosc.* **37** 20–8

[19] Perez-Jimenez A, Lyu D, Lu Z, Liu G and Ren B 2020 Surface-enhanced Raman spectroscopy: benefits, trade-offs and future developments *Chem. Sci.* **11** 4563–77

[20] Boardman A *et al* 2016 Rapid detection of bacteria from blood with surface-enhanced Raman spectroscopy *Anal. Chem.* **88** 8026–35

[21] Tadesse L *et al* 2020 Toward rapid infectious disease diagnosis with advances in surface-enhanced Raman spectroscopy *J. Chem. Phys.* **152** 240902

[22] Bodelón G, Montes-García V, Fernández-López C, Pastoriza-Santos I, Pérez-Juste J and Liz-Marzán L 2015 Au@pNIPAM SERRS tags for multiplex immunophenotyping cellular receptors and imaging tumor cells *Small* **11** 4149–57

[23] Casado-Rodriguez M *et al* 2016 Synthesis of vinyl-terminated Au nanoprisms and nano-octahedra mediated by 3-butenoic acid: direct Au@pNIPAM fabrication with improved SERS capabilities *Nanoscale* **8** 4557–64

[24] Zhang Y, Mi X, Tan X and Xiang R 2019 Recent progress on liquid biopsy analysis using surface-enhanced Raman spectroscopy *Theranostics* **9** 491–525

[25] Nasseri B, Soleimani N, Rabiee N, Kalbasi A, Karimi M and Hamblin M 2018 Point-of-care microfluidic devices for pathogen detection *Biosens. Bioelectron.* **117** 112–28

[26] D'Apuzzo F, Sengupta R, Overbay M, Aronoff J, Rogacs A and Barcelo S 2019 A generalizable single-chip calibration method for highly quantitative SERS via inkjet dispense *Anal. Chem.* **92** 1372–8

[27] D'Apuzzo F, Sengupta R N, Overbay M, Aronoff J S, Rogacs A and Barcelo S J 2020 A generalizable single-chip calibration method for highly quantitative SERS via inkjet dispense *Anal. Chem.* **92** 1372

[28] Alvarez-Puebla R and Liz-Marzán L 2010 SERS-based diagnosis and biodetection *Small* **6** 604–10

[29] Chan J, Fore S, Wachsmann-Hogiu S and Huser T 2008 Raman spectroscopy and microscopy of individual cells and cellular components *Laser Photonics Rev.* **2** 325–49

[30] Abalde-Cela S *et al* 2009 Loading of exponentially grown LBL films with silver nanoparticles and their application to generalized SERS detection *Angew. Chem. Int. Ed.* **48** 5326–9

[31] Anderson D and Moskovits M 2006 A SERS-active system based on silver nanoparticles tethered to a deposited silver film *J. Phys. Chem.* B **110** 13722–7

[32] Bonham A, Braun G, Pavel I, Moskovits M and Reich N 2007 Detection of sequence-specific protein–DNA interactions via surface enhanced resonance Raman scattering *J. Am. Chem. Soc.* **129** 14572–3

[33] Keating C, Kovaleski K and Natan M 1998 Protein:colloid conjugates for surface enhanced Raman scattering: stability and control of protein orientation *J. Phys. Chem.* B **102** 9404–13

[34] Shanmukh S, Jones L, Zhao Y, Driskell J, Tripp R and Dluhy R 2008 Identification and classification of respiratory syncytial virus (RSV) strains by surface-enhanced Raman spectroscopy and multivariate statistical techniques *Anal. Bioanal. Chem.* **390** 1551–5

[35] Xu K, Zhou R, Takei K and Hong M 2019 Toward flexible surface-enhanced Raman scattering (SERS) sensors for point-of-care diagnostics *Adv. Sci.* **6** 1900925

[36] Liu Y, Deng C, Yi D, Wang X, Tang Y and Wang Y 2017 Silica nanowire assemblies as three-dimensional, optically transparent platforms for constructing highly active SERS substrates *Nanoscale* **9** 15901–10

[37] Mitomo H *et al* 2015 Active gap SERS for the sensitive detection of biomacromolecules with plasmonic nanostructures on hydrogels *Adv. Opt. Mater.* **4** 259–63

[38] Liu X, Wang J, Tang L, Xie L and Ying Y 2016 Flexible plasmonic metasurfaces with user-designed patterns for molecular sensing and cryptography *Adv. Funct. Mater.* **26** 5515–23

[39] Wang Y *et al* 2018 Highly sensitive and automated surface enhanced Raman scattering-based immunoassay for H5N1 detection with digital microfluidics *Anal. Chem.* **90** 5224–31

[40] Gao R, Cheng Z, deMello A and Choo J 2016 Wash-free magnetic immunoassay of the PSA cancer marker using SERS and droplet microfluidics *Lab Chip* **16** 1022–9

[41] Nie S and Emory S 1997 Probing single molecules and single nanoparticles by surface-enhanced Raman scattering *Science* **275** 1102–6

[42] Hering K *et al* 2007 SERS: a versatile tool in chemical and biochemical diagnostics *Anal. Bioanal. Chem.* **390** 113–24

[43] Schlücker S, Küstner B, Punge A, Bonfig R, Marx A and Ströbel P 2006 Immuno-Raman microspectroscopy: *in situ* detection of antigens in tissue specimens by surface-enhanced Raman scattering *J. Raman Spectrosc.* **37** 719–21

[44] Jehn C *et al* 2009 Water soluble SERS labels comprising a SAM with dual spacers for controlled bioconjugation *Phys. Chem. Chem. Phys.* **11** 7499

[45] McAughtrie S, Faulds K and Graham D 2009 Surface enhanced Raman spectroscopy (SERS): potential applications for disease detection and treatment *J. Photochem. Photobiol.* C **2014** 40–53

[46] Schütz M, Steinigeweg D, Salehi M, Kömpe K and Schlücker S 2014 Hydrophilically stabilized gold nanostars as SERS labels for tissue imaging of the tumor suppressor p63 by immuno-SERS microscopy *Chem. Commun.* **47** 4216

[47] Fan Z *et al* 2013 Popcorn-shaped magnetic core–plasmonic shell multifunctional nano-particles for the targeted magnetic separation and enrichment, label-free SERS imaging, and photothermal destruction of multidrug-resistant bacteria *Eur. J. Chem.* **19** 2839–47

[48] Alonso M and Sanchez J 2013 Analytical challenges in breath analysis and its application to exposure monitoring *TrAC Trends Anal. Chem.* **44** 78–89

[49] Neerincx A H, Vijverberg S J H, Bos L D J, Brinkman P, van der Schee M P, de Vries R, Sterk P J and Maitland-van der Zee A H 2017 Breathomics from exhaled volatile organic compounds in pediatric asthma *Pediatr. Pulmonol.* **52** 1616–27

[50] Chen Y *et al* 2016 Breath analysis based on surface-enhanced Raman scattering sensors distinguishes early and advanced gastric cancer patients from healthy persons *ACS Nano* **10** 8169–79

[51] Qiao X *et al* 2017 Selective surface enhanced Raman scattering for quantitative detection of lung cancer biomarkers in superparticle@MOF structure *Adv. Mater.* **30** 1702275

[52] Ahmed M M and Hussein M M A 2017 Neurotoxic effects of silver nanoparticles and the protective role of rutin *Biomed. Pharmacother.* **90** 731–9

[53] Kong K V, Lam Z, Lau W K O, Leong W K and Olivo M 2013 A transition metal carbonyl probe for use in a highly specific and sensitive SERS-based assay for glucose *J. Am. Chem. Soc.* **135** 18028

[54] Huang X and El-Sayed M 2010 Gold nanoparticles: optical properties and implementations in cancer diagnosis and photothermal therapy *J. Adv. Res.* **1** 13–28

[55] Fales A, Yuan H and Vo-Dinh T 2013 Cell-penetrating peptide enhanced intracellular Raman imaging and photodynamic therapy *Mol. Pharm.* **10** 2291–8

[56] Loo C *et al* 2004 Nanoshell-enabled photonics-based imaging and therapy of cancer *Technol. Cancer Res. Treat.* **3** 33–40

[57] Kamińska A *et al* 2017 SERS-based immunoassay in a microfluidic system for the multiplexed recognition of interleukins from blood plasma: towards picogram detection *Sci. Rep.* **7** 10656

[58] Gallo V *et al* 2020 Surface-enhanced Raman scattering (SERS)-based immunosystem for ultrasensitive detection of the 90K biomarker *Anal. Bioanal. Chem.* **412** 7659–766

[59] Howell S C, Haffajee A, Pagonis T C and Guze K A 2011 Laser Raman spectroscopy as a potential chair-side microbiological diagnostic device *J. Endod.* **37** 968–72

[60] Abayasekara L M *et al* 2017 Detection of bacterial pathogens from clinical specimens using conventional microbial culture and 16S metagenomics: a comparative study *BMC Infect. Dis.* **17** 631

[61] Ashton L, Lau K, Winder C L and Goodacre R 2011 Raman spectroscopy: lighting up the future of microbial identification *Future Microbiol.* **6** 991–7

[62] Deurenberg R H *et al* 2017 Application of next generation sequencing in clinical microbiology and infection prevention *J. Biotechnol.* **243** 16–24

[63] Moore T, Joshua A S, Moody T D, Payne G M, Sarabia A R, Daniel and Sharma B 2018 *In vitro* and *in vivo* SERS biosensing for disease diagnosis *Biosensors* **8** 46

[64] Karn-orachai K, Sakamoto K, Laocharoensuk R, Bamrungsap S, Songsivilai S, Dharakul T and Miki K 2016 Extrinsic surface-enhanced Raman scattering detection of influenza A virus enhanced by two-dimensional gold–silver core–shell nanoparticle arrays *RSC Adv.* **6** 97791–9

[65] Zengin A, Tamer U and Caykara T 2017 SERS detection of hepatitis B virus DNA in a temperature-responsive sandwich-hybridization assay *J. Raman Spectrosc.* **48** 668–72

[66] Ma D, Zheng J, Tang P, Xu W, Qing Z, Yang S, Li J and Yang R 2016 Quantitative monitoring of hypoxia-induced intracellular acidification in lung tumor cells and tissues using activatable surface-enhanced Raman scattering nanoprobes *Anal. Chem.* **88** 11852–9

Chapter 2

Overview of infectious diseases and its diagnostic techniques

Sumit, Shagun Gupta and Ankur Kaushal

Infectious diseases are illnesses brought on by bacteria, viruses, fungi, or their toxic products. When Viruses, protozoa, fungi, bacteria, and helminths come into contact with the human body, infectious illnesses develop. COVID-19, polio, influenza, measles, smallpox, and rabies infections are some major examples of infectious diseases. In the age of infectious disease outbreaks and the emergence of novel illnesses, it is critical to identify efficient and widely available diagnostic procedures as well as prompt therapeutic management. The first step toward therapy, as well as illness control and prevention, is to make an accurate and early diagnosis. Effective diagnostic procedures are critical for illness detection, correct treatment, and outbreak management in the general population. In this book chapter, we focused on some major infectious diseases and their diagnosis by traditional methods, biochemical testing, and advanced biotechnology methods. Microscopy and cell culture are frequently used traditional methods for identification of infectious agents like bacteria and parasites. Presently, biochemical testing includes immunoassays and colorimetric testing, and advanced biotechnology methods include PCR testing, DNA microarrays, SERS based diagnostic method and biosensors are utilized to detect infectious pathogens effectively.

2.1 Introduction

Infectious diseases like influenza, poliomyelitis, rabies, dengue, and COVID-19, etc are illnesses brought on by bacteria, viruses, fungi, parasites, or their toxic products [1]. These diseases are typically spread by direct (physical contact) or indirect transmission (through Food, water, insects, and air) of pathogens [2]. The symptoms of infectious disease (fever, headache, sore throat, shortness of breathing, abdominal discomfort, muscle ache, rashes, and fatigue) can range from moderate to severe, and therapy is determined by the illness's origin or causative organisms as bacterial, viral and parasitic illnesses require a different kind of therapy [3].

People with a suppressed or deficient immune system (due to intake of immuno-suppressive drugs or fewer immune cells or diseases like AIDS that cause deficiency of immunity) are more susceptible to certain illnesses. Throughout the world, infectious illnesses are the primary cause of illness and death [4]. In the 21st century, we continue to combat both ancient and new infections, such as the plague and HIV [5]. When an epidemic occurs in 2019, others like coronavirus, swing in both the developing and developed nations [6].

A complex health care system has been established at the global level for the prevention of infection to reduce the risk of infectious disease. The health care system is made up of several official and organizational informal networks that function at various geographical levels, such as local, national, regional, and global [7]. Global agencies like WHO, UNDP, UNICEF, and World Bank, have come up with a special program for tropical diseases research that constituted a panel of expert advisory for planning and implementing standardized evaluations of diagnosis to address tropical disease detection techniques and therapy in developing countries [8].

In this book chapter, we discussed major infectious diseases and their diagnostic techniques existing globally like traditional methods, biochemical testing, and advanced biotechnology methods. Microscopy (a rapid and inexpensive method) and cell culture (the most sensitive and accurate method) are frequently used traditional methods for the identification of infectious agents like bacteria and parasites. Biochemical testing includes immunoassays and colorimetric testing. Immunoassays are biochemical assays that use labeled antibodies as the analytical reagent to identify an analyte to determine the presence of an analyte, such as an immunoglobulin or immunogen [9]. Lateral flow immunoassays, enzyme immuno-assay (EIA), an optical immunoassay test, etc are immunoassay-based methods for the detection of viral proteins, antigens of infectious agents, and antibodies produced against them.

Advanced biotechnology methods include genotyping PCR, DNA microarray, SERS-based diagnosis, and biosensors. Genotyping PCR test detects the genetic constituent/genetic composition 'genotype' of a living organism by evaluating an individual DNA sequence and comparing it to a reference or other individual sequence [10], Microarrays of DNA (a DNA-based microarray contains the collection of solid-surface from DNA spots) technique may be utilized effectively in clinical diagnostics for identification of disease-relevant genes and the diagnosis of disease utilizing biomarkers.

SERS-based diagnostic methods work by enhancing Raman scattering of target analyte that interact or are absorbed by the surface plasmon or rough surface of metals like gold or copper or silver. Generally, it is based on dual principles, the first is the electromagnetic (EM) effect and the second is the chemical (CM) effect. SERS-based determination of biomolecules or analytes can be performed by direct methods or indirect methods. In direct detection, the analyte is absorbed on the substrate or linked to the antibody or antigen or DNA probe or other molecules immobilized on the nanomaterial-based surface. The indirect technique uses reporter molecular associated on SERS substrate.

The SERS-based diagnostic technique can be utilized for the quantification of viral genetic material. Sample preparations are required to improve the specificity of this technique, as viruses of different families and species having the same size can be detected [11].

Biosensors-based methods can be used as the gold standard for the detection of infectious diseases because these techniques detect infectious agent substances such as viral proteins, viral genetic material, antigens, and antibodies [12]. The biosensor detects analytes of interest by combining a sensitive biological recognition component (enzymes, antibodies, etc) with a physical transducer (semi-conducting material/nanomaterial) [13]. The findings of the analysis are exhibited by converting the biological reaction into a quantifiable signal that can be utilized for both qualitative and quantitative measurements Biosensors have shown excellent properties such as flexibility, mobility, and high efficiency [14]. Electrochemical biosensors based on DNA hybridization and immunoassays are frequently used to detect infectious diseases worldwide [15]. Some nanomaterials have shown improved detection speed and reproducibility due to their very small size and larger surface area [16].

2.2 Infectious diseases

Pathogenesis or development of any infectious disease is carried out by the invasion of host tissue or cell by infectious agents whose actions affect the host's tissues and impairs the normal functioning of the body [17]. According to the WHO, infectious diseases are caused by harmful microorganisms like bacteria, viruses, parasites, fungi, and helminths [18] (figure 2.1). Mankind suffered from many infectious

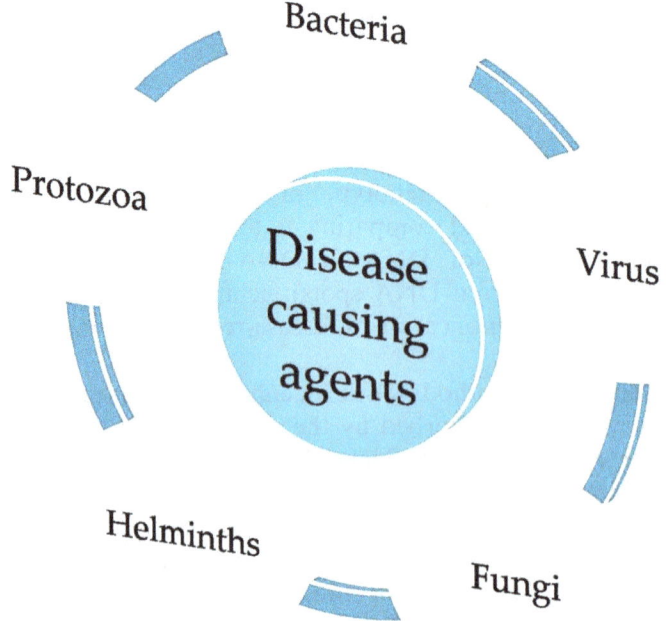

Figure 2.1. Various disease-causing agents.

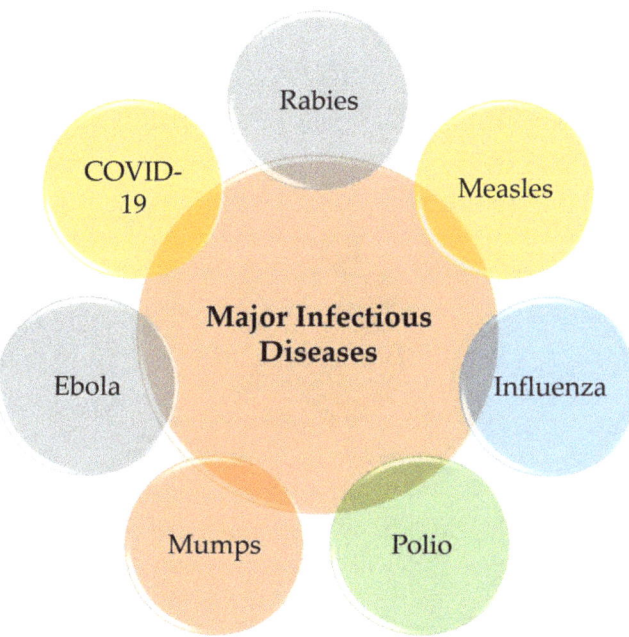

Figure 2.2. Major infectious diseases in the world.

illnesses in ancient times. Many magnificent cultures, like the ancient culture of Rome, Inca culture, Maya culture, and Marine Polynesian culture, were either directly or indirectly decimated by pestilence [19]. There are many examples of novel and emerging infectious illnesses that have harmed localized populations during the past several decades [20]. The public was alarmed by epidemics of infectious illnesses caused by extremely dangerous viruses. Infectious diseases are brought about by extrinsic or external factors. Extrinsic or intrinsic factors can cause organ and/or system function impairment [17]. Intrinsic factors, such as sickle cell anemia, come from inside the host and interfere with the regular functioning of a human organ or system. Extrinsic factors get access to the host's system when the host comes into touch with an external agent, such as malaria [21]. When Viruses, protozoa, fungus bacteria, and helminths come into contact with the human body, infectious illnesses develop [22]. COVID-19, polio, influenza, measles, smallpox, and rabies infections are some major examples of infectious diseases [23] (figure 2.2).

2.2.1 COVID-19

COVID-19, the infectious disease caused by the zoonotic coronavirus (SARS-CoV-2), firstly appeared in Wuhan, China, in late 2019. This virus has not only posed a serious threat to human health but also to the world's economy and lifestyle. The outbreak of COVID-19 was declared a 'Public Health Emergency' at the global level by the world health organization (WHO) on 30 January 2020 which was later recognized as a pandemic in March 2020. There are seven types of human coronavirus (figure 2.3) that

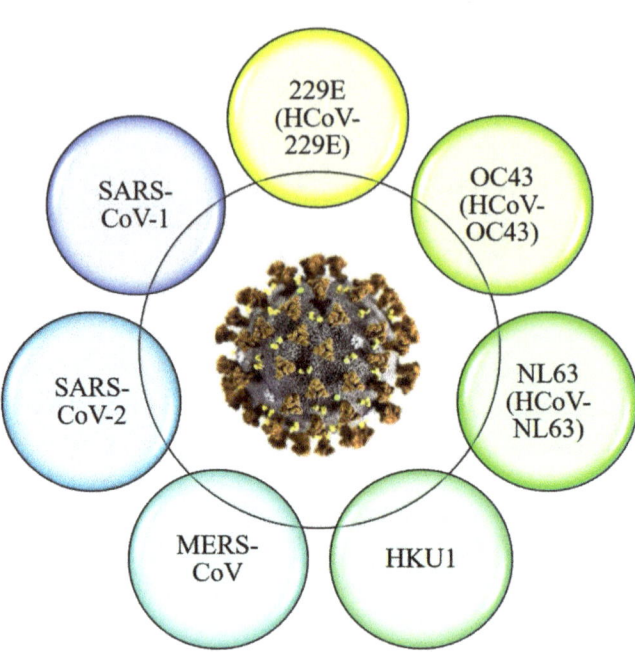

Figure 2.3. Types of coronaviruses.

are known which are responsible for the common cold. Among seven coronavirus species, four viruses are responsible for cold i.e., 229E, OC43, NL63, and HKU1 while the remaining three are responsible for severe acute respiratory problems i.e., SARS-CoV-1, SARS-CoV-2, and MERS-CoV [24, 25].

Presently, COVID-19 patients are considered a medium of transmission for SARS-CoV-2. This virus consists of a protein coat or capsid that protects the nucleus of genomic RNA and phosphorylated nucleocapsid (N) protein that is covered up inside phospholipid bilayers and spike proteins: the spike glycoprotein trimmer (S) and the hemagglutinin-esterase (HE).

The membrane (M) protein (a type III transmembrane glycoprotein) and small envelope (E) protein are at the S proteins that provide the medium for attaching the virus to the host cell surface receiver (Li *et al* 2020) and facilitate viral entry into a host cell [26]. The clinical symptoms in the patients of COVID-19 are observed to be headache, fever, fatigue, cough, and a few patients suffering from gastrointestinal infection [27]. The symptoms in patients suffering from COVID-19 infection were observed after a duration is nearly 5–12 days [28]. The death of a patient depends on various factors like age and immunity of the patient [29]. The period is shorter for the age group >70 years as compared to those under the age of 70 [30]. Systemic and respiratory disorders were observed in the patient due to COVID-19 infection [29].

2.2.2 Ebola

Ebola was declared a public health emergency in West Africa in 2014 and in the Democratic Republic of Congo again in 2018 [31]. The Zaire strain of Ebola kills between 40% and 90% of its victims, with up to 60% of infected persons dying. In 2014, over 14 000 people died as a result of Ebola [32]. According to Barcelona Institute for Global Health, a total of 28 000 cases and 11 300 deaths have been documented by March 2022.

Ebola virus is an RNA virus of single-strand that is non-segmented, negative-sense, and non-segmented. They belong to the family Filoviridae and the genus Ebola virus [33]. Because isolation of the Ebola virus has never been done from any other naturally infected host than humans, its enzootic and epizootic transmission cycles remain unknown [34]. In a single zoonotic spillover event, EBOV is transferred from an animal reservoir or intermediate host to a main human patient [35]. Following that, all human-to-human transmission begins with the initial instance. In contrast, to the spread of other zoonotic hemorrhagic fevers caused by viruses (such as Lassa fever), which are characterized by prolonged spillover and extremely limited spread of infection human-to-human, this is a one-of-a-kind pattern [36].

2.2.3 Influenza

Influenza (commonly called the flu or seasonal flu) is a virus that affects the world in 1918 [37]. Each year, seasonal influenza viruses are spread from one person to another and infect 5%–15% of the human population [38]. Most people do not always consider it to be a serious sickness because it affects the respiratory system which makes people confuse it with a heavy cold [39]. Human influenza's etiology and linkages to avian and swine influenza were unknown in 1918 [40]. According to WHO, influenza is a major hazard to global public health; 650 000 people die each year from influenza across the world. Influenza viruses (also known as H1N1 viruses) are always changing, with new strains emerging by three mechanisms including mutation (antigenic drift), re-assortment (antigenic shift), and recombination [41]. Season, geographic region, context (e.g., closed settings versus community settings), prevalent subtype, and age group all affect influenza attack rates [42]. Influenza Viruses have a spherical or filamentous form with a glycoprotein- and single-stranded RNA gene in the envelope [43]. Influenza viruses are members of the *Orthomyxoviridae* family of viruses, which are RNA-type viruses, categorized into types A, B, and C. Types A and B produce the majority of flu epidemics and outbreaks, with type C being responsible for infrequent mild upper respiratory symptoms [38].

2.2.4 Measles

Measles is a zoonotic disease that has been infecting people since the 4th century BC [44]. It is one of the most contagious viral illnesses; transmit via respiratory secretions, and causes significant sickness, life-long problems, and even death [45]. It is caused by the measles virus (MeV) which is a negative-sense RNA virus of single-strand belonging to the family Paramyxoviridae [46]. Before the advent of the measles vaccine in 1963, there were an estimated 30 million cases of measles per year, with over 2 million fatalities [47]. The number of deaths caused by measles decreased by 79% between 2000 and 2015 [48]. The measles virus can also spread by direct contact with infected secretions, although it does not live long on fomites, since heat and UV rays inactivate it within a few hours [49]. The incubation time for fever is 10 days and for rash is roughly 14 days [50]. A broad maculopapular (non-vesicular) skin rash and a temperature of more than 38.3 °C (101 °F) with cough, coryza (or rhinitis), and/or conjunctivitis are the clinical manifestations of measles [51]. Viral clearance, clinical recovery, and the formation of long-term immunity need host immunological responses to the measles virus [52]. Around 30 million cases of measles were anticipated to occur each year before the invention and widespread use of the measles vaccine, resulting in more than 1 million fatalities [50]. Vaccination against measles is advised for all vulnerable children and adults who are not allergic to the vaccination [53]. Despite advances in lowering measles mortality, the disease continues to be a leading cause of vaccine-preventable death and a significant source of morbidity and mortality in children, especially in Sub-Saharan Africa and Asia [54]. Measles isn't always considered a concern for travelers; therefore, vaccination isn't often included in pre-travel recommendations [55].

2.2.5 Poliomyelitis

Poliomyelitis, or polio, is a disease caused by the poliovirus that is both debilitating and life-threatening. Polio mostly affects children under the age of five and causes nerve damage, which can result in paralysis, breathing difficulties, and death [56]. According to the WHO, one out of every 200 illnesses results in permanent paralysis. 5%–10% of persons die due to immobilization of the paralyzed respiratory muscles [57]. Two of the three wild poliovirus serotypes (types 2 and 3) have been eliminated since the Global Polio Eradication Initiative was formed in 1988. Only Afghanistan and Pakistan continue to have uninterrupted transmission of wild poliovirus type-1 [58].

This virus is communicated from person to person, primarily by the fecal–oral route or, less commonly, through a common vehicle shared among the population (such as contaminated water or food), and multiplies in the gut [59]. The virus enters the body through the mouth or nose and dwells in the throat and intestines of infected people [60]. There is not any permanent therapy for this; it can only be prevented by taking the polio vaccine [61]. The use of advanced epidemiologic and molecular biologic technology, changes in human behavior, a national strategy for early identification and fast response to emerging illnesses, and a plan of action will all become more important to prevent and overcome or reduce the risk of emerging infectious diseases [62].

2.2.6 Rabies

In the 23rd century BC, the pre-mosaic Eshmuna code of Babylon included the earliest legal documentation of rabies. However, it was Louis Pasteur in the 1880s that discovered the viral sickness [63]. Rabies is caused by a fatal virus that is transmitted to humans through the saliva of infected animals, mainly through bites [64]. Rabies virus spread to humans by domestic rabid dogs is responsible for 99% of rabies cases. Rabies is a Rhabdoviridae virus, which means it's a single-stranded RNA virus [63]. Even though rabies is a vaccine-preventable viral zoonosis, it remains a major public health concern in developing countries (mainly in Africa and Asia), as evidenced by the fact that this devastating disease kills over 60 000 people worldwide each year, and around 15 million of the population receive rabies vaccines after possible exposure of infection (post-exposure prophylaxis) [65]. In a rabies-endemic nation, someone is expected to die from rabies every 10–20 min, with 40%–50% of fatalities occurring in youngsters under the age of 15.

2.2.7 Mumps

Mumps is a viral infection caused by the negative-sense RNA virus, Rubulavirus, which mostly affects the saliva-producing (salivary) glands near your ears [66]. Mumps symptoms normally occur two weeks after being exposed to the pathogen [67]. Mumps infections are more common in Asia during the summer months than during other seasons, and outbreaks follow a seasonal pattern [68]. Inflammation and swelling in many parts of the body, such as the testicles, brain, pancreas, and fluid around the brain, are common mumps consequences [69]. Mumps virus is spread by inhalation or oral contact with contaminated respiratory droplets or secretions via the respiratory pathway [70]. Although a single virion is theoretically sufficient to commence infection, numerous additional variables make it improbable that a single virion will be effective in doing so [71]. Before the initiation of the mumps immunization program, mumps was a dangerous illness that caused substantial morbidity and death over the world [72]. It showed 0.04%–7.0% chances of infection in the pre-vaccine period [73]. In 1950, the United States produced and utilized the first inactivated mumps vaccine. Live attenuated mumps virus vaccinations were initially employed in the United States and the Soviet Union in the 1960s [73]. Mump infections were common in congested population centers, such as kindergartens, boarding schools, military barracks, jails, and other crowded places [73]. After the advent of the mumps vaccine, the rate of mumps infection was considerably lowered. The number of immunization doses, age of vaccination, and vaccine coverage all have a role in the shifting epidemiologic pattern of mumps [74].

2.3 Diagnostic techniques

In the age of infectious disease outbreaks and the emergence of novel illnesses, it is critical to identify efficient and widely available diagnostic procedures as well as prompt therapeutic management [75]. The first step toward therapy, as well as illness control and prevention, is to make an accurate and early diagnosis. Effective diagnostic procedures are critical for illness detection, correct treatment, and outbreak management in the general population [76]. Diagnostics in the mainstream can be divided into three categories: (1) traditional, (2) biochemical, and (3) advanced biotechnology methods [77], see figure 2.4.

2.3.1 Traditional methods

  (a) **Microscopy**

   Electron microscopic diagnostics is ideal for identifying infectious agents quickly. It is a critical tool in clinical virus detection and basic viral mechanism research, especially when the agents are unknown or undetected [78]. An experienced virologist or technician can identify a viral pathogen

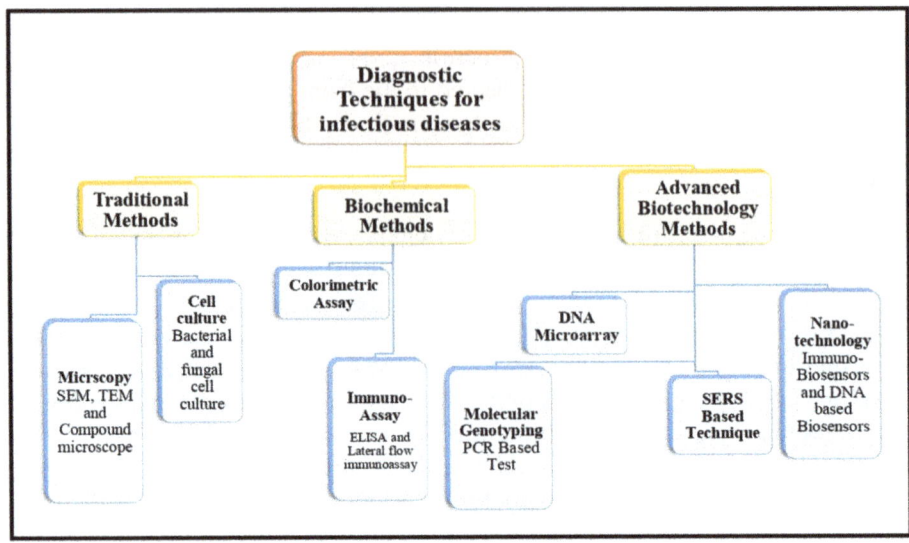

Figure 2.4. Classification of diagnostic techniques.

morphologically using electron microscopy within 10 min [79]. After the development of the first electron micrograph for poxvirus in 1938, immunologic methods were initially employed for the investigations of tobacco mosaic virus in 1941, and in the late 1940s [80]. In 1952, the first photograph of poliovirus was captured, and studies of virus–host connections began in the mid-1950s [81]. Electron microscopy was crucial in identifying the viral agent of the initial Ebola in 1976, as well as the Ebola Reston infection of a monkey colony in 1989, as a filovirus [82, 83]. It enabled the detection of numerous therapeutically relevant infectious organisms in diagnostic cell cultures during the decades of 1970s and 1980s, including various viral agents like adenoviruses, enteroviruses, orthomyxoviruses, paramyxoviruses, and reoviruses [84]. Electron microscopy was successfully adopted in the differential diagnosis of smallpox and chickenpox infections [85]. Microscopy for diagnostic purposes outside of a qualified laboratory is frequently restricted by regulations. The structural features and morphogenesis of viruses from a range of clinical specimens may be seen using electron microscopy [81]. To separate invasive illness from surface colonization, microscopic analysis of tissue may be required—a difference that is difficult to make using culture techniques [86]. Because electron microscopy is ineffective for screening large numbers of samples, alternative immunologic and molecular approaches based on nucleic acid amplification techniques have been developed.

(b) **Cell culture**

Cell culture is a technique that includes isolating cells from their natural environment (specific tissues or organs) and growing them in a controlled artificial environment i.e., *in vitro* [87]. Cell culture offers the necessary environment for the detection and identification of a variety of infection-causing viruses. The research laboratories started viral isolation from animal cell cultures by the early 1960s, but diagnostic services were restricted and frequently not accessible at all [88]. Diagnostic virology had grown considerably by the early 1970s, owing to the availability of highly purified reagents and commercially manufactured cell lines [89]. Vaccinia virus was cultivated in cell cultures as early as 1913 [90], while smallpox and yellow fever viruses were propagated in cell cultures for vaccine manufacturing in the 1930s [91]. However, it wasn't until the 1950s that cell cultures became popular for viral isolation, thanks to the finding that polioviruses could flourish in cell cultures that weren't of neural origin [92].

2.3.2 Biochemical methods

(a) Immunoassay

Immunoassays are biochemical assays that use labeled antibodies as the analytical reagent to identify the presence of an analyte, such as an immunoglobulin or immunogen [9]. Because immunoassays are frequently employed as confirmation tests, their results are rarely meant to be utilized as the sole foundation for a diagnosis [93]. But due to great specificity and sensitivity, immunoassays are the preferred approach for pharmaceutical analysis and drug development sectors [94, 95]. These techniques became the method of choice because of their comparatively inexpensive cost of the apparatus, tools, and reagents [96]. These techniques can measure many substances, including medicines and drugs with low molecular weight, macromolecular macromolecules, metabolites, and/or biomarkers that can help in the diagnosis or prediction of illness [97]. The efficiency of antigen–antibody complex production and the capacity to detect these complexes are two main elements that determine the efficacy of any immunoassay [98].

Using lateral flow immunoassays, direct detection of SARS-CoV-2 viral proteins (antigens) in respiratory secretions and nasopharyngeal swabs provides a faster and less expensive means of testing for SARS-CoV-2 [98]. The suitability of an immunoglobulin M (IgM) antibody-capture immunoassay utilizing peroxidase-labeled mumps antibodies for the practical diagnosis of acute mumps infection is assessed [99]. An indirect enzyme immunoassay (EIA) is used for determining IgG and IgM antibodies to the mumps virus [100], and a solid-phase enzyme immunoassay (EIA) was developed for the detection of poliovirus antigen [101]. To assess IgM antibodies to the measles virus in human sera, researchers utilized a solid-phase enzyme-immunoassay (EIA) using horseradish-peroxidase-conjugated anti-globulin [102]. The flu (influenza) A and B viral antigens may be detected quickly using an optical immunoassay test [103].

(b) Colorimetric testing

Colorimetric approaches have proven to be quick, versatile, less costly, and highly sensitive for detecting a wide range of analytes (in a single test) ranging from dangerous compounds to infections, which may be identified with the naked eye or optical tools [104]. The incorporation of colorimetric assays into portable, versatile, cost-effective, fast, and reliable optical digital detectors with onboard processing capabilities will increase the impact and use of these sensing methods [105]. Colorimetric flu virus biosensor assay was developed by Raji and his co-worker for the rapid detection of flu A and B viruses [106]. In the case of SARS-CoV-2, a gold nanoparticle-based colorimetric biosensor was also developed for detecting viral particles in nasal and throat swabs [107].

2.3.3 Advanced biotechnological methods

(a) Molecular genotyping

Genotyping is the process of evaluating an individual DNA sequence and comparing it to a reference or other individual sequence to determine the genetic constituent/genetic composition 'genotype' of an organism [10]. Rapid molecular approaches have improved laboratories' ability to identify and describe microbial pathogens more thoroughly [108]. COVID-19 is diagnosed predominantly by the identification of RNA from the SARS-CoV-2 virus, the pandemic's primary infectious agent [109]. For faster characterization of mumps virus in clinical samples, nested reverse transcription-PCR technique with higher sensitivity targeting a short portion of the gene encoding the small hydrophobic protein (SH gene) was created [110]. Mumps virus RNA was isolated directly from CSF samples and extracted from mumps virus isolates from individuals with a variety of clinical symptoms [111]. In the diagnosis and monitoring of influenza viruses, molecular approaches employed directly on clinical material play an essential role. The combination of automated nucleic acid purification with real-time PCR might allow for much faster detection of viral infections like influenza viruses in clinical samples [112].

(b) DNA array

A DNA microarray is a solid-surface collection of tiny DNA spots. Each DNA patch includes thousands of probes, which are copies of a certain DNA sequence. DNA array technology advanced quickly in the late 1990s and early 2000s when novel techniques of manufacture and fluorescence detection were suited to the task [113]. DNA microarrays may be utilized effectively in clinical diagnostics, from the identification of disease-relevant genes to the diagnosis of disease utilizing biomarkers [114]. The examination of RNA or DNA aids in the diagnosis of infectious illnesses as well as the identification of hereditary abnormalities and cancer [115]. The performance of DNA microarray-based diagnostics is always increasing as more instruments are included. As a result, microarrays of DNA will become popular as a gold standard technique for illness detection and will play an important role in clinical diagnostics [116].

(c) **Nanotechnology**

Nanotechnology is highly effective in the diagnosis of infectious diseases [117]. Metallic, fluorescent, and magnetic nanoparticles have been used successfully to diagnose infectious diseases [117, 118]. Nanoparticles and their uses in viral detection and tracking are shown in figure 2.5 to better understand infection processes [119]. Fluorescent nanoparticles are applicable for innovative methods of performing real-time diagnostic tests using bioimaging or sensory functions [120]. Quantum dots are semiconductor-based fluorescent nanostructures with a size of about 2–10 nm, with many novel properties, and play crucial roles in disease diagnosis and monitoring [121, 122].

Metal nanoparticles (<100 nm) have unique advantages in the development of new reporting technologies to improve the sensitivity of detection and specification of certified biomarkers in the clinic [123]. Due to their small sizes, metallic nanoparticles show excellent interaction with biomolecules within the cell and on the cell surface [124]. Silver nanoparticles are one of the most efficient antimicrobials against bacteria and viruses among metallic nanoparticles since they are effective against a wide range of pathogens even at low concentrations [125]. The real-time immuno-PCR amplification procedure for HIV detection was improved by employing gold magnetic particles functionalized with antibodies against the HIV capsid protein p24 with oligonucleotides, barcodes, and antibodies [126].

Sandwich hybridization model based on gold nanoparticles used for the detection of target DNA in patient sera using 'gene chips.' A similar methodology was used to

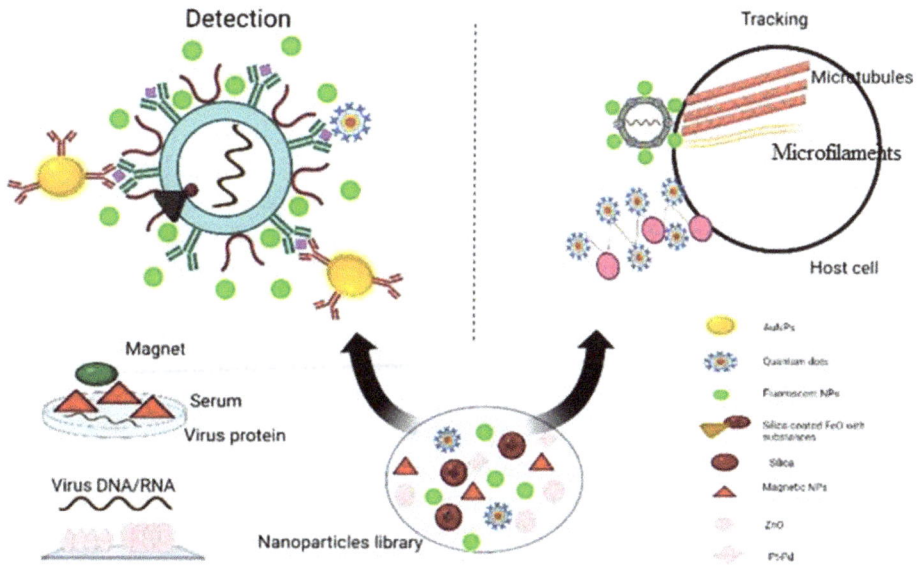

Figure 2.5. Application of nanoparticles in virus detection and tracking.

detect hepatitis B and C using silver nanoparticles [127]. Several materials like gold nanoparticles, magnetic nanoparticles, carbon nanotubes, and mesoporous silica nanoparticles are used for the detection of influenza [128]. The amperometric detection of H5N1 virus using gold nanoparticle modified electrodes in a gold nanoparticle/DNA-aptamer/H5N1/antiH5N1-Alkaline-phosphatase   sandwich model was able to detect H5N1 concentrations in the Femto molar range [129]. Furthermore, due to their high electrical conductivity, metallic nanoparticles are used as a core component in a variety of electrochemical biosensors to detect infectious diseases [130].

(d) **Biosensors**

Biosensors-based methods can be used as the gold standard for the detection of infectious diseases because these techniques detect infectious agent substances such as viral proteins, viral genetic material, antigens, and antibodies [12]. The biosensor detects analytes of interest such as an antigen, antibody, viral protein, DNA, etc by combining a sensitive biological recognition component (enzymes, antibodies, etc) with a physical transducer of semi-conducting material or nanomaterial like graphene quantum dots, graphene oxide nanoparticles and gold nanoparticles, etc [13]. The findings of the analysis are exhibited by converting the biological reaction (oxidation or reduction) into a quantifiable signal (current, voltage, or impedance) that can be utilized for both qualitative and quantitative measurements. Biosensors have shown excellent properties such as flexibility, mobility, and high efficiency [14]. Electrochemical biosensors based on DNA hybridization and immunoassays are frequently used to detect infectious diseases worldwide [15]. Some nanomaterials showed improved detection speed and reproducibility due to their very small size and larger surface area [16].

(e) **SERS-based technique**

Surface-enhanced Raman scattering (SERS) based diagnostic technique is highly reliable for the detection of certain molecular species and has the potential to detect a single molecule [131]. These diagnostic methods are based on the enhancement of Raman scattering of an analyte that interacts or is absorbed by the surface plasmon or rough surface of metals like gold or copper or silver. Generally, it is based on dual principles, the first is the electromagnetic (EM) effect and the second is the chemical (CM) effect. SERS-based detection of analytes can be performed by direct methods or indirect methods [11].

In direct detection, the analyte is absorbed on the substrate or linked to the antibody or antigen or DNA probe or other molecules immobilized on the nano-material-based surface as shown in figure 2.6. This type of detection is useful for analytes having a higher Raman scattering cross-section. This detection approach has the merits of accuracy and control over quantification and the possible identification and determination of chemical properties of the analyte [11, 131]. The indirect technique uses a reporter molecule associated with the SERS substrate. The SERS-based diagnostic techniques can be utilized for the quantification of viral

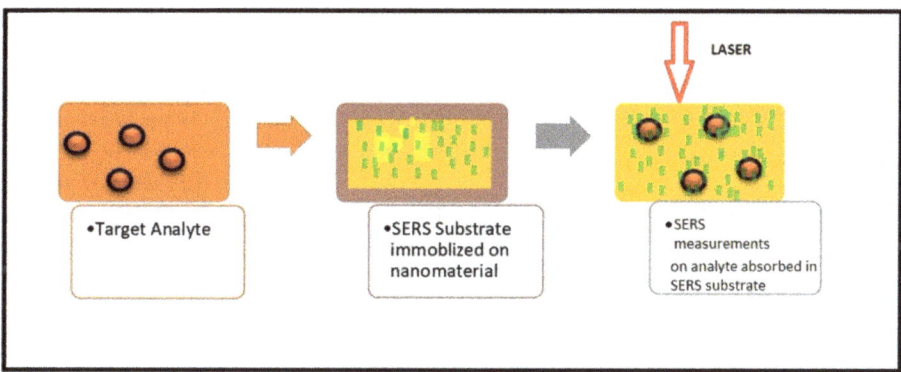

Figure 2.6. SERS-based direct detection of target analyte for diagnosis of infectious disease.

genetic material. The indirect method compares the SERS spectrum variations of reporter molecule and target analyte concentration for diagnosis. Reporter molecules are very tiny and have large Raman cross sections. Sample preparations are required to improve the specificity of this technique, as viruses of different families and species having the same size can be detected [11, 131].

2.4 Conclusion

This chapter summarizes different aspects of infectious diseases viz. spread of disease, prevalence, and diagnosis. The spread of Infectious diseases arises from an infected person, an infected animal, or a contaminated inanimate object to a susceptible host. It is responsible for a huge global issue of disease that impacts public health systems and economies worldwide. Control and prevention of infectious diseases rely on a thorough understanding of the factors determining the spread of infection. The diagnostic techniques evaluated in the population were classical like cell culture and microscopy, immunoassays like ELISA and colorimetric assay, and advanced methods of biotechnology including SERS-based techniques and biosensors. The SERS-based diagnostic technique is highly reliable for the detection of certain molecular species and has the potential to detect a single molecule. Infectious disease diagnosis using SERS based approach is highly recommended due to its higher sensitivity and accuracy.

Acknowledgments

Thanks to the Department of Biotechnology, Central research Cell MM(DU), Mullana for their continuous support and help.

References

[1] van Seventer J M and Hochberg N S 2017 Principles of infectious diseases: transmission, diagnosis, prevention, and control *International Encyclopedia of Public Health* (New York: Academic) pp 22–39

[2] Tellier R, Li Y, Cowling B J and Tang J W 2019 Recognition of aerosol transmission of infectious agents: a commentary *BMC Infect. Dis.* **19** 101

[3] Watson D A and Hester J 2008 Infectious disease ed R Ballweg, E M Sullivan and D Brown *Vetrosky DBT-PA* 4th edn (Philadelphia, PA: W.B. Saunders) ch 27 pp 515–25

[4] Salleh M R 2008 Life event, stress and illness *Malays. J. Med. Sci.* **15** 9–18

[5] Piret J and Boivin G 2021 Pandemics throughout history *Front. Microbiol.* **11** 631736

[6] Harapan H, Itoh N, Yufika A, Winardi W, Keam S, Te H, Megawati D, Hayati Z, Wagner A L and Mudatsir M 2020 Coronavirus disease 2019 (COVID-19): a literature review *J. Infect. Public Health* **13** 667–73

[7] Bloom D E and Cadarette D 2019 Infectious disease threats in the twenty-first century: strengthening the global response *Front. Immunol.* **10** 549

[8] Srivastava S, Singh P K, Vatsalya V and Karch R C 2018 Developments in the diagnostic techniques of infectious diseases: rural and urban prospective *Adv. Infect. Dis.* **8** 121–38

[9] Theel E S, Carpenter A B and Binnicker M J 2015 Immunoassays for diagnosis of infectious diseases *Manual of Clinical Microbiology* (New York: Wiley) pp 91–105

[10] Gorakshakar A, Gogri H and Ghosh K 2017 Evolution of technology for molecular genotyping in blood group systems *Indian J. Med. Res.* **146** 305–15

[11] Saviñon-Flores F, Méndez E, López-Castaños M, Carabarin-Lima A, López-Castaños K A, González-Fuentes M A and Méndez-Albores A 2021 A review on SERS-based detection of human virus infections: influenza and coronavirus *Biosensors (Basel)* **11** 66

[12] Castillo-Henríquez L, Brenes-Acuña M, Castro-Rojas A, Cordero-Salmerón R, Lopretti-Correa M and Vega-Baudrit J R 2020 Biosensors for the detection of bacterial and viral clinical pathogens *Sensors* **20** 6926

[13] Naresh V and Lee N 2021 A review on biosensors and recent development of nano-structured materials-enabled biosensors *Sensors (Basel)* **21** 1109

[14] Mathew M, Radhakrishnan S, Vaidyanathan A, Chakraborty B and Rout C S 2021 Flexible and wearable electrochemical biosensors based on two-dimensional materials: recent developments *Anal. Bioanal. Chem.* **413** 727–62

[15] Mehrotra P 2016 Biosensors and their applications—a review *J. Oral Biol. Craniofac. Res.* **6** 153–59

[16] Huang X, Zhu Y and Kianfar E 2021 Nano biosensors: properties, applications and electrochemical techniques *J. Mater. Res. Technol.* **12** 1649–72

[17] Nii-Trebi N I 2017 Emerging and neglected infectious diseases: insights, advances, and challenges *Biomed. Res. Int.* **2017** 5245021

[18] Ranjita S 2013 Nanosuspensions: a new approach for organ and cellular targeting in infectious diseases *J. Pharm. Investig.* **43** 1–26

[19] Brachman P S 2003 Infectious diseases—past, present, and future *Int. J. Epidemiol.* **32** 684–6

[20] JONES J R 2008 Bioactive glass ed T B T-B Kokubo and C A their *Woodhead Publishing Series in Biomaterials* (Cambridge: Woodhead Publishing) ch 12 pp 266–83

[21] Lovera R, Fernández M S, Jacob J, Lucero N, Morici G, Brihuega B, Farace M I, Caracostantogolo J and Cavia R 2017 Intrinsic and extrinsic factors related to pathogen infection in wild small mammals in intensive milk cattle and swine production systems *PLoS Negl. Trop. Dis.* **11** e0005722

[22] Makarov V v, Love A J, Sinitsyna O v, Makarova S S, Yaminsky I v, Taliansky M E and Kalinina N O 2014 'Green' nanotechnologies: synthesis of metal nanoparticles using plants *Acta Nat.* **6** 35–44

[23] Burrell C J, Howard C R and Murphy F A 2017 Epidemiology of viral infections *Fenner and White's Medical Virology* (New York: Academic) pp 185–203

[24] Cui J, Li F and Shi Z-L 2019 Origin and evolution of pathogenic coronaviruses *Nat. Rev. Microbiol.* **17** 181–92

[25] Su S, Wong G, Shi W, Liu J, Lai A C K, Zhou J, Liu W, Bi Y and Gao G F 2016 Epidemiology, genetic recombination, and pathogenesis of coronaviruses *Trends Microbiol.* **24** 490–502

[26] Cascella M, Rajnik M, Cuomo A, Dulebohn S C and Napoli di R 2020 *Features, Evaluation and Treatment Coronavirus (COVID-19)* [updated 2020 Mar 20] (Tampa, FL: StatPearls)

[27] Guo Y-R, Cao Q-D, Hong Z-S, Tan Y-Y, Chen S-D, Jin H-J, Tan K-S, Wang D-Y and Yan Y 2020 The origin, transmission and clinical therapies on coronavirus disease 2019 (COVID-19) outbreak—an update on the status *Mil. Med. Res.* **7** 11

[28] Li Q, Guan X and Wu P *et al* 2020 Early transmission dynamics in Wuhan, China, of novel coronavirus-infected pneumonia *New Engl. J. Med.* **382** 1199–207

[29] Rothan H A and Byrareddy S N 2020 The epidemiology and pathogenesis of coronavirus disease (COVID-19) outbreak *J. Autoimmun.* **109** 102433

[30] Wang W, Tang J and Wei F 2020 Updated understanding of the outbreak of 2019 novel coronavirus (2019-nCoV) in Wuhan, China *J. Med. Virol.* **92** 441–47

[31] Matson M J, Chertow D S and Munster V J 2020 Delayed recognition of Ebola virus disease is associated with longer and larger outbreaks *Emerg. Microbes Infect.* **9** 291–301

[32] Wilder-Smith A 2021 COVID-19 in comparison with other emerging viral diseases: risk of geographic spread via travel *Trop. Dis. Travel Med. Vaccines* **7** 3

[33] Mühlberger E 2007 Filovirus replication and transcription *Future Virol.* **2** 205–15

[34] Mekibib B and Ariën K K 2016 Aerosol transmission of filoviruses *Viruses* **8** 148

[35] Plowright R K, Parrish C R, McCallum H, Hudson P J, Ko A I, Graham A L and Lloyd-Smith J O 2017 Pathways to zoonotic spillover *Nat. Rev. Microbiol.* **15** 502–10

[36] Jacob S T, Crozier I and Fischer W A 2nd *et al* 2020 Ebola virus disease *Nat. Rev. Dis. Primers* **6** 13

[37] Taubenberger J K and Morens D M 2006 1918 Influenza: the mother of all pandemics *Emerg. Infect. Dis.* **12** 15–22

[38] Moghadami M 2017 A narrative review of influenza: a seasonal and pandemic disease *Iran. J. Med. Sci.* **42** 2–13

[39] Pelletier J P R and Mukhtar F 2020 Passive monoclonal and polyclonal antibody therapies ed R W B T Maitta *Immunologic Concepts in Transfusion Medicine* (Amsterdam: Elsevier) ch 16 pp 251–348

[40] Taubenberger J K 2006 The origin and virulence of the 1918 'Spanish' influenza virus *Proc. Am. Philos. Soc.* **150** 86–112

[41] Shao W, Li X, Goraya M U, Wang S and Chen J-L 2017 Evolution of influenza A virus by mutation and re-assortment *Int. J. Mol. Sci.* **18** 1650

[42] Tokars J I, Olsen S J and Reed C 2018 Seasonal incidence of symptomatic influenza in the United States *Clin. Infect. Dis.* **66** 1511–18

[43] Noda T and Kawaoka Y 2010 Structure of influenza virus ribonucleoprotein complexes and their packaging into virions *Rev. Med. Virol.* **20** 380–91

[44] Düx A, Lequime S and Patrono L V *et al* 2019 The history of measles: from a 1912 genome to an antique origin *bioRxiv* https://doi.org/10.1101/2019.12.29.889667

[45] Azap A and Pehlivanoglu F 2014 Measles ed Ö Ergönül, F Can and L Madoff *Akova MBT Emerging Infectious Diseases* (Amsterdam: Academic) ch 26 pp 347–57

[46] Rota P A, Moss W J, Takeda M, de Swart R L, Thompson K M and Goodson J L 2016 Measles *Nat. Rev. Dis. Primers* **2** 16049

[47] Hendriks J and Blume S 2013 Measles vaccination before the measles-mumps-rubella vaccine *Am. J. Public Health* **103** 1393–401

[48] Moss W J 2017 Measles *Lancet* **390** 2490–502

[49] Leung N H L 2021 Transmissibility and transmission of respiratory viruses *Nat. Rev. Microbiol.* **19** 528–45

[50] Moss W J, Griffin D E and Feinstone W H 2009 Measles *Vaccines for Biodefense and Emerging and Neglected Diseases* (New York: Academic) pp 551–65

[51] Husada D, Kusdwijono , Puspitasari D, Kartina L, Basuki P S and Ismoedijanto 2020 An evaluation of the clinical features of measles virus infection for diagnosis in children within a limited resources setting *BMC Pediatr.* **20** 5

[52] Griffin D E 2016 The immune response in measles: virus control, clearance and protective immunity *Viruses* **8** 282

[53] Khakoo G A and Lack G 2000 Recommendations for using MMR vaccine in children allergic to eggs *Br. Med. J.* **320** 929–32

[54] Rodrigues C M C and Plotkin S A 2020 Impact of vaccines; health, economic and social perspectives *Front. Microbiol.* **11** 1526

[55] Ventola C L 2016 Immunization in the United States: recommendations, barriers, and measures to improve compliance: part 1: childhood vaccinations P T**41** 426–36

[56] Bai J and Cheng J 2015 *Poliomyelitis BT—Radiology of Infectious Diseases* vol 1 ed H Li (Dordrecht: Springer) pp 549–60

[57] Tseha S T 2021 Polio: the disease that reemerged after six years in Ethiopia *Ethiop. J. Health Sci.* **31** 897–902

[58] Chard A N, Datta S D, Tallis G, Burns C C, Wassilak S G F, Vertefeuille J F and Zaffran M 2020 Progress toward polio eradication—worldwide, January 2018–March 2020 *Morb. Mortal. Wkly. Rep.* **69** 784–89

[59] Adebisi Y A, Eliseo-Lucero P D and Nuga B B 2020 Last fight of wild polio in Africa: Nigeria's battle *Public Health Pract.* **1** 100043

[60] Mehndiratta M M, Mehndiratta P and Pande R 2014 Poliomyelitis: historical facts, epidemiology, and current challenges in eradication *Neurohospitalist* **4** 223–29

[61] H V W 2014 Before the vaccines: medical treatments of acute paralysis in the 1916 new york epidemic of poliomyelitis *Open Microbiol. J.* **8** 144–47

[62] Jones K E, Patel N G, Levy M A, Storeygard A, Balk D, Gittleman J L and Daszak P 2008 Global trends in emerging infectious diseases *Nature* **451** 990–93

[63] Singh R, Singh K P, Cherian S, Saminathan M, Kapoor S, Manjunatha Reddy G B, Panda S and Dhama K 2017 Rabies—epidemiology, pathogenesis, public health concerns and advances in diagnosis and control: a comprehensive review *Vet. Q.* **37** 212–51

[64] Rose S R, Keystone J S, Connor B A, Hackett P, Kozarsky P E and Quarry D 2006 Vaccines for travel ed S R Rose, J S Keystone, B A Connor, P Hackett and P E Kozarsky *Quarry DBT-ITHG 2006–2007* 13th edn ed (Philadelphia: Mosby) ch 3 pp 35–62

[65] Rehman S, Rantam F A, Rehman A, Effendi M H and Shehzad A 2021 Knowledge, attitudes, and practices toward rabies in three provinces of Indonesia *Vet. World* **14** 2518–26

[66] Rubin S, Eckhaus M, Rennick L J, Bamford C G G and Duprex W P 2015 Molecular biology, pathogenesis and pathology of mumps virus *J. Pathol.* **235** 242–52

[67] Wu H, Wang F, Tang D and Han D 2021 Mumps orchitis: clinical aspects and mechanisms *Front. Immunol.* **12** 582946

[68] Grassly N C and Fraser C 2006 Seasonal infectious disease epidemiology *Proc. Biol. Sci.* **273** 2541–50

[69] Yung C F, Andrews N, Bukasa A, Brown K E and Ramsay M 2011 Mumps complications and effects of mumps vaccination, England and Wales, 2002–2006 *Emerg. Infect Dis.* **17** 661–766

[70] Louten J 2016 Virus transmission and epidemiology *Essential Human Virology* (New York: Academic) pp 71–92

[71] Klasse P J 2015 Molecular determinants of the ratio of inert to infectious virus particles *Prog. Mol. Biol. Transl. Sci.* **129** 285–326

[72] Greenwood B 2014 The contribution of vaccination to global health: past, present and future *Philos. Trans. R. Soc. Lond.* B **369** 20130433

[73] Su S-B, Chang H-L and Chen A K-T 2020 Current status of mumps virus infection: epidemiology, pathogenesis, and vaccine *Int. J. Environ. Res. Public Health* **17** 1686

[74] Connell A R, Connell J, Leahy T R and Hassan J 2020 Mumps outbreaks in vaccinated populations—is it time to re-assess the clinical efficacy of vaccines? *Front. Immunol.* **11** 2089

[75] Ong C W M, Migliori G B and Raviglione M *et al* 2020 Epidemic and pandemic viral infections: impact on tuberculosis and the lung *Eur. Respir. J.* **56** 2001727

[76] Wijerathna T, Gunathilaka N, Gunawardana K and Rodrigo W 2017 Potential challenges of controlling leishmaniasis in Sri Lanka at a disease outbreak *BioMed Res. Int.* **2017** 6931497

[77] Dwivedi S, Purohit P, Misra R, Pareek P, Goel A, Khattri S, Pant K K, Misra S and Sharma P 2017 Diseases and molecular diagnostics: a step closer to precision medicine *Indian J. Clin. Biochem.* **32** 374–98

[78] Burrell C J, Howard C R and Murphy F A 2017 Laboratory diagnosis of virus diseases *Fenner and White's Medical Virology* (New York: Academic) pp 135–54

[79] Hazelton P R and Gelderblom H R 2003 Electron microscopy for rapid diagnosis of infectious agents in emergent situations *Emerg. Infect. Dis.* **9** 294–303

[80] Zhang Y, Hung T, Song J D and He J S 2013 Electron microscopy: essentials for viral structure, morphogenesis and rapid diagnosis *Sci. China Life Sci.* **56** 421–30

[81] Goldsmith C S and Miller S E 2009 Modern uses of electron microscopy for detection of viruses *Clin. Microbiol. Rev.* **22** 552–63

[82] Escudero-Pérez B, Ruibal P and Rottstegge M *et al* 2019 Comparative pathogenesis of Ebola virus and Reston virus infection in humanized mice *JCI Insight* **4** e126070

[83] Broadhurst M J, Brooks T J G and Pollock N R 2016 Diagnosis of Ebola virus disease: past, present, and future *Clin. Microbiol. Rev.* **29** 773–93

[84] Schramlová J, Arientová S and Hulínská D 2010 The role of electron microscopy in the rapid diagnosis of viral infections—review *Folia Microbiol. (Praha)* **55** 88–101

[85] Roingeard P, Raynal P-I, Eymieux S and Blanchard E 2019 Virus detection by transmission electron microscopy: still useful for diagnosis and a plus for biosafety *Rev. Med. Virol.* **29** e2019

[86] Bowler P G, Duerden B I and Armstrong D G 2001 Wound microbiology and associated approaches to wound management *Clin. Microbiol. Rev.* **14** 244–69

[87] Verma A, Verma M and Singh A 2020 Animal tissue culture principles and applications *Anim. Biotechnol.* 269–93

[88] Leland D S and Ginocchio C C 2007 Role of cell culture for virus detection in the age of technology *Clin. Microbiol. Rev.* **20** 49–78

[89] Hematian A, Sadeghifard N, Mohebi R, Taherikalani M, Nasrolahi A, Amraei M and Ghafourian S 2016 Traditional and modern cell culture in virus diagnosis *Osong Public Health Res. Perspect.* **7** 77–82

[90] Steinhardt E and Lambert R A 1914 Studies on the cultivation of the virus of vaccinia. II *J. Infectious Dis.* **14** 87–92

[91] Cong Y, McArthur M A, Cohen M, Jahrling P B, Janosko K B, Josleyn N, Kang K, Zhang T and Holbrook M R 2016 Characterization of yellow fever virus infection of human and non-human primate antigen presenting cells and their interaction with CD4+ T cells *PLoS Negl. Trop. Dis.* **10** e0004709

[92] Wadell G 1983 Cultivation of viruses *Textbook of Medical Virology* (Oxford: Butterworth-Heinemann) pp 38–44

[93] Darwish I A 2006 Immunoassay methods and their applications in pharmaceutical analysis: basic methodology and recent advances *Int. J. Biomed. Sci.* **2** 217–35

[94] Gübitz G and Schmid M G 2005 Immunoassays, techniques ed P Worsfold and A Townshend Poole CBT-E of AS 2nd edn *Luminescence Immunoassays* (Oxford: Elsevier) pp 352–60

[95] Pandey K 2019 Advancement in analytical and bioanalytical techniques as a boon to medical sciences ed V Bobbarala, G S Zaman, M N M Desa and A M Akim *Biochemical Testing – Clinical Correlation and Diagnosis* (Rijeka: IntechOpen) ch 3

[96] Hesterberg L K and Crosby M A 1996 An overview of rapid immunoassays *Lab. Med.* **27** 41–6

[97] Stenken J A and Poschenrieder A J 2015 Bioanalytical chemistry of cytokines—a review *Anal. Chim. Acta* **853** 95–115

[98] Reverberi R and Reverberi L 2007 Factors affecting the antigen–antibody reaction *Blood Transfus.* **5** 227–40

[99] Glikmann G, Pedersen M and Mordhorst C-H 1986 Detection of specific immunoglobulin m to mumps virus in serum and cerebrospinal fluid samples from patients with acute mumps infection, using an antibody-capture enzyme immunoassay *Acta Pathol. Microbiol. Scand.* C **94C** 145–56

[100] Ollimeurman H P, Krishna R v and Ziegler T 1982 Determination of IgG- and IgM-class antibodies to mumps virus by solid-phase enzyme immunoassay *J. Virol. Methods* **4** 249–56

[101] Ukkonen P, Huovilainen A and Hovi T 1986 Detection of poliovirus antigen by enzyme immunoassay *J. Clin. Microbiol.* **24** 954–58

[102] Tuokko H and Salmi A 1983 Detection of IgM antibodies to measles virus by enzyme-immunoassay *Med. Microbiol. Immunol.* **171** 187–98

[103] Mitamura K, Sugaya N, Shimizu H, Nirasawa M, Takahashi K, Hirai Y and Takeuchi Y 1999 Optical immunoassay test for rapid detection of influenza A and B viruses: an evaluation *J. Japan. Assoc. Infect. Dis.* **73** 1069–73

[104] Vasala A, Hytönen V P and Laitinen O H 2020 Modern tools for rapid diagnostics of antimicrobial resistance *Front. Cell Infect. Microbiol.* **10** 308

[105] Luka G S, Nowak E, Kawchuk J, Hoorfar M and Najjaran H 2017 Portable device for the detection of colorimetric assays *R. Soc. Open Sci.* **4** 171025

[106] Raji M A, Aloraij Y, Alhamlan F, Suaifan G, Weber K, Cialla-May D, Popp J and Zourob M 2021 Development of rapid colorimetric assay for the detection of influenza A and B viruses *Talanta* **221** 121468

[107] Ventura B, della, Cennamo M, Minopoli A, Campanile R, Censi S B, Terracciano D, Portella G and Velotta R 2020 Colorimetric test for fast detection of SARS-CoV-2 in nasal and throat swabs *ACS Sens.* **5** 3043–8

[108] Sibley C D, Peirano G and Church D L 2012 Molecular methods for pathogen and microbial community detection and characterization: current and potential application in diagnostic microbiology *Infect. Genet. Evol.* **12** 505–21

[109] Feng W, Newbigging A M and Le C *et al* 2020 Molecular diagnosis of COVID-19: challenges and research needs *Anal. Chem.* **92** 10196–209

[110] Palacios G, Jabado O and Cisterna D *et al* 2005 Molecular identification of mumps virus genotypes from clinical samples: standardized method of analysis *J. Clin. Microbiol.* **43** 1869–78

[111] Boddicker J D, Rota P A, Kreman T, Wangeman A, Lowe L, Hummel K B, Thompson R, Bellini W J, Pentella M and Desjardin L E 2007 Real-time reverse transcription-PCR assay for detection of mumps virus RNA in clinical specimens *J. Clin. Microbiol.* **45** 2902–8

[112] Ellis J S and Zambon M C 2002 Molecular diagnosis of influenza *Rev. Med. Virol.* **12** 375–89

[113] Bumgarner R 2013 Overview of DNA microarrays: types, applications, and their future *Current Protocols in Molecular Biology* (New York: Wiley) ch 22, unit 22.1

[114] Lemuth K and Rupp S 2015 Microarrays as research tools and diagnostic devices *RNA and DNA Diagnostics* (Cham: Springer) pp 259–80

[115] Yang S and Rothman R E 2004 PCR-based diagnostics for infectious diseases: uses, limitations, and future applications in acute-care settings *Lancet Infect. Dis.* **4** 337–48

[116] Yoo S, Choi J, Lee S Y and Yoo N 2009 Applications of DNA microarray in disease diagnostics *J. Microbiol. Biotechnol.* **19** 635–46

[117] Wang Y, Yu L, Kong X and Sun L 2017 Application of nanodiagnostics in point-of-care tests for infectious diseases *Int. J. Nanomed.* **12** 4789–803

[118] Jat S K, Gandhi H A, Bhattacharya J and Sharma M K 2021 Magnetic nanoparticles: an emerging nano-based tool to fight against viral infections *Mater. Adv.* **2** 4479–96

[119] Kang J, Tahir A, Wang H and Chang J 2021 Applications of nanotechnology in virus detection, tracking, and infection mechanisms *Wiley Interdiscip. Rev. Nanomed. Nanobiotechnol.* **13** e1700

[120] Xiao D, Qi H, Teng Y, Pierre D, Kutoka P T and Liu D 2021 Advances and challenges of fluorescent nanomaterials for synthesis and biomedical applications *Nanoscale Res. Lett.* **16** 167

[121] Mukherjee A, Shim Y and Myong Song J 2016 Quantum dot as probe for disease diagnosis and monitoring *Biotechnol. J.* **11** 31–42

[122] Rizvi S B, Ghaderi S, Keshtgar M and Seifalian A M 2010 Semiconductor quantum dots as fluorescent probes for *in vitro* and *in vivo* bio-molecular and cellular imaging *Nano Rev.* **1** 5161

[123] Ventola C L 2012 The nanomedicine revolution: part 1: emerging concepts P T**37** 512–25

[124] Auría-Soro C, Nesma T, Juanes-Velasco P, Landeira-Viñuela A, Fidalgo-Gomez H, Acebes-Fernandez V, Gongora R, Almendral Parra M J, Manzano-Roman R and Fuentes M 2019 Interactions of nanoparticles and biosystems: microenvironment of nanoparticles and biomolecules in nanomedicine *Nanomaterials (Basel)* **9** 1365

[125] Ferdous Z and Nemmar A 2020 Health impact of silver nanoparticles: a review of the biodistribution and toxicity following various routes of exposure *Int. J. Mol. Sci.* **21** 2375

[126] Wang X, Sun Y, Jing S, Ma X and Zeng Y 2007 Combining gold nanoparticles with real-time immuno-PCR for Analysis of HIV p24 antigens *2007 1st Int. Conf. on Bioinformatics and Biomedical Engineering* pp 1198–201

[127] Wang J, Li J, Baca A J, Hu J, Zhou F, Yan W and Pang D-W 2003 Amplified voltammetric detection of DNA hybridization via oxidation of ferrocene caps on gold nanoparticle/streptavidin conjugates *Anal. Chem.* **75** 3941–45

[128] Mokhtarzadeh A, Eivazzadeh-Keihan R, Pashazadeh P, Hejazi M, Gharaatifar N, Hasanzadeh M, Baradaran B and de la Guardia M 2017 Nanomaterial-based biosensors for detection of pathogenic virus *TrAC Trends Anal. Chem.* **97** 445–57

[129] Diba F S, Kim S and Lee H J 2015 Amperometric bioaffinity sensing platform for avian influenza virus proteins with aptamer modified gold nanoparticles on carbon chips *Biosens. Bioelectron.* **72** 355–61

[130] Choi H K, Lee M-J, Lee S N, Kim T-H and Oh B-K 2021 Noble metal nanomaterial-based biosensors for electrochemical and optical detection of viruses causing respiratory illnesses *Front. Chem.* **9** 672739

[131] Alvarez-Puebla R A and Liz-Marzán L M 2010 SERS-based diagnosis and biodetection *Small* **6** 604–10

Chapter 3

Historical review of SERS in biomedical applications: infectious diseases

Muhammad Usman, Jia-Wei Tang, Zheng-Kang Li, Jin-Xin Lai, Kai-Xuan Yuan, Qing-Hua Liu, Xiao Zhang and Liang Wang[1]

Infectious diseases occur regularly in human populations and have had significant impacts on human history in many aspects, such as social changes and economic developments. It is now well known that infectious diseases are mainly caused by microbial pathogens such as viruses, bacteria, fungi, parasites, etc, the rapid and accurate detection of which is essential in disease prevention and treatment. Many methods and techniques for microbial diagnosis have already been developed and applied in real-world situations, which greatly facilitate the control of most infectious agents. However, current technologies have limitations, and novel methods are constantly needed to face the emerging challenges of microbial detection and identification. Due to its low-cost, label-free nature, and non-invasive features, Raman spectroscopy (RS) is becoming an attractive method for the rapid and accurate detection of microbial pathogens, and the newly developed surface-enhanced Raman spectroscopy (SERS) appears to have the most promising future. In this chapter we provide a historical review of SERS in biomedical applications with a focus on infectious diseases, aiming to gain insight into how SERS can be used in the detection of pathogenic microbes, virulence factor discrimination, and antibiotic resistance profiling. In addition, computational methods, e.g. statistical analysis and machine learning, are also discussed to elucidate powerful combinations of advanced algorithms and SERS spectra in the diagnosis of infectious diseases. Taken together, this study provides a timely overview of the application of the SERS technique in the clinical microbiology field, which holds great potential in the rapid diagnosis and control of infectious diseases in real-world settings.

3.1 Introduction

Infectious diseases, also known as contagious diseases, transmissible diseases, or communicable diseases, are normally caused by microbial pathogens such as viruses,

---

[1] All the authors contributed equally to the study.

bacteria, and fungi, which can be spread from one organism to another through either direct or indirect transmission [1]. Human populations have suffered from infectious diseases for millions of years, but after humans began living in agricultural societies more and more infectious diseases emerged due to the increased density of human populations and the transmission of microbial pathogens from animals to humans [2]. From a historical point of view, infectious diseases such as tuberculosis, polio, smallpox, diphtheria, etc, have had great impacts on human society since ancient times, leading to devastating consequences in human history, such as wars and economic depressions, etc [3]. The currently ongoing COVID-19 pandemic is the newest infectious disease outbreak that human beings are facing, and has caused more than 6 million deaths all over the world and significantly changed the global economy and modern lifestyles [4, 5]. Therefore, effective prevention and control of infectious diseases are important for both the public health of human society and the well-being of individuals.

In clinical laboratories, microbial pathogens were previously mainly discriminated through cultures and biochemical tests, which are time-consuming and labor-intensive despite their high accuracy [6]. As for the advanced molecular methods, such as polymerase chain reaction (PCR) and enzyme-linked immunosorbent assay (ELISA), although these methods are rapid and convenient, they suffer from high false-positive rates due to factors such as sample contamination [7]. Recently, high-throughput sequencing technologies such as next-generation sequencing (NGS) and single-molecule real-time (SMRT) sequencing are emerging as novel tools for microbial identification and species determination; however, the sophisticated preparation procedures and high-level computational analysis methods greatly limited the real-world application of the sequencing methods in clinical laboratories [6]. Due to its rapidity and sensitivity, and the low cost of a single test, matrix-assisted laser desorption ionization-time of flight mass spectrometry (MALDI-TOF MS) has been used widely in medical laboratories for microbial identification and stain typing [8]. However, the instrument itself is rather expensive and is not easily affordable for general users. In addition, the method also suffers from the inability to recognize novel microbial species due to the limitations of the MS database [8].

Raman spectroscopy (RS) is based on the Raman scattering effect which is an inelastic scattering of photons, which was first discovered by the Noble Prize Laureate C V Raman and his student K S Krishnan in 1928 [9]. More than 90 years later, RS has become an established technique that is being used widely for molecular vibration detection in various defined systems [7, 10]. The signals generated via RS form unique and high-resolution fingerprints that can be used to represent particular materials [10]. As a powerful low-cost and non-destructive technique for both quantitative and qualitative characterization of materials, it has found itself with many applications in many biomedical situations [11]. However, it should be emphasized that the Raman scattering effect is very weak when compared to the elastic Rayleigh scattering effect, and only accounts for one in 108 scattered photons [12]. Therefore, regular RS is considered an inefficient, insensitive method with long acquisition times, which greatly limits its real-world applications, although various computational methods have been developed to overcome the low signal-to-noise ratio (SNR) in Raman spectra [11–14].

Luckily, in the 1970s, the discovery and development of surface-enhanced Raman scattering (SERS) by Fleischmann and his group from the University of Southampton, UK, revitalized the RS technique and initiated new directions for its application in the chemistry of interfaces [15]. However, the specific mechanisms for the signal enhancement found in SERS spectroscopy are not clear yet and are highly controversial [15]. In particular, SERS spectroscopy is an advanced technique of RS with highly sensitive structural detection when the analytes are at very low concentrations because of the significant amplification of electromagnetic fields through localized surface plasmon excitations via SERS substrates, that is, metallic nanostructures [16]. Currently, the most frequently used metals for SERS are silver (Ag), gold (Au), and copper (Cu) because they can generate maximal enhancement for visible and near-infrared radiation (NIR), and can be mixed with samples in liquids or on solid surfaces [15].

Through the utilization of the SERS technique in the biomedical fields with a focus on infectious diseases, many clinical samples and microbial pathogens have been identified and determined successfully, which confirms the application potential of this technique in real-world settings such as microbial diagnostics in clinical laboratories. Therefore, to better understand the development and application of the SERS technique in the biomedical field, we examine the discovery and progress of the RS and SERS techniques and reviewed the applications of SERS in microbial identification from the perspective of infectious diseases. The limitations and challenges of the technique are also discussed. Altogether, we provide an overview of the SERS technique in the biomedical field and assessed representative studies involving applications of SERS in infectious diseases, through which we confirm the potential of the SERS technique in the rapid and accurate diagnosis of microbial pathogens in clinical settings.

3.2 The discovery of the Raman effect and its applications

3.2.1 The Raman effect

Spontaneous RS uses a laser source that emits monochromatic light in the visible to near-infrared range. The instrument is used to quantitatively detect inelastically scattered photons generated by the interactions of photons from the laser source with molecules within a sample. The resulting Raman spectra are similar to human fingerprints, unique and specific, and can be used to identify samples. Specifically, the Raman effect is an inelastic collision when a photon collides with a molecule. The molecules in the medium are initially in the ground state, and the excitation light causes the molecules to be excited to a high-energy virtual state, which in turn causes the electrons of the virtual molecules to transition to the excited state, resulting in scattered light. In this process, the energy will be transferred to the molecule by the exciting photon, so that the molecule that transits to the excited state gains energy, resulting in a decrease in the energy of the scattered light. The scattered light measured in the vertical direction is called the Stokes line [17]. Conversely, if the photon gains energy from the sample molecule and receives scattered light at a frequency greater than the incident light, it is called the anti-Stokes line, which is usually weaker [18]. If the photon collides with a molecule and there is no change in energy, but the direction of the collision changes, it is called Rayleigh scattering [19]. In general, Stokes and anti-Stokes lines are symmetrically distributed on either side of the Rayleigh scattering line in the Raman spectrum (figure 3.1(A)), since in each case the energy of vibrational quanta is gained or lost [20]. In addition, Raman shift is defined as the difference in frequency between Raman and Rayleigh scattering.

A typical Raman spectrometer consists of the following five main parts: laser source, filter, sample cell, monochromator, and detector. The most commonly used laser sources are He–Ne lasers (wavelength = 632.8 nm) and Ar lasers (wavelength = 514.5 and 488.0 nm) for visible light. Photomultiplier tubes are the most commonly used detectors, along with charge-coupled devices (CCDs) and indium gallium arsenide (InGaAs) detectors [21]. RS is an optical spectroscopy technique that can probe the vibrational modes associated with chemical bonds in a sample [22]. Because different samples have different chemical compositions, while different chemical compositions correspond to specific characteristic peak combinations, a sample-specific spectral fingerprint or 'Raman spectrum' can thus be generated and this spectral signal, by its uniqueness, provides incredible details about the biochemical composition of a biological sample (figure 3.1(B)). This creates the opportunity to detect multiple biomarkers simultaneously, which cannot be achieved by many diagnostic tests at the current stage. With the upgrade of the Raman spectrometer, its universality and detection speed have been greatly improved, which makes RS more easily applicable to clinical environments [23].

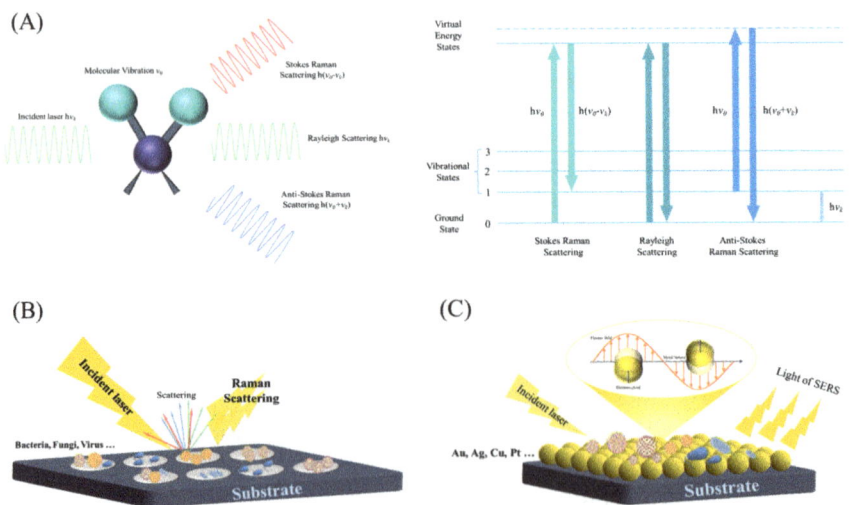

Figure 3.1. A schematic illustration of Raman scattering effects and their application in the detection of microbial pathogens. (A) The principles of the Raman scattering effect. (B) Application of Raman spectroscopy in the detection of pathogenic microbes. (C) Application of SERS in the detection of pathogenic microbes.

3.2.2 Applications of Raman spectrometry

Different cells and tissues are composed of different combinations of proteins, carbohydrates, lipids, and nucleic acids, while each Raman spectrum has many associated vibrational modes to reveal information about the chemical structure and composition of a cell. By searching the PubMed database for the keywords 'Raman' and 'Bacteria', it can be found that, in the 1970s, Thomas used RS to detect RNA extracted from *Escherichia coli* ribosomes in H_2O and $2H_2O$ solutions [24], and Tsuboi observed Raman spectra of purified formyl thioamino acid transfer RNA from *Escherichia coli* in an aqueous solution [25]. In the 1980s resonance Raman spectroscopy was applied to explore intracellular pigment interactions [26, 27], spectral changes in different environments [28], differences in internal structures between similar strains [29, 30], and protein Raman spectra from different strains [31, 32]. By the 1990s research using RS on bacteria gradually increased, and the number of references in the literature exceeds that of the 1970s and 1980s combined.

In addition to the study of the internal structure and chemical composition of various pathogenic bacteria, such as *Bacillus* [33], *Clostridium* [34], and *Escherichia coli* [35], mathematical models have also been introduced into the study of RS. For example, in the work of Jones *et al*, the effect of the mutation of residue tyrosine M210 on the primary donor bacteriochlorophyll was investigated by near-infrared Fourier transform (FT)RS in a reaction center purified from a deficient strain of *Rhodococcus sphaericus*. It was concluded that the effect of the tyrosine M210 mutation on the primary electron transfer rate and asymmetry of the reaction center cannot be attributed to changes in the electron structure of the primary donor [36]. In a study by Mattioli *et al*, specific changes in the hydrogen-bonding states of the primary donor (P), in reaction centers from *Rhodobacter sphaeroides* bearing mutations near P were determined using near-infrared excited FTRS [37]. This study discussed that changes in protein hydrogen bonding to the conjugated carbonyl groups of P alone are not the sole factor that contributes to the sizeable modifications of the P/P+ redox mid-point potentials [37]. Although these studies revealed abundant biological information inside bacteria, these studies only detected the Raman spectra of chemical components inside bacteria through experimental observation but did not analyse the whole biological fingerprint of the bacteria.

For the detection of infectious diseases, we need to be able to distinguish the differences between the Raman spectra of different microbial strains at the species level. In 1998 British scientist Goodacre used dispersive RS to detect Raman spectra of 59 clinical bacterial strains associated with urinary tract infections and used pyrolysis mass spectrometry (PyMS) and Fourier transform infrared spectroscopy to collect data on the same samples. The research team used, for the first time, an artificial neural network (ANN) to train the bacterial spectral data, and the results showed that the ANN model could achieve 80% recognition accuracy on the Raman spectral dataset, showing that RS could distinguish bacterial species with clinical significance [38]. As we entered the new century, the research on RS grew exponentially, and a large number of researchers have focused on the direction of using RS to diagnose infectious diseases. For example, Maquelin *et al* proposed a novel identification method based on confocal Raman microspectroscopy, through which they generated Raman spectra for five bacterial colonies grown on a solid medium for 6 h before comparing the different Raman signals [39]. Correction algorithms were used to reduce the influence of medium and substrate background and uneven sample thickness, while a hierarchical clustering algorithm (HCA) was used to analyse the spectral data of the five strains, and the results showed two main clustering clades, one for *Staphylococcus*, the other for *Enterococcus faecalis* and *Escherichia coli*, and there is a clear difference between *Enterococcus faecalis* and *E. coli* [39]. The study achieved 83% identification accuracy using principal component analysis (PCA) combined with linear discriminant analysis (LDA). The classification results show that RS had great potential as a powerful tool in clinical diagnostic microbiology [39]. This makes the study of the full spectral information of isolated and cultured strains detected by RS popular. As in the study by Mello *et al*, the Raman spectra of bacterial pathogens such as *E. coli*, *Salmonella cholerae*, and *Shigella flexneri* that cause gastroenteritis were collected and distinguished by the partial least squares regression (PLS) algorithm [40]. In a work by Buijtels' team, 63 strains of *Mycobacterium tuberculosis* were detected by RS of eight species, achieving a recognition accuracy of 95.2% [41]. Teh *et al* evaluated the feasibility of applying near-infrared (NIR) RS in the identification of nonneoplastic lesions caused by *Helicobacter pylori* (Hp) infection, which confirmed that intestinal metaplasia (IM) was highly associated with stomach cancer. In the study, the PCA-LDA algorithm achieved 91.7% and 80.0% sensitivity and specificity, respectively [42].

Although RS has been proved to be efficient in distinguishing microbial species, it largely relies on microbial cultures. However, to apply the technique in clinical settings, it needs to be used for the direct analysis of real-world clinical samples such as urine, sputum, blood, alveolar lavage fluid, etc. Sputum is a complex biological sample and contains proteins, nucleic acids, mucins, amino acids, and other components, which, however, are easy to collect. Kumar and collaborators combined *M. tuberculosis* with artificial sputum and collected more than 2500 Raman spectra for identification and evaluation. The PCA-LDA algorithm achieved 98% classification accuracy, demonstrating the ability of RS combined with machine learning to identify *Mycobacterium tuberculosis* and other microbial strains in sputum [43]. Unlike sputum, serum samples do not contain complex proteins and biological metabolites, making them easier to analyse. For efficient and timely diagnosis of hepatitis C virus (HCV), Naseer *et al* used RS to distinguish the differences between HCV-infected sera and healthy sera, and unique characteristic peaks associated with HCV-infected sera were analysed by the analysis of variance (ANOVA) test and *t*-test, and different types of infected samples were also correctly identified using the PCA-LDA algorithm [44]. In another study, Guleken *et al* tested serum samples from 47 patients with the COVID-19 virus. Samples were collected at three different periods of one, three, and six months after infection with the COVID-19 virus. RS was used to identify patients and six different machine learning algorithms were applied to analyse the spectral data at different times. The results showed that the random forest algorithm could achieve a classification accuracy of more than 98% in different stages, and the classification accuracy of all models reached 100% in the analysis of the first and third groups of samples [45]. In conclusion, although RS is still in its infancy, it is believed that the technique has the potential to be developed as a rapid diagnostic tool that can be used as an early prevention and prognostic tool for infectious diseases in the clinical setting.

3.2.3 Disadvantages of Raman spectrometry

As a spectral detection technology, RS has its unique advantages. Whether it is a solid, liquid, or gas, RS can be used to characterize the properties of its substances. Some samples that cannot be extracted can be directly detected by the non-destructive technique. However, the high resolution of the Raman spectral finger-print is often accompanied by the inherent low sensitivity of the Raman scattering effect, which is normally ten orders of magnitude lower in energy than infrared or fluorescence spectroscopy [46], which indicates that the Raman signal itself has a very weak signal intensity. When the instrument detects a sample, the Raman signal can be affected by strong autofluorescence effects from the detection device or the sample itself, which further weakens the Raman spectral features and complicates the analysis. In addition, weak Raman signals involve long acquisition times, slowing down the analysis [47], which makes RS limited in routine macroscopic analysis. Except for the disadvantage of weak signal, for many clinicians, the interpretability of RS is poor, and a large amount of spectral data is often wasted without appropriate computational analysis. Therefore, improvements should be determined for the regular RS technique, which would make it more practical for its real-world applications.

3.3 The development of the SERS techniques

In the 1970s Fleischmann and his research group re-vitalized the RS technique and started new directions for its application in the chemistry of interfaces by discovering the novel SERS effect, which greatly enhanced the signal intensity of Raman effects [15]. SERS enhances the Raman signal by molecules adsorbed on metallic nano-particle surfaces, ensuring data repeatability and reproducibility [160]. Later, SERS and machine learning-based automated spectroscopic diagnostic frameworks have been adopted to analyse and interpret Raman spectral data, which can quickly detect subtle differences between samples, enabling clinicians to interpret Raman results on an individual basis [7]. These methods are discussed in further detail below.

3.3.1 SERS-based on different nanoscale materials

Advanced nanomaterials are frequently used in biomedical applications because of their special physical, chemical, sensing, magnetic, and optical properties. These characteristics of the nanomaterials help to improve the sensitivity and specificity of SERS (figure 3.1(C)). The main significant benefit of these new developments is the ability to modify the properties of nanomaterials by modifying their morphology and composition, as well as their various adsorption capacities by appropriately functionalizing them using surface chemistry and shortening the sensing time through multiplexing. According to a recent study, nanomaterials are increasingly being used in the SERS method to improve the sensitivity and multi-detection capability. The field of pathogen detection is booming due to the variety of bio-sensing techniques as well as the development of nanomaterial fabrication and employment for different applications. In this review, we will focus on the detection of infectious diseases through SERS that use nanomaterials for signal enhancement such as metal nanoparticles (Ag, Au), magnetic nanoparticles, bimetallic nano-particles, silica nanoparticles, graphene, carbon nanotubes, carbon dots, quantum dots, and up-conversion nanoparticles, etc (figure 3.2).

3.3.1.1 Magnetic nanoparticles (MNPs)

Emerging magnetic nanoparticles (MNPs) have attracted increasing attention due to their advantages in sample enrichment. In addition, MNPs have been shown to enhance sensitivity, decrease the time of analysis, and improve the SNR [48, 49]. The size of the MNPs, which is controlled by the preparation technique, determines their function [50]. MNPs smaller than 30 nm are excellent candidates for enhancement applications due to their superparamagnetic properties and rapid responses to an applied magnetic field [51]. MNPs usually have a core–shell structure, with a noble

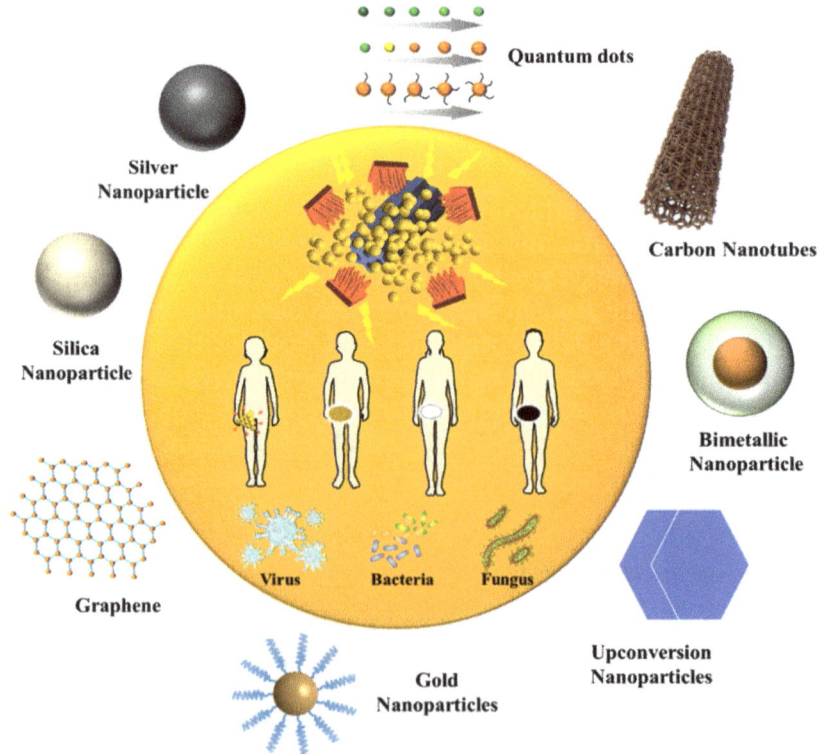

Figure 3.2. The different kinds of nanoparticles used to overcome biological barriers and enhance the sensitivity, speed, and efficiency for early diagnosis and specific detection of infectious diseases.

metal shell outside and a magnetic core inside. Three factors are used to develop functionalized MNPs: production of the magnetic core; coating with a noble metal; and bio/chemical modification [62, 63]. These functionalized MNPs could provide a 'hotspot' and improve SERS sensing performance exceptionally [64]. The prepared MNPs feature high sensitivity, a simple synthesis method, low cost, and excellent control, allowing them to capture and concentrate the target molecules. Taken together, MNPs show significant interest and potential in SERS-based sensing, particularly for rapid pathogen identification through sample enrichment.

3.3.1.2 Gold nanoparticles (AuNPs)
AuNPs are at the forefront of the rapid development of the field of nanomedicine [52]. Over the last half-century, AuNP synthesis methods have been developed with great interest [53] because it is an excellent material to use in the detection of biomolecules at low concentrations due to their uniquely size-dependent physio-chemical properties [54]. The SPR phenomenon, which results in their higher scattering and absorption cross sections, is one of their characteristic features [56]. In addition, the composition of AuNPs can have a significant effect on their optical properties. AuNPs are combined with biomolecules such as antibodies, nucleic acid tags, glycoproteins, etc [54]. There are several different structures of the most commonly used Au nanoparticles for sensor applications, including rods, spheres, and wires [57]. AuNPs are good SERS substrates due to their exceptional biocompatibility, huge surface area, strong chemical and thermal stability, and simplicity of fabrication and modification [55]. As a result, the application of AuNPs in SERS enhancement is a popular approach for detecting pathogens.

3.3.1.3 Silver nanoparticles (AgNPs)
AgNPs were used in the detection of target analytes employing SERS [58]. This method has been used for single-molecule detection due to its high sensitivity [59]. The use of this method for pathogen identification is demonstrated in the following research. The SERS method was employed by Naja *et al* for the detection of *E. coli* bacteria. In this process, protein-A-coated AgNPs and antibodies specific to *E. coli* were employed [60]. The SERS spectra of bacteria were produced by interacting with an *E. coli*–antibody conjugated to protein-A-coated AgNPs. The significance of AgNPs in SERS was revealed by the great molecular selectivity of the SERS spectral fingerprint [60]. A SERS-active silver nanorod array was shown by Driskell *et al* to be capable of detecting and differentiating a variety of significant human pathogens, such as HIV, rotavirus, and the bacterium *Mycoplasma pneumonia* [61]. These methods can detect viruses right down to the strain level.

3.3.1.4 Bimetallic nanoparticles
The components of bimetallic NPs can have a variety of morphologies and structures that are constituted by the core–shell structure. They can be classified as mixed or segregated structures based on their structural makeup [65]. Bimetallic nanoparticles are interesting materials because they have novel features such as tunable surface plasmon bands and optical properties, as well as increased stability

and dispersibility [66, 67]. They have significant exposure to chemical, physical, and biological preparation techniques [68]. Bimetallic Au:Ag core shells in different morphologies have received significant attention from the SERS community [66, 69, 70]. There are several advantages to investigating bimetallic nanostructures for SERS. Due to their chemical and plasmonic properties, they have the potential to combine the best aspects of bimetallic Au:Ag materials [66, 70].

3.3.1.5 Quantum dots (QDs)

QDs are semiconductor nanostructures that have gained popularity recently for multiplex detection because of their broad adsorption and narrow emission band. Furthermore, advantageous features include the ability to tune the emission spectra over a broad range of wavelengths and the resistance to external physicochemical conditions [71]. These typically consist of atoms from the periodic tables IIB–VI, III–V, or IV–VI groups, with diameters ranging from 1 to 10 nm, and their nature determines the quantum-controlled mechanics of their optical properties. There is evidence that the toxicity of QDs depends on their surface characteristics, including their aspect ratio, ligands, and modifications. The applications for quantum dots (QDs) in photo-luminescence (PL) include size-tunable PL and high quantum yield (>20%) [72]. QDs have many exceptional characteristics, including high photostability, great selectivity, and biocompatibility. The combination of these features provides a fantastic opportunity to identify a variety of pathogen recognition components [73]. QDs have a high potential for use in the imaging and detection of infectious diseases [94]. The luminescent QDs serve as practical platforms for rapid and sensitive virus detection, enabling the simultaneous diagnosis of pathogenic viral diseases. Chen *et al* established a QD-based fluoro-immunoassay for the rapid and precise detection of the H5N1 subtype of the avian influenza virus (AIV) [158].

3.3.1.6 Graphene and graphene oxide

Graphene is a single-layer, two-dimensional honeycomb made of densely packed, sp^2-hybridized carbon atoms. It has recently attracted a great deal of interest in the biological field because of its remarkable electrical, optical, and chemical properties. Graphene can be used to make biological recognition components and drug delivery systems because of its polyphenylene ring surface structure and its capacity to stack on to ssDNA and aromatic compounds [74, 75]. Furthermore, graphene has a carrier mobility of around $15\,000$ cm^2 V^{-1} s^{-1}, which has been widely investigated in electrochemistry [76]. Moreover, graphene has excellent optical and thermal con-ductivities [77, 78], enabling applications in biomedical fields such as infectious diseases. Furthermore, graphene and its graphene oxide (GO) derivative have often been described as effective drug carriers with unusually high drug loading abilities because of their large surface area, low cost, and effective electrostatic interactions. [79–81]. It has been demonstrated in the literature that plasmonic nanoparticles can be coated with graphene or GO nanosheets for high-performance SERS applications [82, 83]. Therefore, the combination of plasmonic noble-metallic nanostructures with GO could offer a popular platform for efficient SERS detection.

3.3.1.7 Carbon nanotubes (CNTs)

CNTs are categorized into single-walled carbon nanotubes (SWCNTs) and multi-walled carbon nanotubes (MWCNTs) based on the number of layers of carbon atoms [84]. The superior mechanical strength of CNTs is primarily due to the sp^2 hybridization of the carbon atoms [85]. When CNTs are used to diagnose infectious diseases, they typically contain several surface functional groups, including carboxyl and hydroxyl groups, on their surface. This results in a vast number of 'hotspot' sites that produce an order of magnitude greater local electromagnetic field strength. Furthermore, CNTs appear to be biocompatible, which is required for effective SERS sensing of biological objects [159]. The application of CNTs in SERS sensors is currently a hot topic of discussion in the research community because of the observed charge transfer carried on by the chemical amplification of SERS.

3.3.1.8 Carbon dots (CDs) or carbon particles

Carbon dots (CDs), a novel class of nanomaterials, exhibit excellent optical properties, excellent light durability, low cytotoxicity, excellent biocompatibility, and ease of synthesis [95, 96]. CDs are novel members of the zero-dimensional family with a size of less than 10 nm [95]. They are primarily made of carbon, have an sp^2 or sp^3 carbon skeleton, and have a large number of functional groups or polymer chains [95]. Furthermore, the oxygen-containing functional groups that can encapsulate CDs make their water solubility and biocompatibility superior. Carbon-based nanomaterials can be used as a component in SERS-based biosensors because of their superior physicochemical properties. In particular, the high electrical conductivity and large surface area of carbon-based nanomaterials enhance the sensitivity of the SERS-based sensors [160]. These advantages have led to a significant emergence in the use of CDs in the diagnosis of infectious diseases in recent years.

3.3.1.9 Up-conversion nanoparticles (UCNPs)

Fluorescent inorganic nanomaterials called lanthanide-doped UCNPs can absorb two or more low-energy photons to create higher-energy photons and release fluorescence signals [97]. A type of very promising fluorescent probe for the detection of infectious diseases, UCNPs have a number of benefits over typical fluorescent materials, including low toxicity, long luminescence lifetimes, good SNRs, and strong resistance to photobleaching. Due to their unique fluorescence mechanism, which absorbs 980 nm near-infrared (NIR) light and up-converts it to high-energy visible photons, UCNPs have recently gained a lot of interest in biological applications [98]. They are able to get beyond several restrictions such as photostability, photo-blinking, and cytotoxicity. UCNPs still have some disadvantages, including their limited photostability, photo-blinking, and cytotoxicity [99, 100]. Recent studies have shown that UCNP probes have outstanding power for the accurate and fast detection of analytes (such as bacteria, viruses, biotinylated antibodies, and human IgG and IgM antibodies) [86–89]. UCNP material was employed in prior studies to quantify individual bacteria [90, 91]. In addition, multiplex pathogenic bacterial detection using up-conversion nanoparticles with particular recognition components (aptamers and antibodies) has been advanced [92, 93]. Due to these benefits, UCNPs are excellent candidates for the development of multifunctional theranostic nanoplatforms, which combine optical imaging, drug delivery, and photodynamic therapy at the level of living cells and small animals [101, 102].

3.3.1.10 Silica nanoparticles

Fluorescent silica NPs (FSNPs) have attracted a great deal of interest in bio-imaging and bio-sensing due to their numerous appealing properties in recent years. First, the silica NP matrix can encapsulate substances to significantly change their physical or chemical properties. Second, the optical transparency of the silica NP matrix enables the excitation and emission of light to pass over it [103]. Third, the surface of hydroxylated silica NPs can be significantly enhanced using a variety of silane-based compounds to boost biocompatibility. Fourth, hydrophilic silica NPs readily disperse in an aqueous solution. Lastly, the mechanical and chemical stability of silica NPs is excellent [104, 105]. These characteristics have led to the fabrication of various FSNP types for the diagnosis of infectious diseases. The advantages of silica NPs are that they perform better than conventional fluorescent dyes in terms of sensitivity, multiplexing potential, photostability, and ease of functionalization. Silica nanoparticles can hold tens of thousands of fluorescent dye molecules, which also results in a highly improved and repeatable signal. Silica NPs are attractive for the detection, real-time tracking, and monitoring of infectious diseases because of their distinctive optical properties. Tan *et al* established triple-dye-doped silica NPs for multiplexed bacteria identification [161]. These nanoparticles were conjugated to monoclonal antibodies for the sensitive detection of different bacterial pathogens such as *E. coli*, *S. typhimurium*, and *Staphylococcus aureus* at low concentrations [184]. These improved features make silica NPs appealing for the detection of infectious diseases.

3.3.2 Computational analysis of SERS spectra

Biological samples are highly complex and heterogeneous, and their Raman spectra contain a large number of Raman vibrational modes. Therefore, extracting useful information from feature-rich mass spectral data is a key hurdle to overcome [106]. However, it is important to note that the variation that occurs between the spectra of different biological samples is often small and visual detection alone or univariate statistical methods can lead to a large loss of information. Typically, Raman datasets in biological research are large and high-dimensional, requiring more efficient multivariate methods, such as chemometrics, for truly exploratory and comprehensive analysis.

Due to the fluorescence, the effect of the sample itself, and interferences such as cosmic rays, dark currents, ambient noise, etc, that are generated within Raman or from other sources [192–194], fast and efficient Raman spectral data analysis could be hindered greatly. Various spectral processing algorithms have been developed for this, often involving operations such as quality control, spike removal, curve smoothing, baseline correction, and normalization [107]. Spectral signal preprocessing is the first stage in the introduction of chemometrics. The preprocessed data means that the influence of external factors on the spectral data during the analysis process is greatly reduced [108]. For example, in the collected Raman spectral data, the noise signal completely covers the original Raman signal [108], and the spectral data can be regarded as outliers and eliminated at this time [147]. For cosmic spikes caused by interfering electrons in the detector, we can eliminate the effects of extreme outliers on the overall spectrum by visual inspection, average spectral comparisons, and/or thresholding [108]. Since spikes are usually characterized by high intensity, sharpness, and random locations in Raman spectra, an algorithm is developed to distinguish the peak and normal Raman bands from the Raman spectra collected from white blood cells in the study of Ryabchykov *et al* [109]. By setting the threshold value proportional to the maximum normalization of the Laplacian operator of each Raman spectrum, the algorithm can perform peak removal without setting the parameters in advance, and the sensitivity can reach 99% [109]. For Raman spectra with unpredictable intensities generated by the internal components of the spectrometer during spectrometry, smoothing denoising algorithms such as median filtering, wavelet transform, and Savitzky–Golay (S–G) are used to improve the quality of spectral data. Among them, the S–G algorithm is one of the most commonly used spectral preprocessing methods [110, 111]. In a recent study by Liu *et al*, the polynomial fitting order of the S–G algorithm was set to 2 to smooth the SERS spectral data of *Klebsiella pneumonia* [112]. For the uncontrollable noise generated by the SERS substrate or the sample itself, baseline correction is used to deal with the continuous distortion in spectrum acquisition [108]. Kashi *et al* used polynomial fitting baseline correction to remove the AgNPs spectral background on aluminum plates before further analysing SERS spectra of bacteria commonly distributed in four types of food [113]. Normalization is the last step of the preprocessing procedures [114], which is used to justify the signals at each of the Raman shifts in a group of spectra from the same sample [110]. All the Raman signal intensities are mapped to the range of 0–1 to control the differences among Raman signal intensity levels. In the work of Liu *et al*, single-cell Raman spectra of ten marine actinomycetes were normalized to remove the effects of differences in sample thickness and laser power [115].

Based on preprocessed Raman spectra, chemometrics was used for the classification and prediction of microbial species. In general, chemometric methods can be divided into unsupervised and supervised machine learning methods (figure 3.3) [116]. Unsupervised methods are exploratory. By clustering the positional relationships between sample data, the model can autonomously discover hidden relationships within the data without any prior knowledge [117]. Commonly used unsupervised machine learning algorithms are principal components analysis (PCA) and hierarchical clustering analysis (HCA). Shahzad *et al* used the PCA algorithm to classify healthy people and TB patients, healthy people and TB patients with type 1 diabetes mellitus (T1DM) patients, and healthy people and TB patients with type 2 diabetes mellitus (T2DM) when analysing the SERS spectra of pulmonary tuberculosis patients [118]. The results showed that the PCA algorithm

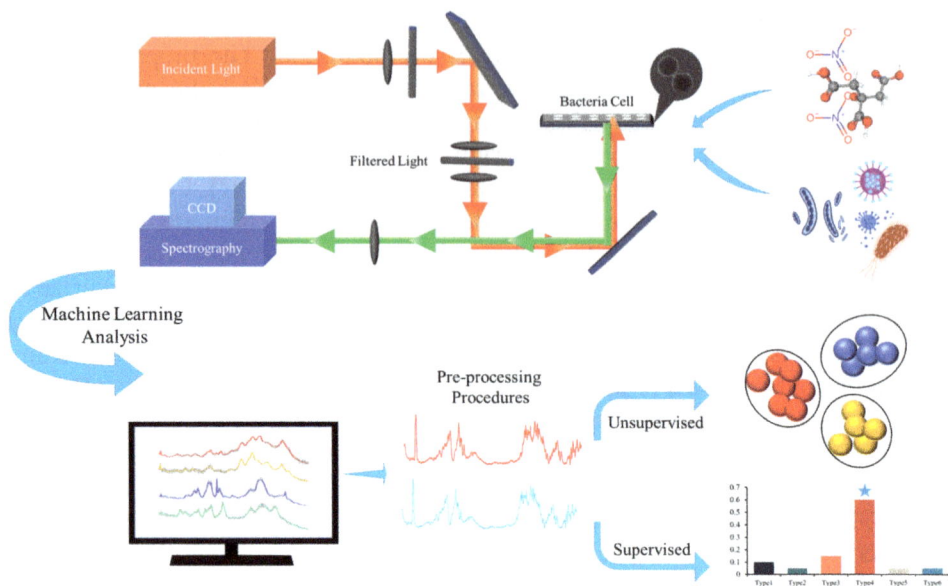

Figure 3.3. Schematic illustration of the combination of machine learning algorithms with SERS spectroscopy for microbial pathogen detection.

could distinguish the SERS spectra of serum samples from different types of patients better [118]. As a clustering algorithm, hierarchical clustering creates a hierarchical nested clustering tree by calculating the similarity between data points of different categories, using a tree structure to describe the organization of the sample [119]. In a study by Bashir *et al*, SERS was used to identify and distinguish tigecycline-resistant *E. coli* (TREC) from tigecycline-sensitive *E. coli* (TSEC). The clustering results identified three main clusters, that is, TREC, TSEC, and carbapenemase-resistant TSEC, respectively, which indicated that the HCA algorithm could effectively classify drug-resistant and drug-sensitive strains [111].

As the supervised machine learning algorithm, it divides the dataset into a training set, validation set, and test set. By learning the similarities and differences between the spectral data categories of the training set, the known data are used to establish an analysis model, which can be better applied to the classification and prediction of the new unknown test set [111]. In this way, these algorithms can be used for specific and accurate screening and diagnosis of microbial pathogens in infectious diseases. Commonly used supervised learning methods include but are not limited to partial least squares discriminant analysis (PLS-DA), support vector nachines (SVMs), and neural networks . The PLS-DA algorithm solves the classification and prediction of Raman spectral data by introducing the idea of discriminant analysis [113, 120]. When studying the SERS data of bacterial samples from three genera and six different species, Villa *et al* used PLS-DA as a multivariate supervision model to classify and identify the SERS spectra of all test samples, and the sensitivity and specificity of classification results were 100% [120]. Then the model was used to analyse a potentially new species of bacterium, and the experimental results were verified with 16S sequencing analysis, further confirming that PLS-DA is a valuable spectral analysis tool [120]. As a powerful discriminant algorithm, the SVM shows many unique advantages in solving sample issues such as small samples, nonlinear samples, high-dimensional pattern recognition, etc [121]. In the work of Cheng *et al*, human serum Raman spectroscopy was combined with an SVM algorithm to identify multiple hepatitis C patients. First of all, the serum Raman spectra of healthy people, hepatitis C virus cluster 1 (HCV1) and hepatitis C virus cluster 2 (HCV2) patients were analysed, and the model could achieve a recognition accuracy of 91.1% [122]. Additionally, the hepatitis C virus genotype 3B (HCV3b) and hepatitis C virus cluster 4 (HCV4) patient sera were classified into one group to discriminate them from hepatitis C virus gene 3A (HCV3a) patients, and the model was combined with the normalized Raman spectrum data to identify the serum of the two groups with 90% accuracy [122].

To reduce the shortcomings of complex preprocessing and complicated manual parameter adjustment in the process of machine learning, deep learning is used widely in the identification of Raman spectral signals due to its excellent computing power [123, 124]. Ciloglu and his team proposed a deep neural network (DNN) based on stacked autoencoder (SAE) to quickly identify SERS spectral data of methicillin-resistant *Staphylococcus aureus* (MRSA) and methicillin-sensitive *Staphylococcus aureus* (MSSA). Compared with traditional machine learning algorithms, the results showed that the SAE+DNN algorithm could learn features from the original data and classify the two types of *S. aureus* with 97.66% accuracy, and the performance was better than the traditional machine learning classifiers [125]. In another study, Fu *et al* used SERS to quickly diagnose the resistance of urinary tract infection (UTI) bacteria and collected a total of 54 000 SERS spectra from 18 kinds of isolates of six common UTI bacteria [126]. A convolutional neural network (CNN) was used to identify bacterial species, antibiotic sensitivity, and multidrug resistance (MDR). This method significantly simplified Raman data processing procedures by surpassing the background removal and smoothing steps and achieved over 96% recognition accuracy [126]. This work further assured the potential application of combining SERS and deep learning techniques for the rapid identification of pathogens and their associated antibiotic susceptibility.

3.4 SERS in microbial identification

How to achieve rapid identification of pathogenic microorganisms, in particular selected types of bacteria, viruses, and fungi that can cause infectious diseases in humans, has been a critical point of concern for microbiologists and clinicians. Traditional procedures such as cultures and biochemical tests are time-consuming, requiring one to five days from the clinical laboratory to the bedside of the patients [127], which causes infectious diseases to continue to sicken millions of people worldwide with high fatality rates every year. Therefore, rapid and accurate diagnosis of microbial pathogens could help to save millions of lives annually. As a non-invasive, label-free, and low-cost optical technology that can potentially allow for rapid pathogenic identification directly from patient samples, the method has attracted increasing attention from both the academic and industrial fields [128–134]. Some of the recent applications of the SERS technique in the field of infectious diseases are introduced below to show the recent progress in the technique and its great potential in the future.

3.4.1 Viruses

During pandemics, rapid diagnosis of infectious diseases is essential. The most severe influenza pandemic (Spanish flu, H1N1 subtype) occurred in 1918–20 and the most recent influenza pandemic (swine flu, H1N1 subtype) occurred in 2009–10. Human immunodeficiency virus (HIV, primarily the HIV-1 strain) caused another significant pandemic, this time lasting the longest and resulting in the greatest number of fatalities among recent viral pandemics [181]. The severe acute respiratory syndrome coronavirus (SARS-CoV) initially appeared in China in 2019 [179]. The first case of coronavirus (COVID-19) was detected in China in December 2019 and it has since spread throughout the world, causing major health issues and socioeconomic difficulties [180, 197]. The emergence of COVID-19 has highlighted the significance of rapid and sensitive diagnostics for identifying and monitoring infectious diseases [135, 195]. Many infectious diseases caused by viruses pose a significant risk to the economy and public health [196]. The COVID-19 pandemic has infected over 571 million people and claimed the lives of nearly 6 387 009 people worldwide as of 3 October 2022 according to the Johns Hopkins University (JHU) website. The detection of COVID-19 by SERS can be extended to many other viral pathogens such as rhinovirus, influenza, and parainfluenza within minutes with samples as small as 102 EID50/l at 90% specificity. This precision is comparable to quantitative reverse transcription (PCR), but with the additional advantages of rapid diagnostics and enrichment [136–139]. Similarly, SERS has been used for the diagnosis of HIV, with a sensitivity and specificity of 97.5% and 95%, respectively, and a limit of detection (LOD) of 95–100 copies/ml [140]. These developments are crucial for examining patient samples that can contain a variety of pathogens.

3.4.1.1 Label-free virus detection and spectral interpretation

Label-free SERS could also improve the diagnosis of viral infections from patient samples, allowing for the differentiation of several influenza viruses without the requirement to extract viral nucleic acids [141–145]. In the detection of complex biological macromolecules such as viruses, bacteria, and protein biomarkers, SERS spectra acquired from label-free detection are usually complex and it is difficult to extract the peaks of the analytes. As a result, Raman spectrum differences between biological groups can be subtle and it can be challenging to distinguish, for example, seasonal coronavirus and COVID-19, H5N1 influenza and H3N2 influenza, and methicillin-resistant susceptible *Staphylococcus aureus*. However, there are exceptions to this case, even though it has been reported to be easy to detect some viruses using the label-free SERS method, this could be due to the composition and structure of the virus. Influenza strains were successfully identified despite the absence of any Raman reporters on Au/Ag nanorods. In the study, the peaks in the

SERS spectra were connected to the spike proteins identified on the viral envelope proteins hemagglutinin and neuraminidase. The interpretation and classification of spectra in label-free SERS can benefit from sophisticated data analysis. SERS spectral data and visualization of spectral variations in principal component analysis (PCA) can discover unknown features without prior knowledge of classification groups [146]. PCA and SERS have been used to analyse spectral data for the diagnosis of viral infections including HIV and hepatitis B virus (HBV). The PCA-LDA diagnostic algorithm can distinguish HBV from normal samples based on derivative SERS spectra with high diagnostic sensitivity and specificity of 83.0% and 91.4%, which is around a 10.2% enhancement in diagnostic accuracy compared to SERS spectra [140, 141]. This development could be due to the capacity of derivative SERS spectra to identify subtle spectral properties and collect additional data from the overlapping Raman bands in the serum sample.

3.4.1.2 Rapid and sensitive label-based virus detection

Most infectious diseases, including COVID-19, influenza A, and HIV, require assays to determine a specific virus rather than screening for a broad range of pathogens. In this circumstance, labeled SERS methods can offer improved specificity and sensitivity as well as quantitative analysis for virus identification. The virus load in a patient sample varies based on the infectious stage, the source of the sample, and disease diagnostic approaches, which require the detection of low virus concentrations across infectious diseases [148]. For other novel infections, such as the recently discovered COVID-19, the relationship between viral load and disease severity is not entirely explained, highlighting the need for a diagnostic method capable of detecting substantially lower viral loads [182]. Furthermore, labeled SERS also allows the detection of complex body fluid samples including whole blood, urea, and sputum. As a result, sensitivity and specificity are greatly enhanced, and a large number of biomarkers can be detected simultaneously [182]. In addition, labeled SERS has also been used in other applications, most notably for the diagnosis of influenza by employing affinity agents such as antibodies, aptamers, and polymers. While it is possible to directly detect SERS spectra from biomolecules using affinity agents, SERS signals can be increased by using Raman signal reporters such as resonant fluorescent dyes or aromatic thiols. These reporters are integrated into the affinity agent or the SERS substrate, making it much easier to detect and quantify viral pathogens, particularly in samples with low viral concentrations [182]. However, due to cross-reactivity, conjugation with affinity agents can increase the chance of false-positive results.

To target and bind particular antigens, immune cells naturally create proteins known as antibodies. The functionalized Au NPs with monoclonal antibody fragments against gp120, a characteristic HIV surface protein, were used to detect the SERS of HIV-1 virus-like particles. Viral particle concentrations as low as 35 fg ml^{-1} were readily detected [149]. SERS has also been successfully applied to identifying mosquito-borne flavivirus by using an anti-flavivirus 4G2 antibody on Au NPs [150].

When antibodies bind to plasmonic surfaces, their orientations are random, affecting the packing density on SERS substrates and hence the possible SERS improvements. Furthermore, antibodies have low temperature stability, a signal that interferes with the SERS signal, and the potential to produce false-positive results because of antigen cross-reactivity. These problems have been addressed by new techniques, such as weakening the disulfide bond of the antibody and incorporating single-stranded DNA or synthetic peptides [151–153]. Synthetic antibody fragments have also been used to overcome some of the drawbacks of monoclonal antibodies due to their being simpler to produce, small in size, and very simple to bind to SERS substrates [154, 155]. Aptamers, unlike antibodies, promise a high packing density on SERS substrates and a more flexible, focused, and tight target binding. Aptamers are sections of nucleotides or peptides that have a particular affinity for binding to a target molecule. Furthermore, aptamers fold in three dimensions around targets, giving them a tunable orientation and improved selectivity [156]. Recently, influenza viruses were detected using an aptamer-based SERS that focused on the viral hemagglutinin at concentrations of 10^{-4} units/probe [156].

3.4.2 Bacteria

3.4.2.1 SERS detection of bacteria

Human beings frequently contract pathogenic bacterial infections, which can be treated successfully with antibiotics in otherwise healthy individuals. However, the long-term consequences of broad-spectrum antibiotics are a severe concern, which is having a minimal effect on the treatment of certain pathogens for a variety of reasons. This requires the advancement of best prescription practices, which is possible under the condition that the infection-causing bacteria can be identified precisely and rapidly. At the very least, this would allow for the provision of a targeted treatment for the illness, lowering the risk of the emergence of resistant strains in the future and increasing the duration of effectiveness of some treatments. Furthermore, it would be ideal to identify a pathogen before a patient experiences symptoms of a disease. This would require analysing biomass concentrations as low as 1 CFU ml^{-1} [183].

Jarvis *et al* were the first researchers to use SERS studies to discriminate between *E. coli*, *Klebsiella oxytoca*, *Klebsiella pneumoniae*, *Citrobacter freundii*, *Enterococcus* spp., and *Proteus mirabilis* in 2004 [157]. The emergence of SERS-based methods for the identification of bacteria has received a lot of attention over the past ten years. More recent research in the area of bacterial SERS has made use of methods for identifying vegetative bacteria and bacterial spores that are phenotypically comparable to pathogens that potentially represent a bioterrorism threat [162]. There have also been reports of applications for managing manufacturing processes, which require high sensitivity and quantitative reproducibility [16]. Another significant amount of research reporting on the application of SERS for the identification of different bacterial species has emerged in recent years [163]. Two Raman-based methods have been developed, one of which was optimized to analyse suspension [165], while the other was focused on single-bacterial analysis [129]. The bacteria from the urine sample are washed and placed on a piece of nickel foil to dry for single-cell analysis. Raman spectra are used to record single bacterial cells from the patient's sample. The database determines the identification of the pathogen for every single-cell measurement. For each specimen, a species was assigned to anywhere between 66% and 98% of the measured cells. It was found that the first seven patient samples contained *E. coli*, and the next three samples had *Enterococcus faecalis* as the predominant species [165]. These findings are in agreement with the benchmark of urine culture. Each of the patient samples analysed may be appropriately assigned using a threshold of 60% abundance in the single-cell Raman spectra. Notably, an inhibitor test result was positive in five out of ten samples that were examined. Thus, despite the presence of antibiotics or other growth inhibitors, Raman spectroscopic analysis can still detect pathogens in urine [129]. The applications for the simultaneous detection of non-cultivatable bacteria from patient body fluids are particularly promising [130, 131].

The second method performs the Raman spectroscopic examination directly in suspension after using dielectrophoretic forces to gather bacteria in specific spatial locations. For the examination of conventional urine samples, only minimal sample preparation is required. One drop of the filtered and cleaned urine is employed on a dielectrophoresis chip with four gold electrodes (figure 3.4). RS analyses bacteria when they are moved into the middle of the electrodes by an alternating electric field. Similar to the first method, a database developed from Raman spectra and patient samples are used to identify the bacteria in the urine sample. The differentiation of *E. coli* and *E. faecalis* has been demonstrated to have a high prediction accuracy [165]. Furthermore, it was demonstrated that the electric field has no impact on the viability of the confined bacteria, which is critical if the method is enhanced to be used for rapid spectroscopy-based antibiotic susceptibility testing. Additionally, centrifugal forces can be employed to directly extract bacteria from suspension for RS analysis rather than dielectrophoresis [166].

3.4.2.2 Bacterial imaging and mapping with SERS

A basic understanding of how the chemical imaging of bacterial pathogens can reveal information about sample heterogeneity and the dispersion of physiologically significant biomarkers in the sample is described here. SERS provides a novel and

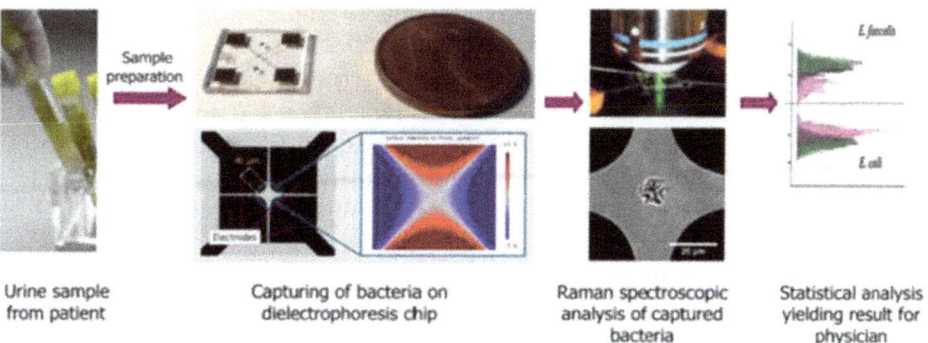

| Urine sample from patient | Capturing of bacteria on dielectrophoresis chip | Raman spectroscopic analysis of captured bacteria | Statistical analysis yielding result for physician |

Figure 3.4. Rapid pathogen detection using a Raman and dielectrophoresis system was performed from urine samples. (Reproduced with permission from [165]. Copyright 2013 American Chemical Society.)

non-destructive method of chemical imaging because each spectrum contains a wealth of vibrational data [167]. This chapter will also briefly discuss the significant advancements in SERS-based mapping of bacterial samples. Wang *et al* chemically mapped pure and mixed samples of *S. enterica* and *E. coli* using Ag dendrites [71]. The bacterial suspensions and Ag dendrites were combined before SERS mapping, and the resulting mixture was then dried on a hydrophobic substrate. The mapping of *S. enterica* was carried out using SERS by collecting 225 data points in 5 μm increments from a 75 μm × 75 μm sample area and generating a SERS image using the intensity of the 1332 cm^{-1} band. The SERS mapping procedure revealed an LOD of 10^4 CFU ml^{-1} in comparison to the conventional detection method that resulted in an LOD of 10^6 CFU ml^{-1}. Importantly, the researchers revealed the ability to determine individual concentrations of *E. coli and S. enterica* [71]. The SERS maps were analysed with PCA after collection to determine the individual concentrations and distribution of the two bacterial species.

3.4.3 Fungi

Fungi are heterotrophic organisms with a nucleus and a cell wall. They are a large group in the biological kingdom and are usually divided into three categories: yeast, mold, and fungi. In recent years, with the widespread use of broad-spectrum antibiotics, glucocorticoids, immunosuppressants, and the use of various interventional medical technologies, the number and types of clinical fungal infections have increased year by year, and fungal infection are becoming one of the main causes of nosocomial infections [191]. For example, *Candida albicans* accounts for about 60% of all infections, resulting in a mortality rate close to 40% [168]. The infection can kill organ transplant patients, cancer patients, and AIDS patients [191]. Therefore, methods and technologies for the efficient identification and monitoring of fungi have attracted much attention.

Based on previous studies and investigations, we found that RS, in particular SERS, is very promising in the field of fungal identification and detection. As early as 1995 Edwards *et al* first used FT-Raman spectroscopy to detect the cell walls of three fungi, *Agaricus bisporus*, *Mortierella* genus, and *Mucor* genus, and assigned the Raman characteristic peaks to these fungal genera and species [169]. In the early 2000s Gussem *et al* confirmed that the collected RS signals were mainly from polysaccharides, chitin, and amylopectin on the fungal cell wall and lipids and phospholipids on the cell membrane [170]. So far, only a few reports have revealed SERS imaging of fungi, all of which have focused on a single species [185, 186]. Although SERS has previously been used to identify clinically significant bacteria and viruses, it has never been used to detect or identify pathogenic fungi [187–190]. In 2016 Witkowska *et al* performed the first SERS experiments used for the differentiation and identification of four different pathogenic fungi [171]. In this study, the pathogenic species *Aspergillus flavus*, *Trichophyton rubrum*, *Scopulariopsis brumptii*, and *Candida krusei* were detected and identified using the SERS method. The SERS spectra of the four fungal pathogens, which were deposited on SERS-active substrates as aqueous solutions of clean fungal cells, were then examined further. Each fungal pathogen spectrum has unique spectral properties that create a species-specific fingerprint. Additionally, the purpose of this study was to evaluate the efficiency of SERS and PCA analysis in identifying fungal pathogens from clinical skin samples, and the effective identification of different subspecies of the common dermatophyte *Trichophyton* was realized, which made it possible to identify fungi of the same genus and different subspecies [171]. Dina *et al* used the chemical reduction method to synthesize AgNPs and successfully generated SERS spectra to discriminate *Aspergillus fumigatus*, *Aspergillus cryptosporum*, and *Rhizopus powdery* based on analyses via the PCA and linear discriminant method (PCA-LDA) [172]. The whole process took only 5 min, which greatly shortened the time to confirm the diagnosis of invasive fungal infection. It can be seen that the SERS spectral detection technology integrated with nanotechnology shows very good development potential and application prospects in the identification of fungal species and the rapid diagnosis of clinical diseases.

However, there are relatively few studies and applications of SERS in fungal detection. The core issues faced when applying SERS technology to fungal detection are sensitivity, reproducibility, and specificity. The characteristics of the fungal samples themselves restrict their efficient quantitative testing by SERS spectroscopy. To solve this problem, detection strategies and methods using SERS tags have been proposed. In the study of Mabbott *et al*, single-stranded thioDNA-modified silver hydroxylamine nanoparticles were used as SERS tags, combined with principal component analysis, to successfully detect *Candida albicans*, *Candida glabrata*, *Candida cruzi*, and *Aspergillus fumigatus* for identification and classification [173]. Based on this, we believe that the combination of microfluidic technology is expected to solve and break through the bottleneck problems of low detection efficiency, poor signal stability, and narrow application range of current SERS analysis technology, and provide higher precision and more reliable testing methods for fungal detection

3.5 Limitations and challenges

SERS spectroscopy provides an efficient, rapid, and non-destructive method for the detection of microbial pathogens that is suitable for clinical diagnostics of infectious diseases. In comparison to traditional molecular approaches, sample preparation is a simple method and does not require expensive equipment. Furthermore, a wide range of methods for isolating or enriching microorganisms has been proposed, allowing single-cell studies as well as non-culture-based recognition and detection. Nevertheless, it might take some time before SERS spectroscopy is applied in real-world clinical settings. According to Wang *et al*, there are currently no well-annotated commercial databases of microbial Raman signatures [7]. When comparing collected Raman spectra from different instruments, keep in mind that the quantum efficiency of the specific detector and optical components is wavelength-dependent. Therefore, obtained data needs to be adjusted following an instrument response profile [174]. As a result, the Raman spectra reported in different investigations are group-specific and specially designed, making data standardization challenging [175]. However, no extensive research has been completed to investigate the Raman spectra of different microbial groups. The SERS method is often used in studies of microbes. The ability to regulate SERS microbial detection methods remains a major obstacle [176, 177]. The techniques used to prepare samples, the types of culture media, and the interactions between certain microbial cells and the SERS substrate are a few examples of these [176, 177]. Currently, other issues are the requirement for sophisticated instrumentation and specialist users, which have relatively high input costs. If those issues are resolved, SERS might spark a revolution in clinical diagnostic microbiology. Despite its wide range of medical applications, a given device outfitted with numerous diagnostic databases might develop into a complicated diagnostic tool. SERS could be used to rapidly identify pathogens and characterize their virulence factors, resulting in personalized antimicrobial treatment, dramatically reduced healthcare financial burdens, and, most crucially, improved patient management and decreased infection mortality.

SERS is sensitive and efficient, but it often lacks a user-friendly component in sample processing and spectrum interpretation. For instance, before Raman interrogation, purification and isolation processes are typically required to isolate pathogens and other biomarkers from complicated biological samples, including sputum, blood, saliva, and urine [178]. After purification, Raman spectrum datasets from patient samples could be difficult to translate into clinically valuable information, requiring the use of advanced data analysis tools. Raman diagnostics are rapid to perform, although stability can be challenging. Furthermore, the fluctuating signal enhancement brought on by NP aggregation and analyte distribution on the SERS substrate complicates quantitative analysis. Raman spectral set-ups are also usually benchtop-scale platforms that need substantial capital investment. All these issues should be borne in mind and urgent solutions sought by both the academic and industrial fields for the technique to gain more real-world applications in the diagnosis of infectious diseases.

3.6 Conclusion

Surface-enhanced Raman spectroscopy is known as one of the most sensitive analytical techniques and has been widely investigated for its capacities in the diagnosis of infectious diseases. Metallic nanoparticles sit at the center of the SERS technique, which not only plays an important role in the enhancement of Raman scattering effects but also makes it possible for the technique to simultaneously identify mixed pathogens such as viruses, bacteria, fungi, etc, in clinical samples. However, due to the lack of standard instruments and consistent performance procedures during sample preparation and Raman spectral collection, there is still a huge gap between laboratory research and clinical applications. In addition, the lack of a standard SERS spectral database in the field also limits the usage of the technique in clinical laboratories, which needs to be solved urgently. In conclusion, the SERS technique holds great potential for fast and accurate identification of clinical pathogens, which could revolutionize the diagnosis of infectious diseases in real-world settings.

Conflict of interest

The authors declare that the research was conducted in the absence of any commercial or financial relationships that could be construed as a potential conflict of interest.

Authorship contributions

LW conceived the structure of the manuscript and was responsible for project administration. LW, FL, QHL, and JWT wrote the original manuscript. MU, XDZ, and CYW revised the manuscript. All authors read and approved the final manuscript.

Funding statement

LW was financially supported by the National Natural Science Foundation ofChina (Grant No. 31900022), University Young Science and TechnologyInnovation Team (Grant No. TD202001), and Jiangsu Qinglan Project (year 2020), Guangdong Basic and Applied Basic Research Foundation (Grant No. 2022A1515220023), Xuzhou Key R&D Plan Social Development Project (Grant No. KC22300).

References

[1] Van Seventer J M and Hochberg N S 2017 Principles of infectious diseases: transmission, diagnosis, prevention, and control *International Encyclopedia of Public Health* (Boston, MA: Boston University School of Public Health) pp 22–39

[2] Wolfe N D, Dunavan C P and Diamond J 2007 Origins of major human infectious diseases *Nature* **447** 279–83

[3] Baker R E *et al* 2021 Infectious disease in an era of global change *Nat. Rev. Microbiol.* **20** 193–205

[4] Scapaticci S, Neri C R, Marseglia G L, Staiano A, Chiarelli F and Verduci E 2022 The impact of the COVID-19 pandemic on lifestyle behaviors in children and adolescents: an international overview *Ital. J. Pediatr.* **48** 22

[5] Mou J 2020 Research on the impact of COVID19 on global economy *IOP Conf. Ser.: Earth Environ. Sci.* **546** 032043

[6] Tang J W, Li J Q, Yin X C, Xu W W, Pan Y C, Liu Q H, Gu B, Zhang X and Wang L 2022 Rapid discrimination of clinically important pathogens through machine learning analysis of surface enhanced Raman spectra *Front. Microbiol.* **13** 843417

[7] Wang L, Liu W, Tang J-W, Wang J-J, Liu Q-H, Wen P-B, Wang M-M, Pan Y-C, Gu B and Zhang X 2021 Applications of Raman spectroscopy in bacterial infections: principles, advantages, and shortcomings *Front. Microbiol.* **12** 683580

[8] Singhal N, Kumar M, Kanaujia P K and Virdi J S 2015 MALDI-TOF mass spectrometry: an emerging technology for microbial identification and diagnosis *Front. Microbiol.* **6** 791

[9] Mallik D C V 2000 The Raman effect and Krishnan's diary *Notes Rec. R. Soc. Lond.* **54** 67–83

[10] Tang J-W, Liu Q-H, Yin X-C, Pan Y-C, Wen P-B, Liu X, Kang X-X, Gu B, Zhu Z-B and Wang L 2021 Comparative analysis of machine learning algorithms on surface enhanced Raman spectra of clinical *Staphylococcus* species *Front. Microbiol.* **12** 696921

[11] Chen S, Lin X, Yuen C, Padmanabhan S, Beuerman R W and Liu Q 2014 Recovery of Raman spectra with low signal-to-noise ratio using Wiener estimation *Opt. Express* **22** 12102–14

[12] Orlando A, Franceschini F, Muscas C, Pidkova S, Bartoli M, Rovere M and Tagliaferro A 2021 A comprehensive review on Raman spectroscopy applications *Chemosensors* **9** 262

[13] Zhao X Y, Liu G Y, Sui Y T, Xu M and Tong L 2021 Denoising method for Raman spectra with low signal-to-noise ratio based on feature extraction *Spectrochim. Acta* A **250** 119374

[14] Fan X, Zeng Y, Zhi Y L, Nie T, Xu Y and Wang X 2021 Signal-to-noise ratio enhancement for Raman spectra based on optimized Raman spectrometer and convolutional denoising autoencoder *J. Raman Spectrosc.* **52** 890–900

[15] Sur U K 2017 Surface-enhanced Raman scattering *Raman Spectroscopy and Applications* (Vienna: Intech Open)

[16] Sharma B, Frontiera R R, Henry A-I, Ringe E and Van Duyne R P 2012 SERS: materials, applications, and the future *Mater. Today* **15** 16–25

[17] Widjaja E, Zheng W and Huang Z 2008 Classification of colonic tissues using near-infrared Raman spectroscopy and support vector machines *Int. J. Oncol.* **32** 653–62

[18] Li S, Zhang Y, Xu J, Li L, Zeng Q, Lin L, Guo Z, Liu Z, Xiong H and Liu S 2014 Noninvasive prostate cancer screening based on serum surface-enhanced Raman spectroscopy and support vector machine *Appl. Phys. Lett.* **105** 091104

[19] Lyng F M, Traynor D, Nguyen T N, Meade A D, Rakib F, Al-Saady R, Goormaghtigh E, Al-Saad K and Ali M H 2019 Discrimination of breast cancer from benign tumours using Raman spectroscopy *PLoS One* **14** 0212376

[20] Li Y S and Church J S 2014 Raman spectroscopy in the analysis of food and pharmaceutical nanomaterials *J. Food Drug Anal.* **22** 29–48

[21] Wang W T, Zhang H, Yuan Y, Guo Y and He S X 2018 Research progress of Raman spectroscopy in drug analysis *AAPS PharmSciTech* **19** 2921–8

[22] Li S X, Zeng Q Y, Li L F, Zhang Y J, Wan M M, Liu Z M, Xiong H L, Guo Z Y and Liu S H 2013 Study of support vector machine and serum surface-enhanced Raman spectroscopy for noninvasive esophageal cancer detection *J. Biomed. Opt.* **18** 027008

[23] Ralbovsky N M and Lednev I K 2020 Towards development of a novel universal medical diagnostic method: Raman spectroscopy and machine learning *Chem. Soc. Rev.* **49** 7428–53

[24] Thomas G J Jr 1970 Raman spectral studies of nucleic acids: III. Laser-excited spectra of ribosomal RNA *Biochim. Biophys. Acta Proteins Proteom.* **213** 417–23

[25] Tsuboi M, Takahashi S, Muraishi S, Kajiura T and Nishimura S 1971 Raman spectrum of a transfer RNA *Science* **174** 1142–4

[26] Fee J A, Kuila D, Mather M W and Yoshida T 1986 Respiratory proteins from extremely thermophilic, aerobic bacteria *Biochim. Biophys. Acta* B **1853** 153–85

[27] Adar F, Dixit S and Erecinska M 1981 Resonance Raman spectra of cytochromes c and b in *Paracoccus denitrificans* membranes: evidence for heme–heme interactions *Biochemistry* **20** 7528–31

[28] Woodruff W H, Norton K A, Swanson B I and Fry H A 1984 Temperature dependence of the resonance Raman spectra of plastocyanin and azurin between cryogenic and ambient conditions *Proc. Natl Acad. Sci. USA* **81** 1263–7

[29] Meyer J, Moulis J M and Lutz M 1984 Structural differences between [2Fe-2S] clusters in spinach ferredoxin and in the 'red paramagnetic protein' from *Clostridium pasteurianum*. A resonance Raman study *Biochem. Biophys. Res. Commun.* **119** 828–35

[30] Moulis J M, Meyer J and Lutz M 1984 Characterization of $[4Fe-4S]^{2+}$, $[4Fe-4Se]^{2+}$ and hybrid (S, Se) clusters in *Clostridium pasteurianum* ferredoxin. A resonance Raman study *Biochem. J.* **219** 829–32

[31] Szalontai B, Gombos Z and Csizmadia V 1985 Resonance Raman spectra of phycocyanin, allophycocyanin and phycobilisomes from blue-green alga *Anacystis nidulans Biochem. Biophys. Res. Commun.* **130** 358–63

[32] Ainscough E W, Bingham A G, Brodie A M, Ellis W R, Gray H B, Loehr T M, Plowman J E, Norris G E and Baker E N 1987 Spectrochemical studies on the blue copper protein azurin from *Alcaligenes denitrificans Biochemistry* **26** 71–82

[33] Choma C T, Surewicz W K, Carey P R, Pozsgay M and Kaplan H 1990 Secondary structure of the entomocidal toxin from *Bacillus thuringiensis* subsp. kurstaki HD-73 *J. Protein Chem.* **9** 87–94

[34] Fu W, Morgan T V, Mortenson L E and Johnson M K 1991 Resonance Raman studies of the [4Fe-4S] to [2Fe-2S] cluster conversion in the iron protein of nitrogenase *FEBS Lett.* **284** 165–8

[35] Cooper R A, Knowles P F, Brown D E, McGuirl M A and Dooley D M 1992 Evidence for copper and 3, 4, 6-trihydroxyphenylalanine quinone cofactors in an amine oxidase from the Gram-negative bacterium *Escherichia coli* K-12 *Biochem. J.* **288** 337–40

[36] Jones M R, Heer-Dawson M, Mattioli T A, Hunter C N and Robert B 1994 Site-specific mutagenesis of the reaction centre from *Rhodobacter sphaeroides* studied by Fourier transform Raman spectroscopy: mutations at tyrosine M210 do not affect the electronic structure of the primary donor *FEBS Lett.* **339** 18–24

[37] Mattioli T A, Williams J C, Allen J P and Robert B 1994 Changes in primary donor hydrogen-bonding interactions in mutant reaction centers from *Rhodobacter sphaeroides*: identification of the vibrational frequencies of all the conjugated carbonyl groups *Biochemistry* **33** 1636–43

[38] Goodacre R, Timmins E M, Burton R, Kaderbhai N, Woodward A M, Kell D B and Rooney P J 1998 Rapid identification of urinary tract infection bacteria using hyperspectral whole-organism fingerprinting and artificial neural networks *Microbiology* **144** 1157–70

[39] Maquelin K, Choo-Smith L P, van Vreeswijk T, Endtz H P, Smith B, Bennett R, Bruining H A and Puppels G J 2000 Raman spectroscopic method for identification of clinically relevant microorganisms growing on solid culture medium *Anal. Chem.* **72** 12–9

[40] Mello C, Ribeiro D, Novaes F and Poppi R J 2005 Rapid differentiation among bacteria that cause gastroenteritis by use of low-resolution Raman spectroscopy and PLS discriminant analysis *Anal. Bioanal. Chem.* **383** 701–6

[41] Buijtels P C, Willemse-Erix H F, Petit P L, Endtz H P, Puppels G J, Verbrugh H A, van Belkum A, van Soolingen D and Maquelin K 2008 Rapid identification of mycobacteria by Raman spectroscopy *J. Clin. Microbiol.* **46** 961–5

[42] Teh S K, Zheng W, Ho K Y, Teh M, Yeoh K G and Huang Z 2010 Near-infrared Raman spectroscopy for optical diagnosis in the stomach: identification of helicobacter-pylori infection and intestinal metaplasia *Int. J. Cancer* **126** 1920–7

[43] Kumar S, Gopinathan R, Chandra G K, Umapathy S and Saini D K 2020 Rapid detection of bacterial infection and viability assessment with high specificity and sensitivity using Raman microspectroscopy *Anal. Bioanal. Chem.* **412** 2505–16

[44] Naseer K, Saleem M, Ali S, Mirza B and Qazi J 2019 Identification of new spectral signatures from hepatitis C virus infected human sera *Spectrochim. Acta* A **222** 117181

[45] Guleken Z, Tok Y T, Jakubczyk P, Paja W, Pancerz K, Shpotyuk Y, Cebulski J and Depciuch J 2022 Development of novel spectroscopic and machine learning methods for the measurement of periodic changes in COVID-19 antibody level *Measurement* **196** 111258

[46] Liu G K, Zheng H and Lu J L 2017 Recent progress and perspective of trace antibiotics detection in aquatic environment by surface-enhanced Raman spectroscopy *Trends Environ. Anal. Chem.* **16** 16–23

[47] Eberhardt K, Stiebing C, Matthäus C, Schmitt M and Popp J 2015 Advantages and limitations of Raman spectroscopy for molecular diagnostics: an update *Expert Rev. Mol. Diagn.* **15** 773–87

[48] Rocha-Santos T A 2014 Sensors and biosensors based on magnetic nanoparticles *Trends Environ. Anal. Chem.* **62** 28–36

[49] Bonnet R *et al* 2018 Highly labeled methylene blue-ds DNA silica nanoparticles for signal enhancement of immunoassays: application to the sensitive detection of bacteria in human platelet concentrates *Analyst* **143** 2293–303

[50] Li Q, Kartikowati C W, Horie S, Ogi T, Iwaki T and Okuyama K 2017 Correlation between particle size/domain structure and magnetic properties of highly crystalline Fe_3O_4 nanoparticles *Sci. Rep.* **7** 9894

[51] Noqta O A, Aziz A A, Usman I A and Bououdina M 2019 Recent advances in iron oxide nanoparticles (IONPs): synthesis and surface modification for biomedical applications *J. Supercond. Nov. Magn.* **32** 779–95

[52] Salata O V 2004 Applications of nanoparticles in biology and medicine *J. Nanobiotechnol.* **2** 3

[53] Giljohann D A, Seferos D S, Daniel W L, Massich M D, Patel P C and Mirkin C A 2020 Gold nanoparticles for biology and medicine *Angew. Chem.* **49** 3280–94

[54] Wilson R 2008 The use of gold nanoparticles in diagnostics and detection *Chem. Soc. Rev.* **37** 2028–45

[55] Radwan S H and Azzazy H M 2009 Gold nanoparticles for molecular diagnostics *Expert Rev. Mol. Diagn.* **9** 511–24

[56] Huo Q and Worden J G 2007 Monofunctional gold nanoparticles: synthesis and applications *J. Nanoparticle Res.* **9** 1013–25

[57] Xiao T, Huang J, Wang D, Meng T and Yang X 2020 Au and Au-based nanomaterials: synthesis and recent progress in electrochemical sensor applications *Talanta* **206** 120210

[58] Tallury P, Malhotra A, Byrne L M and Santra S 2010 Nanobioimaging and sensing of infectious diseases *Adv. Drug Deliv. Rev.* **62** 424–37

[59] Wong K K and Liu X 2010 Silver nanoparticles—the real 'silver bullet' in clinical medicine? *MedChemComm* **1** 125–31

[60] Naja G, Bouvrette P, Hrapovic S and Luong J H 2007 Raman-based detection of bacteria using silver nanoparticles conjugated with antibodies *Analyst* **132** 679–86

[61] Driskell J D, Shanmukh S, Liu Y J, Hennigan S, Jones L, Zhao Y P, Dluhy R A, Krause D C and Tripp R A 2008 Infectious agent detection with SERS-active silver nanorod arrays prepared by oblique angle deposition *IEEE Sens. J.* **8** 863–70

[62] Deng H, Li X, Peng Q, Wang X, Chen J and Li Y 2005 Monodisperse magnetic single-crystal ferrite microspheres *Angew. Chem.* **117** 2842–5

[63] Xuan S, Wang F, Wang Y X, Jimmy C Y and Leung K C 2010 Facile synthesis of size-controllable monodispersed ferrite nanospheres *J. Mater. Chem.* **20** 5086–94

[64] Liu J, Che R, Chen H, Zhang F, Xia F, Wu Q and Wang M 2012 Microwave absorption enhancement of multifunctional composite microspheres with spinel Fe_3O_4 cores and anatase TiO_2 shells *Small* **8** 1214–21

[65] Sharma G, Kumar A, Sharma S, Naushad M, Dwivedi R P, ALOthman Z A and Mola G T 2019 Novel development of nanoparticles to bimetallic nanoparticles and their composites: a review *J. King Saud Univ. Sci.* **31** 257–69

[66] Cui Y, Ren B, Yao J L, Gu R A and Tian Z Q 2006 Synthesis of $Ag_{core}Au_{shell}$ bimetallic nanoparticles for immunoassay based on surface-enhanced Raman spectroscopy *J. Phys. Chem.* B **110** 4002–6

[67] Dehghani Z, Hosseini M, Mohammadnejad J, Bakhshi B and Rezayan A H 2018 Colorimetric aptasensor for *Campylobacter jejuni* cells by exploiting the peroxidase like activity of Au@Pd nanoparticles *Microchim. Acta* **185** 448

[68] Mandal R, Baranwal A, Srivastava A and Chandra P 2018 Evolving trends in bio/chemical sensor fabrication incorporating bimetallic nanoparticles *Biosens. Bioelectron.* **117** 546–61

[69] Jana N R 2003 Silver coated gold nanoparticles as new surface enhanced Raman substrate at low analyte concentration *Analyst* **128** 954–6

[70] Kumar G P, Shruthi S, Vibha B, Reddy B A, Kundu T K and Narayana C 2007 Hot spots in Ag core–Au shell nanoparticles potent for surface-enhanced Raman scattering studies of biomolecules *J. Phys. Chem.* C **111** 4388–92

[71] Lesiak A, Drzozga K, Cabaj J, Bański M, Malecha K and Podhorodecki A 2019 Optical sensors based on II–VI quantum dots *J. Nanomater.* **9** 192

[72] Michalet X, Pinaud F F, Bentolila L A, Tsay J M, Doose S J, Li J J, Sundaresan G, Wu A M, Gambhir S S and Weiss S 2005 Quantum dots for live cells, *in vivo* imaging, and diagnostics *Science* **307** 538–44

[73] Kaittanis C, Santra S and Perez J M 2010 Emerging nanotechnology-based strategies for the identification of microbial pathogenesis *Adv. Drug Deliv. Rev.* **62** 408–23

[74] Zhang Z, Xiang X, Hu Y, Deng Y, Li L, Zhao W and Wu T 2021 A sensitive biomolecules detection device with catalytic hairpin assembly and cationic conjugated polymer-assisted dual signal amplification strategy *Talanta* **223** 121716

[75] Liu Z, Robinson J T, Sun X and Dai H 2008 PEGylated nanographene oxide for delivery of water-insoluble cancer drugs *J. Am. Chem. Soc.* **130** 10876–7

[76] Wu X, Chuang Y, Contino A, Sorée B, Brems S, Tokei Z, Heyns M, Huyghebaert C and Asselberghs I 2018 Boosting carrier mobility of synthetic few layer graphene on SiO_2 by interlayer rotation and decoupling *Adv. Mater. Interfaces* **5** 1800454

[77] Li S *et al* 2021 A HiPAD integrated with rGO/MWCNTs nano-circuit heater for visual point-of-care testing of SARS-CoV-2 *Adv. Funct. Mater.* **31** 2100801

[78] Zhao Y, Li K, He Z, Zhang Y, Zhao Y, Zhang H and Miao Z 2016 Investigation on fluorescence quenching mechanism of perylene diimide dyes by graphene oxide *Molecules* **21** 1642

[79] Wang P, Xia M, Liang O, Sun K, Cipriano A F, Schroeder T, Liu H and Xie Y H 2015 Label-free SERS selective detection of dopamine and serotonin using graphene-Au nano-pyramid heterostructure *J. Anal. Chem.* **87** 10255–61

[80] Chen S, Li X, Zhao Y, Chang L and Qi J 2015 Graphene oxide shell-isolated Ag nanoparticles for surface-enhanced Raman scattering *Carbon* **81** 767–72

[81] Qiu X, You X, Chen X, Chen H, Dhinakar A, Liu S, Guo Z, Wu J and Liu Z 2017 Development of graphene oxide-wrapped gold nanorods as robust nanoplatform for ultrafast near-infrared SERS bioimaging *Int. J. Nanomed.* **12** 4349

[82] Yu X, Cai H, Zhang W, Li X, Pan N, Luo Y, Wang X and Hou J G 2011 Tuning chemical enhancement of SERS by controlling the chemical reduction of graphene oxide nanosheets *ACS Nano* **5** 952–8

[83] Xu W, Ling X, Xiao J, Dresselhaus M S, Kong J, Xu H, Liu Z and Zhang J 2012 Surface enhanced Raman spectroscopy on a flat graphene surface *Proc. Natl Acad. Sci. USA* **109** 9281–6

[84] Yadav N, Tyagi M, Wadhwa S, Mathur A and Narang J 2020 Few biomedical applications of carbon nanotubes *Meth. Enzymol* **630** 347–63

[85] Roldo M and Fatouros D G 2013 Biomedical applications of carbon nanotubes *Annu. Rev. Phys. Chem.* **109** 10–35

[86] Yliharsila M, Valta T, Karp M, Hattara L, Harju E, Holsa J, Saviranta P, Waris M and Soukka T 2011 Oligonucleotide array-in-well platform for detection and genotyping human adenoviruses by utilizing upconverting phosphor label technology *Anal. Chem.* **83** 1456–61

[87] Yan Q, Ding X Y, Chen Z H, Xue S F, Han X Y, Lin Z Y, Yang M, Shi G and Zhang M 2018 pH-regulated optical performances in organic/inorganic hybrid: a dualmode sensor array for pattern-recognition-based biosensing *Anal. Chem.* **90** 10536–42

[88] Pakkila H, Yliharsila M, Lahtinen S, Hattara L, Salminen N, Arppe R, Lastusaari M, Saviranta P and Soukka T 2012 Quantitative multianalyte microarray immunoassay utilizing upconverting phosphor technology *Anal. Chem.* **84** 8628–34

[89] Kale V, Pakkila H, Vainio J, Ahomaa A, Sirkka N, Lyytikainen A, Talha S M, Kutsaya A, Waris M and Julkunen I 2016 Spectrally and spatially multiplexed serological array-in-well assay utilizing two-color upconversion luminescence imaging *Anal. Chem.* **88** 4470–7

[90] Xin H, Li Y, Xu D, Zhang Y, Chen C H and Li B 2017 Single upconversion nanoparticle-bacterium cotrapping for single-bacterium labeling and analysis *Small* **13** 1603418

[91] Yin M, Wu C, Li H, Jia Z, Deng Q, Wang S and Zhang Y 2019 Simultaneous sensing of seven pathogenic bacteria by guanidine-functionalized upconversion fuorescent nanoparticles *ACS Omega* **4** 8953–9

[92] Wu S, Duan N, Shi Z, Fang C and Wang Z 2014 Simultaneous aptasensor for multiplex pathogenic bacteria detection based on multicolor upconversion nanoparticles labels *Anal. Chem.* **86** 3100–7

[93] Zhang B, Li H, Pan W, Chen Q, Ouyang Q and Zhao J 2016 Dual-color upconversion nanoparticles (UCNPs)-based fuorescent immunoassay probes for sensitive sensing food-borne pathogens *Food Anal. Methods* **10** 2036–45

[94] Zrazhevskiy P and Gao X 2013 Quantum dot imaging platform for single-cell molecular profiling *Nat. Commun.* **4** 1619

[95] Xu X, Ray R, Gu Y, Ploehn H, Gearheart L, Raker K and Scrivens W A 2004 CDs were prepared from single-walled carbon nanotubes (SWCNTs) using arc-discharge soot by electrophoresis *J. Am. Chem. Soc.* **126** 12736

[96] Ji C, Zhou Y, Leblanc R M and Peng Z 2020 Recent developments of carbon dots in biosensing: a review *ACS Sens.* **5** 2724–41

[97] Gu Z, Yan L, Tian G, Li S, Chai Z and Zhao Y 2013 Recent advances in design and fabrication of upconversion nanoparticles and their safe theranostic applications *Adv. Mater.* **25** 3758–79

[98] Wang F and Liu X 2009 Recent advances in the chemistry of lanthanide-doped upconversion nanocrystals *Chem. Soc. Rev.* **38** 976–89

[99] Gorris H H and Wolfbeis O S 2013 Photon-upconverting nanoparticles for optical encoding and multiplexing of cells, biomolecules, and microspheres *Angew. Chem. Int. Ed.* **52** 3584–600

[100] Cheng L, Wang C and Liu Z 2013 Upconversion nanoparticles and their composite nanostructures for biomedical imaging and cancer therapy *Nanoscale* **5** 23–37

[101] Cui S, Chen H, Zhu H, Tian J, Chi X, Qian Z, Achilefu S and Gu Y 2012 Amphiphilic chitosan modified upconversion nanoparticles for *in vivo* photodynamic therapy induced by near-infrared light *J. Mater. Chem.* **11** 4861–73

[102] Cheng L, Yang K, Li Y, Chen J, Wang C, Shao M, Lee S T and Liu Z 2011 Facile preparation of multifunctional upconversion nanoprobes for multimodal imaging and dual-targeted photothermal therapy *Angew. Chem.* **123** 7523–8

[103] Tallury P, Payton K and Santra S 2008 Silica-based multimodal/multifunctional nano-particles for bioimaging and biosensing applications *Nanomedicine* **3** 579–92

[104] Wang L, Zhao W and Tan W 2008 Bioconjugated silica nanoparticles: development and applications *Nano Res.* **1** 99–115

[105] Wang L, Wang K, Santra S, Zhao X, Hilliard L R, Smith J E, Wu Y and Tan W 2006 Watching silica nanoparticles glow in the biological world *Anal. Chem.* **78** 646–54

[106] Brozek-Pluska B, Musial J, Kordek R and Abramczyk H 2019 Analysis of human colon by Raman spectroscopy and imaging-elucidation of biochemical changes in carcinogenesis *Int. J. Mol. Sci.* **20** 3398

[107] Kumar Y and Karne S C 2017 Spectral analysis: a rapid tool for species detection in meat products *Trends Food Sci. Technol.* **62** 59–67

[108] Guo S, Popp J and Bocklitz T 2021 Chemometric analysis in Raman spectroscopy from experimental design to machine learning-based modeling *Nat. Protoc.* **16** 5426–59

[109] Li N and Yang Y 2016 Using semi-nonnegative matrix underapproximation for statistical process monitoring *Chemom. Intell. Lab. Syst.* **153** 126–39

[110] Ullah R, Khan S, Chaudhary I I, Shahzad S, Ali H and Bilal M 2020 Cost effective and efficient screening of tuberculosis disease with Raman spectroscopy and machine learning algorithms *Photodiagnosis Photodyn. Ther.* **32** 101963

[111] Bashir S *et al* 2021 Surface-enhanced Raman spectroscopy for the identification of tigecycline-resistant *E. coli* strains *Spectrochim. Acta* A **258** 119831

[112] Liu W, Tang J W, Lyu J W, Wang J J, Pan Y C, Shi X Y, Liu Q H, Zhang X, Gu B and Wang L 2022 Discrimination between carbapenem-resistant and carbapenem-sensitive *Klebsiella pneumoniae* strains through computational analysis of surface-enhanced Raman spectra: a pilot study *Microbiol. Spectr* **10** 02409–21

[113] Kashif M *et al* 2021 Surface-enhanced Raman spectroscopy for identification of food processing bacteria *Spectrochim. Acta* A **261** 119989

[114] Kothari R, Fong Y and Storrie-Lombardi M C 2020 Review of laser Raman spectroscopy for surgical breast cancer detection: stochastic backpropagation neural networks *Sensors* **20** 6260

[115] Liu Y, Xu J, Tao Y, Fang T, Du W and Ye A 2020 Rapid and accurate identification of marine microbes with single-cell Raman spectroscopy *Analyst* **145** 3297–305

[116] Gautam R, Vanga S, Ariese F and Umapathy S 2015 Review of multidimensional data processing approaches for Raman and infrared spectroscopy *EPJ Techn. Instrum.* **2** 8

[117] El Bouchefry K and de Souza R S 2020 Learning in big data: introduction to machine learning *Knowledge Discovery in Big Data from Astronomy and Earth Observation* (New York: Elsevier) pp 225–49

[118] Shahzad K *et al* 2022 Classification of tuberculosis by surface-enhanced Raman spectroscopy (SERS) with principal component analysis (PCA) and partial least squares–discriminant analysis (PLS-DA) *Anal. Lett.* **55** 1731–44

[119] Granato D, Santos J S, Escher G B, Ferreira B L and Maggio R M 2018 Use of principal component analysis (PCA) and hierarchical cluster analysis (HCA) for multivariate association between bioactive compounds and functional properties in foods: a critical perspective *Trends Food Sci. Technol.* **72** 83–90

[120] Villa J E, Quiñones N R, Fantinatti-Garboggini F and Poppi R J 2019 Fast discrimination of bacteria using a filter paper-based SERS platform and PLS-DA with uncertainty estimation *Anal. Bioanal. Chem.* **411** 705–13

[121] Botta R, Chindaudom P, Eiamchai P, Horprathum M, Limwichean S, Chananonnawathorn C, Patthanasettakul V, Kaewseekhao B, Faksri K and Nuntawong N 2018 Tuberculosis determination using SERS and chemometric methods *Tuberculosis* **108** 195–200

[122] Cheng H, Xu C, Zhang D, Zhang Z, Liu J and Lv X 2020 Multiclass identification of hepatitis C based on serum Raman spectroscopy *Photodiagnosis Photodyn. Ther.* **30** 101735

[123] Thrift W J, Cabuslay A, Laird A B, Ranjbar S, Hochbaum A I and Ragan R 2019 Surface-enhanced Raman scattering-based odor compass: locating multiple chemical sources and pathogens *ACS Sens.* **4** 2311–9

[124] Ding J, Lin Q, Zhang J, Young G M, Jiang C, Zhong Y and Zhang J 2021 Rapid identification of pathogens by using surface-enhanced Raman spectroscopy and multi-scale convolutional neural network *Anal. Bioanal. Chem.* **413** 3801–11

[125] Ciloglu F U, Caliskan A, Saridag A M, Kilic I H, Tokmakci M, Kahraman M and Aydin O 2021 Drug-resistant *Staphylococcus aureus* bacteria detection by combining surface-enhanced Raman spectroscopy (SERS) and deep learning techniques *Sci. Rep.* **111** 18444

[126] Fu Q, Zhang Y, Wang P, Pi J, Qiu X, Guo Z, Huang Y, Zhao Y, Li S and Xu J 2021 Rapid identification of the resistance of urinary tract pathogenic bacteria using deep learning-based spectroscopic analysis *Anal. Bioanal. Chem.* **413** 7401–10

[127] Neugebauer U, Rösch P and Popp J 2015 Raman spectroscopy towards clinical application: drug monitoring and pathogen identification *Int. J. Antimicrob. Agents* **46** S35–9

[128] Pahlow S, Meisel S, Cialla-May D, Weber K, Rösch P and Popp J 2015 Isolation and identification of bacteria by means of Raman spectroscopy *Adv. Drug Deliv. Rev.* **15** 105–20

[129] Kloß S, Kampe B, Sachse S, Rösch P, Straube E, Pfister W, Kiehntopf M and Popp J 2013 Culture independent Raman spectroscopic identification of urinary tract infection pathogens: a proof of principle study *Anal. Chem.* **85** 9610–6

[130] Kloß S, Lorenz B, Dees S, Labugger I, Rösch P and Popp J 2015 Destruction-free procedure for the isolation of bacteria from sputum samples for Raman spectroscopic analysis *Anal. Bioanal. Chem.* **407** 8333–41

[131] Kloß S, Rösch P, Pfister W, Kiehntopf M and Popp J 2015 Towards culture-free Raman spectroscopic identification of pathogens in ascitic fluid *Anal. Chem.* **87** 937–43

[132] Stöckel S, Meisel S, Elschner M, Rösch P and Popp J 2012 Raman spectroscopic detection of anthrax endospores in powder samples *Angew. Chem., Int. Ed. Engl.* **51** 5339–42

[133] Kusić D, Kampe B, Ramoji A, Neugebauer U, Rösch P and Popp J 2015 Raman spectroscopic differentiation of planktonic bacteria and biofilms *Anal. Bioanal. Chem.* **407** 6803–13

[134] Silge A, Abdou E, Schneider K, Meisel S, Bocklitz T, Lu-Walther H W, Heintzmann R, Rösch P and Popp J 2015 Shedding light on host niches: label-free *in situ* detection of *Mycobacterium gordonae* via carotenoids in macrophages by Raman microspectroscopy *Cell. Microbiol.* **176** 832–42

[135] World Health Organization 2019 *Top 10 Causes of Death* (Geneva: World Health Organization)

[136] Yeh Y T *et al* 2020 A rapid and label-free platform for virus capture and identification from clinical samples *Proc. Natl Acad. Sci. USA* **117** 895–901

[137] Shanmukh S, Jones L, Driskell J, Zhao Y, Dluhy R and Tripp R A 2006 Rapid and sensitive detection of respiratory virus molecular signatures using a silver nanorod array SERS substrate *Nano Lett.* **6** 2630–6

[138] Luo S C, Sivashanmugan K, Liao J D, Yao C K and Peng H C 2014 Nanofabricated SERS-active substrates for single-molecule to virus detection *in vitro*: a review *Biosens. Bioelectron.* **61** 232–40

[139] Driskell J D, Kwarta K M, Lipert R J, Porter M D, Neill J D and Ridpath J F 2005 Low-level detection of viral pathogens by a surface-enhanced Raman scattering based immuno-assay *Anal. Chem.* **77** 6147–54

[140] Otange B, Birech Z, Rop R and Oyugi J 2019 Estimation of HIV-1 viral load in plasma of HI-1-infected people based on the associated Raman spectroscopic peaks *J. Raman Spectrosc.* **50** 620–8

[141] Lu Y *et al* 2018 Label free hepatitis B detection based on serum derivative surface enhanced Raman spectroscopy combined with multivariate analysis *Biomed. Opt. Express* **9** 4755–66

[142] Lin Y Y, Liao J D, Yang M L and Wu C L 2012 Target-size embracing dimension for sensitive detection of viruses with various sizes and influenza virus strains *Biosens. Bioelectron.* **35** 447–51

[143] Ganbold E O, Kang T, Lee K, Lee S Y and Joo S W 2012 Aggregation effects of gold nanoparticles for single-base mismatch detection in influenza A (H1N1) DNA sequences using fluorescence and Raman measurements *Colloids Surf.* B **93** 148–53

[144] Chang C W, Liao J D, Shiau A L and Yao C K 2011 Non-labeled virus detection using inverted triangular Au nano-cavities arrayed as SERS-active substrate *Sens. Actuators* B **156** 471–8

[145] Lin Y Y, Liao J D, Ju Y H, Chang C W and Shiau A L 2011 Focused ion beam-fabricated Au micro/nanostructures used as a surface enhanced Raman scattering-active substrate for trace detection of molecules and influenza virus *Nanotechnology* **18** 185308

[146] Novelli-Rousseau A, Espagnon I, Filiputti D, Gal O, Douet A, Mallard F and Josso Q 2018 Culture-free antibiotic-susceptibility determination from single-bacterium Raman spectra *Sci. Rep.* **8** 3957

[147] Brownfield B and Kalivas J H 2017 Consensus outlier detection using sum of ranking differences of common and new outlier measures without tuning parameter selections *Anal. Chem.* **89** 5087–94

[148] Granados A, Peci A, McGeer A and Gubbay J B 2017 Influenza and rhinovirus viral load and disease severity in upper respiratory tract infections *J. Clin. Virol.* **86** 14–9

[149] Lee J H, Kim B C, Byeung-Keun O H and Choi J W 2015 Rapid and sensitive determination of HIV-1 virus based on surface enhanced Raman spectroscopy *J. Biomed. Nanotechnol.* **11** 2223–30

[150] Paul A M, Fan Z, Sinha S S, Shi Y, Le L, Bai F and Ray P C 2015 Bioconjugated gold nanoparticle based SERS probe for ultrasensitive identification of mosquito-borne viruses using Raman fingerprinting *J. Phys. Chem.* C **119** 23669–75

[151] Tort N, Salvador J P, Avino A, Eritja R, Comelles J, Martínez E, Samitier J and Marco M P 2012 Synthesis of steroid–oligonucleotide conjugates for a DNA site-encoded SPR immunosensor *Bioconjugate Chem.* **23** 2183–91

[152] Tsai C W, Jheng S L, Chen W Y and Ruaan R C 2014 Strategy of Fc-recognizable peptide ligand design for oriented immobilization of antibody *Anal. Chem.* **86** 2931–8

[153] Baniukevic J, Boyaci I H, Bozkurt A G, Tamer U, Ramanavic A and Ramanaviciene A 2013 Magnetic gold nanoparticles in SERS-based sandwich immunoassay for antigen detection by well oriented antibodies *Biosens. Bioelectron.* **43** 281–8

[154] Wang Y, Tang L J and Jiang J H 2013 Surface-enhanced Raman spectroscopy-based, homogeneous, multiplexed immunoassay with antibody-fragments-decorated gold nanoparticles *Anal. Chem.* **85** 9213–20

[155] Kumada Y 2014 Site-specific immobilization of recombinant antibody fragments through material-binding peptides for the sensitive detection of antigens in enzyme immunoassays *Biochim. Biophys. Acta Proteins Proteom.* **1844** 1960–9

[156] Kukushkin V I, Ivanov N M, Novoseltseva A A, Gambaryan A S, Yaminsky I V, Kopylov A M and Zavyalova E G 2019 Highly sensitive detection of influenza virus with SERS aptasensor *PLoS One* **14** 0216247

[157] Jarvis R M and Goodacre R 2004 Discrimination of bacteria using surface-enhanced Raman spectroscopy *Anal. Chem.* **76** 40–7

[158] Chen L, Sheng Z, Zhang A, Guo X, Li J, Han H and Jin M 2010 Quantum-dots-based fluoroimmunoassay for the rapid and sensitive detection of avian influenza virus subtype H5N1 *Luminescence* **25** 419–23

[159] Liu C, Wang L, Guo Y, Gao X, Xu Y, Wei Q, Man B and Yang C 2019 Suspended 3D AgNPs/CNT nanohybrids for the SERS application *Appl. Surf. Sci.* **487** 1077–83

[160] Liang X, Li N, Zhang R, Yin P, Zhang C, Yang N, Liang K and Kong B 2021 Carbon-based SERS biosensor: from substrate design to sensing and bioapplication *NPG Asia Mater.* **13** 8

[161] Wang L, Zhao W, O'Donoghu M B and Tan W 2007 Fluorescent nanoparticles for multiplexed bacteria monitoring *Bioconjugate Chem.* **18** 297–301

[162] Yan F and Vo-Dinh T 2007 Surface-enhanced Raman scattering detection of chemical and biological agents using a portable Raman integrated tunable sensor *Sensors Actuators* B **121** 61–6

[163] Jarvis R M and Goodacre R 2004 Discrimination of bacteria using surface enhanced Raman spectroscopy *Anal. Chem.* **76** 40–7

[164] Clarke S J, Littleford R E, Smith W E and Goodacre R 2005 Rapid monitoring of antibiotics using Raman and surface enhanced Raman spectroscopy *Analyst* **130** 1019–26

[165] Schröder U C *et al* 2013 Combined dielectrophoresis–Raman setup for the classification of pathogens recovered from the urinary tract *Anal. Chem.* **85** 10717–24

[166] Schröder U C, Bokeloh F, O'Sullivan M, Glaser U, Wolf K, Pfister W, Popp J, Ducrée J and Neugebauer U 2015 Rapid, culture-independent, optical diagnostics of centrifugally captured bacteria from urine samples *Biomicrofluidics* **9** 044118

[167] Wang P, Pang S, Chen J, McLandsborough L, Nugen S R, Fan M and He L 2016 Label-free mapping of single bacterial cells using surface-enhanced Raman spectroscopy *Analyst* **141** 1356–62

[168] Jamil S, Jamil N, Saad U, Hafiz S and Siddiqui S 2016 Frequency of *Candida albicans* in patients with funguria *J. Coll. Physicians Surg. Pak.* **26** 113–6

[169] Edwards H G, Russell N C, Weinstein R and Wynn-Williams D D 1995 Fourier transform Raman spectroscopic study of fungi *J. Raman Spectrosc.* **26** 911–6

[170] De Gussem K, Vandenabeele P, Verbeken A and Moens L 2009 Use of dendrograms of slice spectra as a new graphical tool for the interpretation of two-dimensional correlation spectra *Appl. Spectrosc.* **63** 73–80

[171] Witkowska E, Jagielski T, Kamińska A, Kowalska A, Hryncewicz-Gwóźdź A and Waluk J 2016 Detection and identification of human fungal pathogens using surface-enhanced Raman spectroscopy and principal component analysis *Anal. Methods* **8** 8427–34

[172] Dina N E, Gherman A M, Chiş V, Sârbu C, Wieser A, Bauer D and Haisch C 2018 Characterization of clinically relevant fungi via SERS fingerprinting assisted by novel chemometric models *Anal. Chem.* **90** 2484–92

[173] Mabbott S, Thompson D, Sirimuthu N, McNay G, Faulds K and Graham D 2016 From synthetic DNA to PCR product: detection of fungal infections using SERS *Faraday Discuss.* **187** 461–72

[174] Rebrošová K, Šiler M, Samek O, Růžička F, Bernatová S, Holá V, Ježek J, Zemánek P, Sokolová J and Petráš P 2017 Rapid identification of staphylococci by Raman spectroscopy *Sci. Rep.* **7** 14846

[175] Lorenz B, Wichmann C, Stöckel S, Rösch P and Popp J 2017 Cultivation-free Raman spectroscopic investigations of bacteria *Trends Microbiol.* **25** 413–24

[176] Witkowska E, Niciński K, Korsak D, Dominiak B, Waluk J and Kamińska A 2020 Nanoplasmonic sensor for foodborne pathogens detection. Towards development of ISO-SERS methodology for taxonomic affiliation of *Campylobacter* spp *J. Biophotonics* **13** 201960227

[177] Samek O, Bernatová S and Dohnal F 2021 The potential of SERS as an AST methodology in clinical settings *Nanophotonics* **10** 2537–61

[178] Langer J *et al* 2019 Present and future of surface-enhanced Raman scattering *ACS Nano* **14** 28–117

[179] Zhong N S *et al* 2003 Epidemiology and cause of severe acute respiratory syndrome (SARS) in Guangdong, People's Republic of China, in February *Lancet* **362** 1353–8

[180] Wang L, Ji F, Li C, Pan X, Yan X, Wang R and Gu B 2020 Re-appearance of the SARS-CoV-2 virus nucleic acid in patients recovering from COVID-19 *Ann. Trans. Med.* **8** 656

[181] Gribanyov D, Zhdanov G, Olenin A, Lisichkin G, Gambaryan A, Kukushkin V and Zavyalova E 2021 SERS-based colloidal aptasensors for quantitative determination of influenza virus *Int. J. Mol. Sci.* **22** 1842

[182] Qin Z, Peng R, Baravik I K and Liu K 2020 Fighting COVID-19: integrated micro-and nanosystems for viral infection diagnostics *Matter* **3** 628–51

[183] Kahraman M, Müge Yazici M, Şahİn F, Bayrak Ö F, Topcu E and Culha M 2007 Towards single-microorganism detection using surface-enhanced Raman spectroscopy *Int. J. Environ. Anal. Chem.* **87** 763–70

[184] Wang L, Yang C and Tan W 2005 Dual-luminophore-doped silica nanoparticles for multiplexed signaling *Nano Lett.* **5** 37–43

[185] Prusinkiew M A, Farazkhorasani F, Dynes J J, Wang J, Gough K M and Kaminskyj S G 2012 Proof-of-principle for SERS imaging of *Aspergillus nidulans* hyphae using *in vivo* synthesis of gold nanoparticles *Analyst* **137** 4934–42

[186] Szeghalmi A, Kaminskyj S, Rösch P, Popp J and Gough K M 2007 Time fluctuations and imaging in the SERS spectra of fungal hypha grown on nanostructured substrates *J. Phys. Chem.* B **111** 12916–24

[187] Petersen L M, Martin I W, Moschetti W E, Kershaw C M and Tsongalis G 2019 Third-generation sequencing in the clinical laboratory: exploring the advantages and challenges of nanopore sequencing *J. Clin. Microbiol.* **58** e01315

[188] Szymborski T, Witkowska E, Adamkiewicz W, Waluk J and Kamińska A 2014 Electrospun polymer mat as a SERS platform for the immobilization and detection of bacteria from fluids *Analyst* **139** 5061–4

[189] Kamińska A, Witkowska E, Winkler K, Dzięcielewski I, Weyher J L and Waluk J 2015 Detection of hepatitis B virus antigen from human blood: SERS immunoassay in a microfluidic system *Biosens. Bioelectron.* **66** 461–7

[190] Isola N R, Stokes D L and Vo-Dinh T 1998 Surface-enhanced Raman gene probe for HIV detection *Anal. Chem.* **70** 1352–6

[191] Ling L, Xin-yu H, Shi-fang L, Chuang G and Yi X 2021 Research progress in identification and detection of fungi based on SERS spectroscopy *Spectrosc. Spectr. Anal.* **41** 1661–8

[192] Dewi H A, Meng F, Sana B, Guo C, Norling B, Chen X and Lim S 2014 Investigation of electron transfer from isolated spinach thylakoids to indium tin oxide *RSC Adv.* **4** 48815–20

[193] Bonnier F *et al* 2011 Erratum: *In vitro* analysis of immersed human tissues by Raman microspectroscopy *J. Raman Spectrosc.* **42** 1711

[194] Ali S M, Bonnier F, Lambkin H, Flynn K, McDonagh V, Healy C, Lee T C, Lyng F M and Byrne H J 2013 A comparison of Raman, FTIR and ATR-FTIR micro spectroscopy for imaging human skin tissue sections *Anal. Methods* **5** 2281–91

[195] Parihar A, Ranjan P, Sanghi S K, Srivastava A K and Khan R 2020 Point-of-care biosensor-based diagnosis of COVID-19 holds promise to combat current and future pandemics *ACS Appl. Bio Mater.* **3** 7326–43

[196] Yadav S, Sadique M A, Ranjan P, Kumar N, Singhal A, Srivastava A K and Khan R 2021 SERS based lateral flow immunoassay for point-of-care detection of SARS-CoV-2 in clinical samples *ACS Appl. Bio Mater.* **4** 2974–95

[197] Ji F *et al* 2021 Clinical findings in a group of COVID-19 patients: a single-center retrospective study *Ann. Transl. Med.* **9** 44

IOP Publishing

SERS-Based Advanced Diagnostics for Infectious Diseases

Raju Khan, Shalu Yadav and Mohd Abubakar Sadique

Chapter 4

Use of nanotechnology in SERS-based diagnostics

Shagun Gupta, Surbhi Sharma, Puja Adhikari, Shadan Raza and Ankur Kaushal

Surface-enhanced Raman scattering (SERS) is one of the cutting-edge technologies used in label-free bio-analytical assays to enhance the sensitivity of molecular assemblies adsorbed or attached to nanostructured metallic surfaces. SERS utilizes different colloidal nanoparticles to monitor the biological interactions on the solid surfaces, enhances the sensitivity, and shortens the turn-around time of bio-analytical assays. Since nanotechnology was first discovered in 1959, it has expanded its astonishing applications in diagnostics and nano-fabrication on sensor surfaces by improving the sensitivity, specificity, and customizable compatibility. Because of the breakthroughs made in the development of SERS-based *in vitro* assays using nano-technology, SERS-based technology is now able to meet the 'ASSURED' (Affordable, Sensitive, Specific, User-friendly, Rapid, Equipment-free, and Deliverable) criteria of the World Health Organization (WHO). The discovery of the SERS effect revolutionized the Raman technique for trace analysis. The SPR phenomenon enables single-molecule identification which was impossible with the earlier Raman technique, and nanoparticles such as gold, carbon, and silver considerably amplify the Raman effect. It is a useful technique for the development of point-of-care detection of diverse infectious diseases, malignancies, and neurological disorders due to its ability to cope with small sample quantities, quick reactivity, and hypersensitivity. This chapter describes the use of nanomaterials for the development of SERS and its fabrication processes. The recent utilization of SERS-based biosensors is also examined, which includes *ex vivo* fluids and biomolecules such as proteins, microRNAs, and DNA with the monitoring of cellular attributes such as temperature, pH, and ion concentrations.

4.1 Introduction

Biosensors are predominantly used for quantitatively measuring, identifying, and detecting biomolecules in biological process studies and medical diagnosis. One of the most potent and sensitive spectroscopic methods, SERS stands out for its million-fold increase in Raman emissions when employing the right substrates (silver, copper, and gold). After being discovered for the first time in the 1970s on a roughened silver metal surface, SERS quickly gained popularity in the domains of chemistry, materials science, biochemistry, and life science. SERS-based biosensors offer various advantages in bio-analysis [1]: (i) the magnitude of reflecting the intrinsic fingerprint molecular information of biomolecules and ultra-sensitivity at the one-molecule level; (ii) narrow peak bandwidth with good resistance to photo-bleaching and photo-degradation when in combination with fluorescence spectro-scopy; (iii) numerous choices for signal enhancement substrates with various sizes and shapes to serve diverse applications; and (iv) huge laser penetration depth assisting both *in vitro* and *in vivo* diagnosis and imaging. The research areas for SERS focus on bio-analysis, mostly fabrication and its application in biosensors. Fabrication of SERS-based biosensor using nanoparticles to detect bio-molecular interactions [2–5].

Raman scattering depends on the loss of energy, known as Stokes, or its gain, known as anti-Stokes, of photons which are scattered inelastically due to a molecule's vibration events, reflecting the molecular structure data and permitting *in situ* and real-time detection. Surface-enhanced Raman scattering (SERS) is a subgroup of Raman scattering and provides million-fold enhancement by employing plasmonic nanostructures, reducing the detection sensitivity down to the single-atom level. The enhancement is attained via two well-defined mechanisms, namely electromagnetic enhancement (EM) [6] and chemical enhancement (CE). Concerning electromagnetic enhancement, the main idea is to integrate approaching light with the localized surface plasmon resonances (LSPRs) of plasmonic

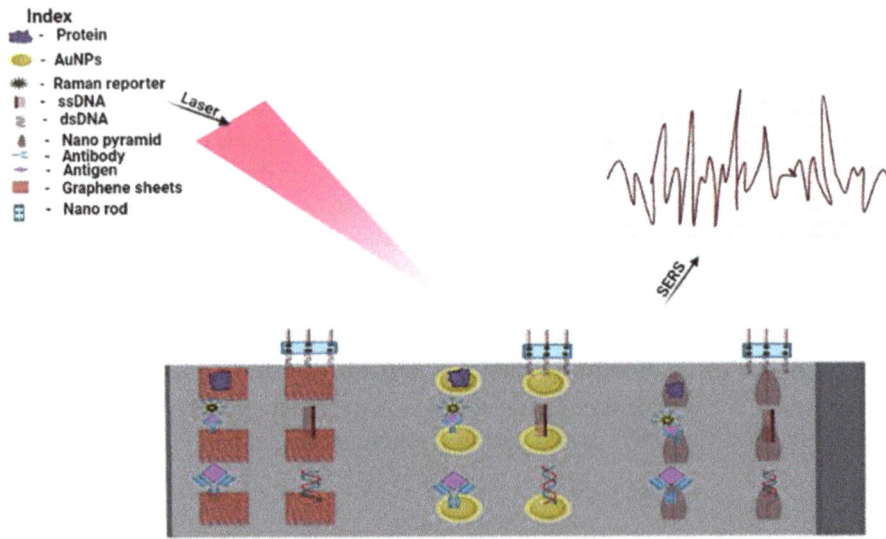

Figure 4.1. An overview of the fabrication of a SERS-based biosensor using nanoparticles to detect bio-molecular interactions.

nanostructures so that the secondary electric field effectively directs the electromagnetic field. The enhanced EM field amplifies the intensity of SERS when the molecules are near the plasmonic nanostructures (10 nm distance). Electromagnetic enhancement is regarded as the main contributor to signal enhancement with a 10^4–10^7 enhancement factor. Chemical enhancement occurs at times when the molecules are bonded directly to the plasmonic surface for generating a charge-transfer structure. Even though it is associated with the underlying analyte molecule's chemical structure and their affinity to the surface, the chemical enhancement's contribution to chemical enhancement is smaller than that of electromagnetic enhancement, within the range of a 10–100 enhancement factor [1, 2, 6].

Nanotechnology combined with SERS provides a better performance in terms of reproducibility, high sensitivity, and improved instrumental capabilities [7]. Both the scientific and technological fields require ultrasensitive detection of analytes present at the trace or molecular level. The most promising approach for the monitoring of analytes in the vicinity of a nanostructured surface has benefits such as high specificity, high sensitivity, narrow line width, multiplexed testing (detection of multiple labels) capability of on-site detection of analytes, and target localization [8]. SERS addresses the enhancement of Raman scattering intensity by different molecules when a nanostructured metallic surface is present. In the fabrication of SERS substrates, nanostructures help by enhancing the electromagnetic field for molecules near or on their surface, and the size, shape, dielectric parameters, composition, and interparticle gap spacing of the nanostructures (aggregated, self-assembled, uniform-plasmonic, alloyed, magnetic carbon-based, etc) influence the properties of the SERS substrates effectively as they have the specific surface plasmon resonance property compared to their bulk materials [9, 10].

The gold and silver nanoparticles are considered to be the first-generation SERS substrates [11]. Anisotropic nanoparticles are the second-generation SERS substrates and include rod-, triangle-, cubic-, and star-shaped plasmonic nanoparticles with a higher electromagnetic field concentration leading to higher SERS enhancement [12]. Three-dimensional nanoscale plasmonic substrates and nanoparticle assemblies are the next generations, containing hot spots with greater SERS enhancement factors [13]. Silver nanoparticles, gold nanowires, silver nanorods, gold nanorods with gold-coated magnetic nanoparticles, gold and silver nanowires, gold nanostars, etc, are SERS-active substrates reported in the detection of various bacterial infections, urinary tract infections, keratoconjunctivitis, dengue, Zika, malaria, etc [14].

The emergence of plasmonic nanomaterials represents a paradigm shift in addressing the capabilities of SERS biosensing platforms. These nanomaterials proved to be effective as the signal amplification substrates for sensing as they have an excellent enhancement efficiency between 10^{10}–10^{11} (sufficient for detecting a single molecule) [15]. The graphene-based materials possess the ability to act as a protective layer against oxidation, and have flexibility, excellent optical permeability, SERS enhancement via the charge-transfer mechanism, and better mechanical strength. Celik and Kurt fabricated three-dimensional porous expanded graphite with a silver nanoparticle nanocomposite to produce a SERS platform for rhodamine 6G [16]. Metal nanoparticle self-assembly has gained attention because of its applications in sensors, plasmonics, surface-enhanced optics, and catalysts. Guo *et al* fabricated gold nanoparticle monolayer film using polyvinyl-pyrrolidone as a surfactant at the air–water interface with interparticle gaps smaller than 2 nm. Further, the monolayer film was transferred onto the glassy carbon electrode which produced an Au electrode making it suitable for electrochemical SERS measurements [17]. Various SERS substrates including metal nanoshells, porous templates coated with metal films, electrochemically roughened metal surfaces, and nanoporous gold films with self-organized nanoscale surface morphologies also enable high detection sensitivity and detection up to a single-molecule level. The nanofabricated SERS templates prevent the exploration of the hot spot (location observed due to maximum signal enhancement) [18]. The fabrication of gold nanoshurikens and nanocylinders is also promising for the enhancement of sensitivity and LSPR signal. Gold and silver nanoparticles overcome the limitations of the plasmonic colorimetric assays which include a lack of low-level sensitivity which is required for the early detection of viral and bacterial pathogens [19].

Among the many approaches, lateral flow assays, microfluidic devices, lab-on-a-chip assays, and paper-based immunoassays are the most frequent SERS diagnostic platforms developed for testing infectious diseases [13]. To establish strong SERS signals, hot spot contriving has become the basis for the fabrication of enhancing substrates for mounting zero-dimensional to three-dimensional structures [20]. The zero- or one-dimensional substrates focus on generating single particles with wide curvature regions by systematizing complex nanoparticle morphology or post-synthetic morphological modifications. The two-dimensional enhancing structures are arrays with regular narrow gaps fabricated by top-down or bottom-up processes. Three-dimensional SERS platforms are for the most part large-area structures and closely packed super-crystals organized by the self-assembly of integrating colloidal nanoparticles. The various structures produce strong electromagnetic field enhancements and offer a diverse range of enhancing approaches for SERS-based biosensors with varying sensing purposes.

In this chapter, the basics of SERS and recent advances in the design and fabrication of SERS-based biosensors are introduced, and applications such as *in vitro* bio-analysis, *ex vivo* determination of bio-fluids or cellular systems, the detection of biomolecules such as proteins and nucleic acids, as well as the observation of cellular pH, temperature, and ionic environment are discussed.

4.2 Construction of SERS-based biosensors

Recent developments in improving the structures and substrates have inspired an increase in SERS applications, particularly in the medicinal and biological sciences [21, 22]. There are commonly two type of techniques for SERS-based biosensors: direct, also called label-free, detection and indirect detection, necessitating SERS tags. Direct detection in SERS-based biosensors provides the molecular fingerprint information of biomolecules as they track the inherent vibrations directly without a need for label molecules [23]. Since the biomolecules are constrained close to the EM field of the enhancing substrates, SERS sensing is possible [24].

Affinity agents bound to the surface are required for biomolecules that are unable to stay in this region or have a low concentration. The inherent detecting mechanism is what causes direct SERS sensing to be limited. Some biomolecules emit signals that are relatively weak, complicated, and vulnerable to interference from other molecules which are present in the matrix. In indirect SERS sensing, particular SERS signals are marked as SERS tags on the boosting substrates. When the targets or ligands are bonded or retaliated with SERS tags to environmental factors such as pH, temperature, or ionic concentration occurs, it indicates that the presence of target biomolecules or changes in the biological surroundings can be observed in SERS signals (SERS read-outs). Due to the distinctive and consistent signals of SERS tags and the variety in the design and construction of biosensors, indirect sensing loses the ability to offer molecular information but opens up additional possibilities in qualitative and quantitative sensing.

SERS is a potent tool for biological as well as biomedical sensing, particularly for the detection of biomolecules such as proteins, DNA, and micro-RNA as well as the monitoring of various biological properties. This is due to the careful design and fabrication of the enhancing substrates as well as the variety of construction methods for both direct as well as indirect SERS platforms. We now go into more detail about recent developments and uses of SERS-based biosensing.

4.3 Biological and biomedical applications of SERS-based biosensors

Due to technological advancements, SERS had shown its potential in the varied field of biosciences as well as in geophysics, as illustrated in figure 4.2.

4.3.1 Protein detection

In the biological sciences, particularly in the early identification and treatment of diseases, the sensing and determination of the quantity and structure of proteins play significant roles. To easily and affordably learn about the innate structure of proteins that contain chromophores such as cytochrome C, myoglobin, and hemoglobin, label-free SERS biosensing is used [1]. The intricate chemical structures of proteins and the limited cross sections of Raman scattering, however, make explicit detection challenging. To successfully increase SERS, boosting procedures must be devised.

Label-free methods for repeatable and accurate SERS protein detection using colloidal nanoparticle aggregates and metallic nanostructures were outlined by Kahraman *et al* [25]. While Karadan *et al* built SERS-based biosensors with 2.4×10^8 enhancement factors for thiophenol [26] to distinguish the charge of proteins such as BSA, HSA, and lysozyme as well as the detection of amyloid beta proteins linked to Alzheimer's disease. They did this by decorating Si nanopillar arrays with silver nanoparticles. However, due to various adsorption orientations or protein denaturation, changes in the native SERS spectra of the same protein may be observed. Szekeres *et al* [27] investigated the SERS spectra of BSA with gold nanoparticles without agents causing aggregation at various concentrations. The concentration-

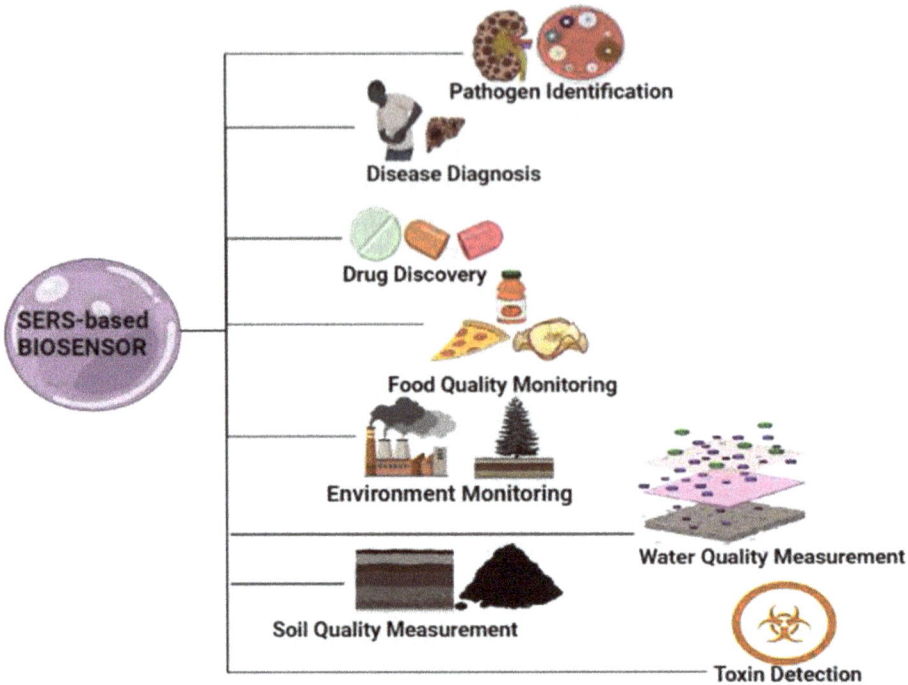

Figure 4.2. Different applications of SERS-based biosensors.

dependent agglomerates of the NPs' distinctive SERS enhancement implied that the BSA molecules might be changed over time. The structure and quantity of proteins can still be determined imprecisely using simple label-free detection methods.

The enzyme-linked immunosorbent assay (ELISA), when used in conjunction with SERS tags as SERS immunoassays, is extensively employed for the indirect detection of proteins due to its low cost, simplicity of use, and specificity [28]. As a result, it has great multiplexing abilities, a low spectrum overlap, and high sensitivity. In the creation of SERS immunoassays, the sandwich-type test with antigen and antibody binding is most frequently employed. Yang *et al* developed the SERS-immunoassay platform using core–shell satellite nanostructures modified with anti-alpha-fetoprotein (AFP) antibodies and as the solid substrate used a nitrocellulose membrane [29]. The thin silica inter-layer of the Au@Ag core–shell-satellite nanostructures is a significant SERS platform, exhibiting long-range plasmon coupling and resulting in a high-enhancement effect. A detection limit as low as 0.3fg/mL in the sandwich-type SERS-immunoassay displays AFP-sensitive detection. These biosensors for protein detection have progressed from traditional to more complex systems which include test strips along with microfluidic chips [30]. These sensors are on the verge of rapid development. It has been shown that dual-reporter SERS immunoassays can detect proteins more precisely and simultane-ously. Accompanied by two distinct SERS labeling tags of prostate-specific antigen (PSA), complexed PSA (c-PSA), and free PSA (f-PSA), Cheng *et al* created magnetic-separation SERS immunoassays. Better accuracy for the f-PSA to total PSA ratio (f/t) in clinical samples was provided by simultaneous detection [31]. Choung *et al* provided a dual-reporter technique in the SERS-immunoassay by pairing affinity reagents tagged with particular Raman reporters employed for the reduction of false positives. This approach is capable of distinguishing between true positives and false positives for thrombin and tumor necrosis factor-alpha (TNF-α) detection, regardless of lower concentrations of target proteins in complex bio-materials.

4.3.2 Nucleic acid detection

Amplification using quantitative polymerase chain reaction (qPCR) in conjunction with fluorescence spectroscopy is the most frequently utilized amplification method in practical analytical procedures for nucleic acids, particularly DNAs [33]. The SERS-PCR method, which combines SERS with PCR, has demonstrated improved efficacy and accuracy but is hindered by its high cost, labor requirements, and time-consuming nature [34]. Direct SERS sensing's reproducibility and sensitivity have recently grown due to an interest in employing SERS to gather intrinsic DNA molecular vibrational information [33]. Tian *et al* created aluminum nano-crystal aggregates for the label-free detection of ssDNA with near-infrared SERS enhance-ment [35]. The aluminum nanocrystals with an intrinsic oxide layer offer a favorable affinity phosphate backbone of ssDNA, thus preventing non-specific adsorption. Identification of 9-mer ssDNA oligomers made up of four bases was possible by measuring the two different 20-mer ssDNA oligomer sequences. Chen *et al* showed the electrokinetic capture of analytes (DNA) in plasmonic nanoslits that were created optically to be lengthened nanopores, which resulted in the regional recognition by direct SERS sensing of four nucleobases [36]. It was shown that different nucleobases have asynchronous spectroscopic activity, whether they are present separately or as a component of DNA strands. Li *et al* produced high-quality SERS hot spots by employing aluminum ions to aggregate AgNPs, which allowed them to monitor the DNA i-motif's formation and estimated the number of planes of the i-motif base pair [37].

MicroRNAs (miRNAs), which are single-stranded, non-coding, short RNA molecules, are crucial parts of numerous biological processes. miRNA analysis has received a lot of attention since miRNAs are essential indicators for the identification and treatment of diseases such as cancer, neurological disorders, and immunological disorders [38]. SERS-based biosensor research has so far focused a lot of attention on the DNA hybridization processes for sensor assembly as well as the ultrasensitive and targeted analysis of miRNAs. Using a complementary dsDNA-aided target-catalyzed hairpin construction and an Au/Ag bimetallic SERS reporter, Sun *et al* developed a SERS sensor which has a sensitivity limit of 0.306 fM for detecting miRNAs associated with acute myocardial infarction (miR-133a).

He *et al* demonstrated very sensitive miRNA detection with 0.121012 M being the detection limit using a SERS sensor made of DNA-conjugated with gold nanoparticles with varied DNA conjugation densities [40]. MiR-223 and AFP were both found by SERS at the same time, and Cheng *et al* recognized both of them as possible liver cancer biomarkers [41]. In this case, the antibody served as the AFP trapping agent, while the branching DNA was used to recognize and collect miRNA. The detection limit of miR-223 is 10 attomolars, supporting the substantial potential of SERS sensing in the early diagnosis of liver cancer.

4.3.3 Biological environment monitoring

In addition to the study of biomolecules, the monitoring of the cellular environment, which depends on biological parameters such as pH, temperature, and ion concentration [42, 43], is the salient application of SERS-based biosensors. This is shown in figure 4.2. Since there are not enough molecules with strong enough Raman scattering cross sections for label-free detection, indirect SERS sensors are typically utilized. These sensors rely on the SERS tags' responses to environmental changes.

Wang *et al* developed a sensing platform for intra- and extracellular pH using Ag nanoparticles embellished with optical fiber tips that contained 4-Mpy (4-mercaptopyridine) due to the response of Raman reporters to pH changes [44]. SERS signals can be obtained directly from optical fiber tips, which are also capable of manipulation and excitation. It was found that among the normal and cancer cell lines, there seems to be a difference in the intracellular pH. SERS performance at single-particle levels for up to 18 different types of gold and silver NPs was investigated by Zhang *et al*, with various forms and architectures using the Raman reporter para-mercaptobenzoic acid to sense the intracellular pH [45]. The time-lapse monitoring of HeLa cells was performed using the SERS sensors relying on p-MBA which connected Au@Ag core/satellites. SERS is employed currently to assess cellular temperature, particularly in photothermal therapy (PTT). Through the use of SERS-guided PTT, Aioub *et al* examined the molecular features of cell death using spherical gold nanoparticle-based SERS biosensors. He observed that a reduction in the disulfide bond in the spectrum at about 500 cm^{-1} is what causes the heat denaturation of proteins [46].

Using indocyanine green (ICG) conjugated Au nanostars, Chen *et al* [47] reported a SERS temperature sensing platform for monitoring the intracellular temperature of glioblastoma cells in real-time during PTT (as SERS tags). Because the alteration in the intensity ratio of the ICG SERS bands at 667 cm^{-1} and 729 cm^{-1} is sensitive to the temperature during PTT, SERS sensing can be employed for a theranostic probe as an intracellular thermometer.

Ion-specific SERS-based sensors have been developed because SERS is an important spectroscopic tool for ion detection [48–51]. For monitoring SERS changes in spectra of N',N-bis(2-hydroxybenzylidene)-4-aminophenyl disulfide, Zhuang *et al* prepared a biosensor after fast chelation of Zn(II) ions, as it is an essential microelement which plays vital biological and physiological roles in humans. Due to its concentration, it can be used as a biomarker for the prior diagnosis of some diseases [52]. This method proffers an ultrasensitive approach for the detection of Zn(II) ions with detection up to the limit of 10–14 M, making it possible to track Zn(II) uptake by HeLa cells. Pramanik *et al* report that Zn(II) produced the aggregation of *p*-(imidazole)-azo-benzenethiol linked gold nanoparticles, which resulted in the generation of a variety of SERS signals [53]. Prostate metastatic cells were found at a concentration of 5 cells/mL using a Zn(II) sensing SERS-based assay, indicating substantial potential for early prostate cancer diagnosis. Zn(II) ions were selectively detected using this method down to 100 ppt.

The SERS methodology provides a nominally invasive, non-destructive technique for testing in living creatures with little sample preparation required. At present, it functions as a helpful analytical tool. Immunoassays of many protein markers in bio-fluids is the fundamental bio-analytical use of the SERS system [30, 54]. Because SERS detection requires a stage of differentiation due to its uniform structure, magnetic nanoparticles are used for the separation of unreacted components and immune complexes which includes the unbound SERS nanotags [56, 57]. Recently, a novel SERS-based biosensor design was published [56] that uses immunocomplex-based manufacturing to synthesize the SERS-active product. When nanoparticles and enzymes are combined, the responsibilities of substrate modification and the transporter of immunoassay active components (such as antibodies and antigens) can be merged [58]. 5-bromo-4-chloro-3-indolyl phosphate (BCIP), the immunoassay's alkaline phosphatase substrate, is broken down to yield inorganic phosphate, the enzyme's sole active component (BCI) [59, 60], and the SERS immunoassay recognizes specific bands within the response material [60].

Pham *et al* reported an enzyme-amplified SERS immunoassay for IgG and prostate-specific antigen detection. The basic principle behind this approach is that an enzyme reduces silver, resulting in a coating of Raman molecules, or modified silica NPs, over AuNPs. When the target analyte was present, the alkaline phosphatase-marked immunological complex initiated the conversion of 2-phospho-L-ascorbic acid into ascorbic acid (AA). Hot spots were produced as a result of Ag^+ being converted by ascorbic acid into Ag, which also amplified the signal from the SERS sample solution. The ratiometric enzyme-linked immunosorbent test's ability to detect allergens with extreme sensitivity is another illustration of the evolution of the SERS-active product [61]. The SERS nanotag used in this investigation was a covalent organic matrix seeded with AuNPs modified with an antibody. This SERS nanotag demonstrated the enzyme's ability and accelerated the conversion of a 4-nitrothiophenol substrate to 4-aminothiophenol in the presence of sodium borohydride. Gold nanostars showed Raman hot spots after they formed the Au–S bond with them. By dividing the signal intensities of the various bands of 4-aminothiophenol and 4-nitrothiophenol, respectively, the analyte concentration under study was determined. The Raman peak may be quantified using the SERS multiplex format since it is narrower than the fluorescence and luminescence peaks [54]. Multiplex SERS-based immunoassays have lately been used to identify pathogens, cancer markers, and poisons [62–64]. The next section discusses the possibilities and advancements that may increase the use of SERS biosensors for fast and point-of-care diagnosis.

Combining detecting devices with microfluidic methods is one way to create SERS technology [67]. By using microfluidics to separate reagent streams and detect numerous analytes simultaneously on a single chip, the researcher can boost analytical productivity. Smaller sample sizes are also obtained when using microchannels, and the complex interlaced channel structure permits controlled flows, uniform reagent mixing, and enhanced repeatability of results [68, 69]. Volume minimization is a useful advancement in analytical methods, on the one hand. On the other hand, it tightens the limitations on the capacity to find sensitive tags. Therefore, it seems that the most sensible choice is to combine microfluidics with a complementary sensitive technique such as SERS. Additionally, in-stream observations decrease the sample heating, adding to one of the main drawbacks of Raman methods, and micro-channel detection creates a high surface-to-volume ratio, both of which are necessary for precise SERS measurements [67, 70]. Due to the seamless integration of the two technologies, microfluidic analytical devices developed with SERS detection are growing in popularity. These analytical methods have so far been used effectively to detect a vast variety of analytes, together with medicines and drugs, pesticides, hormones, antibiotics, various disease markers, nucleic acids, whole cells, and others [68, 69, 71–80]. The four inflammation-related indicators C reactive protein, IL-6, serum amyloid A, and procalcitonin were simultaneously detected using Chen *et al* microfluidic matrix [76]. Through labels with core–surface structures recorded by SERS, they sent out signals. Multiplex detection may be advantageous for other activities as well. For instance, three distinct SERS-labeled molecular probes were used simultaneously by Wang *et al*, targeting various epitopes of the same pathogen for ensuring the precise detection of pathogenic targets at the individual level of cells with its subspecies [80].

Increasingly sophisticated analytical set-ups and the capacity to determine the analyte content utilizing two distinct methods are becoming more widespread. The proposed method, sometimes referred to as a dual detection strategy, combines various methods for determining what is present in the target analyte or cells, enabling a comparison of the methods' sensitivity or detection limits under identical circumstances. Zhang *et al* latest's review of SERS-combined approaches is in [81]. To combine SERS, electrochemical methods [82], fluorescence detection [79], and the polymerase chain reaction (PCR) method [84] were employed. Wang *et al* [83] used nanostars modified with antibodies and aptamers to find circulating tumor cells. The neatly positioned gold nanoflowers on a Au-ITO electrode, which served as the substrate, were changed by an aptamer that interacted with circulating cancer cells. Fluorescent and reporter tags the hairpin trigger DNA molecules, polyethylene glycol-treated nanostars, and antibodies against the pre-selected cells were used to create the SERS nanotag. By evaluating the strength of the fluorescence or the Raman shift after the complex had already formed on the substrate, the quantity of it could be identified. The comparison of the analytical methods of fluorescence and SERS by the authors suggests that the limit of SERS detection may be decreased by a factor of two to find the cancer embryonic antigen. Castao-Guerrero *et al* [82] used concurrent SERS and electrochemical detection of specified antigen–antibody interactions. At first, the capturing antibodies on gold screen printed paper electrode were covalently immobilized and then modified with cysteamine to provide attainable functional groups for cross-linking with antibodies, and then the secondary antibodies were covalently immobilized with a reporter molecule 4-aminothiophenol on gold nanostars. Then, electrochemical impedance spectroscopy was used to evaluate the capabilities of electrochemical detection before attaching the Raman probe to this configuration. The analysis was carried out in two steps because there was a gap in time between the two detection strategies. Along with the buffer to serum carrying the cancer embryonic antigen, the limit of detection was lowered by a factor of ten, which was probably caused by the inability to prevent the blood serum sample's matrix effect. When using SERS, the researchers assert a ten-fold increase in sensitivity.

Escherichia coli, *Salmonella*, and *Staphylococcus aureus* can all be detected in contaminated milk in two different ways, qualitatively and quantitatively, according to Xu *et al* [85]. Both bimetallic gold and silver magnetic nanoparticles modified with 4-mercaptophenylboronic acid (4-MPBA) as the tag for SERS and function-alized up-converting nanoparticles were utilized in this investigation. Interestingly, the authors chose a phenylboronic acid derivative for the interaction because it can be used to connect with the carbohydrate moiety of the wall bacterium. Here, 4-MPBA was employed to produce a Raman probe that served as both a SERS reporter and a bacteria-capturer instead of extra reporters. Despite having distinct SERS reporter spectra, three different bacterial species attached to the phenyl-boronic acid residue similarly. Since the significant differences between the bacteria created changes in their spectral properties, enabling the use of this parameter to identify the bacteria in the combination, these were given the name 'bacterial fingerprints' by scientists. As a result, rather than emphasizing the benefits of fluorescence and SERS, the study mentioned above shows how to use both and also how signal changes depending on whether the bacterium is living or dead. The combination of PCR and paper-based SERS was suggested by Lee *et al* [84] to identify the bacterial DNA of *Mycoplasma pneumonia* (figure 4.3). The paper-based device was coupled with silver nanowires. When the target DNA was present, the EvaGreen dye used was interchangeably incorporated into the DNA structure after several cycles of amplification (0–30). In this instance, a weak SERS signal was picked up. The dye bonded to the silver nanowires on the paper's surface to create so-called 'hot spots', which amplified the signal if the necessary DNA was not created throughout the process. In this case, the SERS signal was obtained from the paper's surface. When contrasting the intensities at the test and control points, it was possible to see the distinction between a positive and a negative outcome, as depicted in figure 4.3.

4.4 Recent applications of SERS-based diagnostics for infectious diseases

Infectious diseases such as malaria, human immunodeficiency virus, tuberculosis, influenza, pneumonia, and diarrhea cause 5–6 million deaths annually and are caused by viruses and bacteria [86]. Thus the early diagnosis of a disease is vital for the prevention of spread of the disease while ensuring epidemic preparedness [87]. Combining nanotechnologies with a SERS-based detection system with more

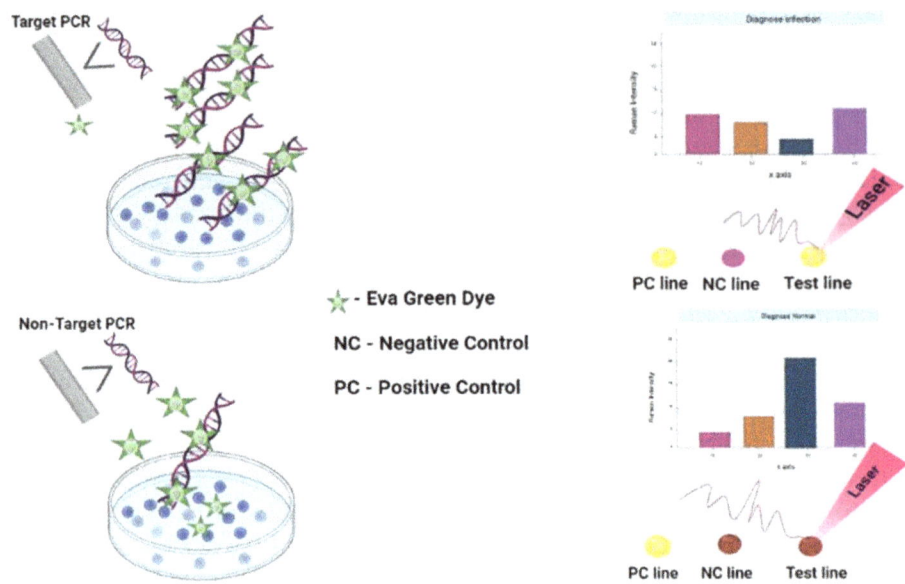

Figure 4.3. Schematic exemplar of the diagnostic process using a paper-based SERS substrate for respiratory bacterial DNA. In the aspect of the target, EvaGreen dye intercalation is dominant in the DNA structure whilst in the case of the non-target, the majority of EvaGreen has adhered to the AgNW hot spot areas. The diagnosis can be made by comparing the Raman intensity between the test line and the control lines.

accuracy and rapid diagnosis of infectious diseases is a good diagnostic approach [88]. Various lateral flow assay techniques using nanomaterials as detection probes are reported for the detection of different infectious diseases. Optical labels such as quantum dots, fluorescence microspheres, carbon nanoparticles, europium nano-particles, and plasmonic nanoparticles have been developed for optical readers [86].

Paper-based lateral flow assay strips are the simplest for the precise detection of a certain target analyte present in a sample and do not require any expertise for their operation. A wide variety of analytes such as nucleic acids, proteins, bacterial pathogens, and infectious viruses can be tested for using LFA strips [86, 87]. The gold nanoparticles conjugated with antibodies as detection probes are most frequently used in conventional colorimetric LFAs [89]. The accumulation of AuNPs induces a color change when observed below the localized surface plasmon effects [89]. Hwang *et al* reported a SERS-based biosensor with hollow gold nanosphere Raman reporters as detection probes for the detection of *Staphylococcal enterotoxin*. The sandwich-type antibody–antigen–antibody conju-gated with hollow gold nanosphere reactions was the governing principle of the SERS-based lateral flow assay strip [90]. Sanchez-Purrá *et al* reported SERS-based multifold detection of dengue and Zika viral biomarkers using gold nanostars conjugated with specific antibodies using 1,2-bis(4-pyridyl) ethylene (BPE) and 4-mercaptobenzoic acid (MBA) for both the diseases with the detection of very low levels of biomarkers [91]. For detecting human deficiency virus type 1 (HIV-1) Fu *et al* developed a SERS-LFA platform using Raman reporters and SERS nanotags of oligonucleotide-functionalized AuNPs [92]. Shen *et al* developed a SERS-LFA for pseudorabies virus, an infectious disease in wild animals with a detection limit of up to 5 ng ml^{-1} [93]. Huang *et al* reported a highly sensitive localized surface plasmon coupled fluorescence (LSPCF) fiber-optic biosensor for the detection of SARS-CoV infection using Au-PA connecting with a fluorophore labeled secondary antibody. The biosensor was suitable for the early diagnosis at the initial stage of SARS patients [94].

A top priority area of study in the biological sciences is the creation of a quick point-of-care approach for the identification of different chemicals. Among the current methods, lateral flow immunoassay (LFIA) tests are in demand because they are based on antigen–antibody interactions on a membrane carrier in a flow of reagents with the production of vividly identifiable immune complexes that have been tagged with nanoparticles. LFIA's low cost and simplicity of testing are unquestionable benefits. The effectiveness of test systems is, however, diminished by insufficient sensitivity and inadequately high-quality ('yes/no') findings. In this respect, the amalgamation of LFIA along with SERS for detection is of ample interest as captured Ab immobilized in the test zone centralize and the lateral flow format of the assay and the SERS nanotag allow the study to be carried out without requiring auxiliary washing or separation steps [87].

Aptamers and antibodies are used as receptor molecules to engage with the desired drug during the construction of SERS-based LFIA. Because they offer highly precise binding to the target analyte, antibodies are a better option. These two analytical techniques are combined by the use of noble metal nanoparticles, most frequently gold nanoparticles, which are utilized in SERS immunoassays as a component of the nanotag and in classical LFIA as a detectable label. This is because the addition of reporter and receptor molecules to nanoparticles causes the development of a SERS nanotag. The increase or decrease in the quantity of SERS nanotags confined in the test zone will be the result of the interaction between receptor molecules and the analyte. During the development of an immune complex, the content of analytes can be determined using the spectra of reporter molecules from SERS nanotags. A review by Khlebtsov *et al* [95] previously provided an overview of the methods for designing high-performance SERS-based LFIA systems as well as the prospects for their use.

The form of the metal nanoparticles in the SERS nanotag is a key component in the constitution of the SERS-based LFIA [84]. For the LFIA's viral detection, Sánchez-Purrà *et al* [96] compared gold nanoparticles of various forms. The work suggests that nanoflowers, nanostars, and other particles with sharp corners and spikes may be advantageous for use in SERS-based LFIA because of their potential for greater signal amplification resulting from the re-ordering of electric fields at the corners. Concerning this, it is advisable to use the created nanoparticles or nano-composites in systems with poor sensitivity to enhance the implementation of the analysis. For instance, Lin *et al* [97] examined the SERS-based LFIA performance for the measurement of bi-phenol A using SERS nanotags rooted on star-shaped and spherical Au nanoparticles of equal size (40 nm). According to the research, using SERS nanotags, such as modified gold nanostars with anti-BPA antibodies and 4-ATP, can raise the ocular and quantitative limits of the detection of phenol A beyond 20 and 205 times, when compared with Au nanospheres.

Star-shaped gold nanoparticles were found to be equally effective in determining the influenza virus's nucleoprotein using the SERS-LFIA approach [98]. As a SERS nanotag, this study used star-shaped nanoparticles of size around 100 nm that had been modified with monoclonal antibodies and 4-ATP against nucleoproteins. The flu virus nucleoprotein had a detection limit that was 37 and 300 times finer than that of fluorescent and conventional LFIA, respectively. The development of SERS-based LFIA is heavily influenced by nanoparticle size. According to Chen et al [66], using particles larger than 40 nm is better because of the stronger surface electromagnetic amplification effect and the increased SERS signal. The nanoparticle's stability, the caliber of the coating, the gap size, and the number of reporter molecules per particle can be identified using Raman spectrometers, and are the most crucial elements in the manufacture and selection of the SERS nanotag.

As a result, Khlebtsov et al created gold nanorods coated in a shell with a gap of 1 nm allying the core and shell. These nanorods also contained the reporter molecule 1,4-nitrobenzenthiole, which, after being conjugated to particular antibodies, was used in the SERS-LFIA of troponin I as a SERS nanotag [99]. The comparison of the sensitivity of the created SERS-LFIA with the standard LFIA built using identical immunoreagents demonstrated a 30-fold boost in sensitivity when employing the SERS nanotag in conjunction with SERS signal striking, thus modifying the theory of electromagnetic SERS [6, 100]. Kneipp et al developed a single-molecule detection platform [101] using silver fabrication. Later, Tian et al integrated the idea of transition metal SERS [102] to build an assembly for sample detection at the nanoscale, which was effective in identifying proteins. To modify SERS, AgNP fabrication was performed using a calcium dipicolinate labeled reporter to detect the presence of bacteria and viruses; similarly, an antigen-labeled probe was used to create a sandwich to improve SERS [103–108]. Yadav et al significantly improved the SERS platform by using a dual-layer DTNB-modified SiO_2@AgNPs LIFA immunoassay to detect SARS-CoV-2 with a limit of detection of 1 pg ml^{-1} [109]. Another study reported the capability of SERS [66] to produce gold 'nanomatreshki', constituting a sphere-shaped Au core and a 4-NBT reporter molecule shell sandwiched between the coatings, corroborating the effectiveness of a 1 nm gap linking the metal core and shell. For the coinciding detection of SARS-CoV-2, the construction of SERS-LFIA with IgM and IgG antibodies and nanoparticles with a recombinant antigen were functionalized together. When the sensitivity was compared to a commercialized test with LFIA for antibodies to SARS-CoV-2, the detection was two orders of magnitude higher for IgM and IgG antibodies.

Sandwiching a SERS immunoassay with LFIA is a novel method proposed by Tang and co-authors [55] for improving the sensitivity of SERS-LFIA and is depicted in figure 4.4. The test and control zones on the analytical membrane created sections made of hydrophobic poly-methyl methacrylate and hydrophilic silver spray, on which the immobilization of antibodies against carcinoembryonic antigen (anti-CEA) was done. The flower-shaped silver nanoplates were altered with a reporter molecule (crystal violet) and antibodies for anti-CEA to function as a

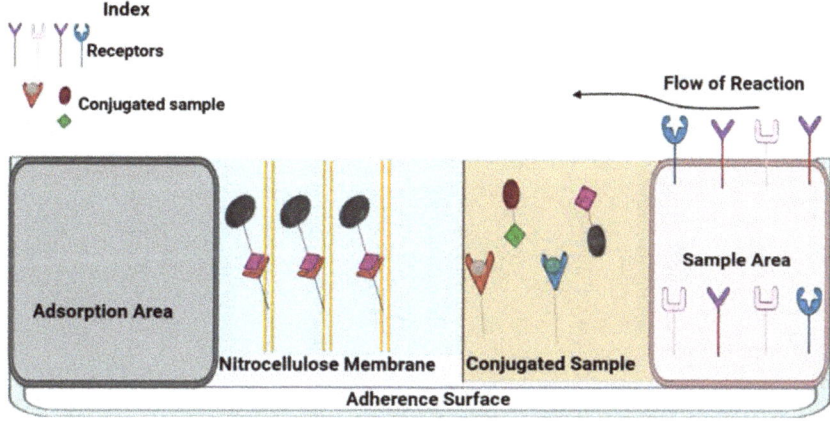

Figure 4.4. An overview of the SERS-LIFA sandwich approach to detecting infectious disease.

nanotag. The new SERS-LFIA made it possible to perform a highly sensitive analysis of the carcinoembryonic antigen. Advancing the SERS platform, Tay *et al* developed a paper-based SERS sensor to detect narcotics using an iodide base [110] whereas Lan *et al* developed flame aerosol deposited Ag–SiO_2 SERS [111] to detect pesticides present on the shell of fruits which was promising with the detection limit of 0.04 ppm (table 4.1).

4.5 Challenges of SERS-based diagnostics

Raman spectroscopy is normally not employed in clinical settings, except for pharmaceutical applications including drug quality assessment and medicine formulation [112]. Medical diagnostics require straightforward hardware and software that can be readily incorporated into the workflow of doctors, microbiologists, and pathologists, whether they are carried out in a hospital, clinical lab, or at the point of care. For Raman to be employed in clinical settings, it requires providing accurate quantitative data with spectral reproducibility, rapid sample preparation, and effective low-cost apparatus [113–115]. These limitations are especially severe in settings with few resources, where diagnostic tools must adhere to the WHO's ASSURED (Affordable, Sensitive, Specific, User-friendly, Rapid and Robust, Deliverable to end-users) standards [116]. Raman spectrometers are sensitive and precise, but frequently lack convenience in their sample processing and spectral interpretation. In particular, the isolation of pathogens and other biomarkers from complex biological samples such as sputum, blood, saliva, and urine typically necessitates purification and isolation steps before Raman interrogation [117]. Raman spectrum datasets obtained from patient samples that have been purified can be challenging to translate into therapeutically valuable information and require sophisticated data analysis methods. Although Raman diagnostics can be quick, robustness can be difficult. In particular, the varied signal enhancement caused by NP aggregation, polydispersity, and/or analyte distribution on the SERS substrate makes quantitative analysis difficult. Additionally, benchtop-scale Raman spectral

Table 4.1. Advancements and modifications of the SERS-based platform.

Serial no.	Technique discovered	Year developed	Material	Detection	Sample	LOD/sensitivity	Reference
1.	Discovery of SERS	1974	Johnson Matthey Specpure rod/polytetrafluoroethylene-coated platinum 'wire'/saturated calomel and pure silver	Studying the role of adsorption of pyridine on the rough surface of a silver electrode	Pyridine	1025 cm^{-1} (associated with nitrogen)	[100]
2.	Electromagnetic theory of the SERS effect	1977	Plasmon incorporated Ag	Mechanism of light scattering and hot spot formation	A different light source	Promising to detect samples on the nanoscale	[6]
3.	SERS enhanced with chemicals	1977	Colloidal silver solution/NaCl where argon was used as the laser	Spectra of a single crystal violet molecule in the aqueous colloidal silver solution	Crystal violet: methanol [1:15]	700 and 1700 cm^{-1}	[101]
4.	SERS enhanced with transition metals	1987	Fe, Co, Ni, Ru, Rh, Pd, and Pt	Surface enhancement	SERS probe labeled with different transition metals	In comparison to 514.5 nm, the enhancement factors for 632.8 nm are roughly 43 and 28 times greater	[102]
5.	SERS enhanced at the tip	2000	Electrochemical etching at the tip using thin wire	Measuring the Raman enhancement	Argon, probe of different magnification	Resolution <55 nm diameter	[103]
6.	SERS with advanced nanostructures	2002	AgNPs/ta-C-nano-crystalline graphite	Dielectric properties	Amorphous carbon	10^3–10^4 nm	[104]
7.	SERS as a sensor	2006	AgNPs nanofilm substrate	Bacillus anthracis	Calcium dipicolinate from Bacillus subtilis	<2.6 × 10^3 spores	[105]
8.	SERS used in viral-antigen detection	2013	AuNPs/(PMPs)/(Pabs)	WNV E and RVFV N antigens	Serum	0.1 ng ml^{-1}	[106]

No.	Application	Year	Method	Target	Sample	Result	Reference
9.	Influenza detection using SERS	2015	AuNps–Ag–proteinG–mAb–RBITC	pAb–Cys3–protein	Serum/blood/ strain-A/CA/ 07/2009p (H1N1)	4.1×10^3 TCID/ml	[107]
10.	SERS modified with LFIA	2016	Fe_3O_4 fabricated magnetic AuNPs modified with antibodies as probes	Pathogenic strain/species	Bacteria	~23 CFU ml^{-1} for *E. coli* *O157:H7* and ~17 CFU ml^{-1} for *Salmonella typhimurium*	[108]
11.	SERS as a biomarker detector in cancer	2017/18	f-PSA antibody/MGITC-labeled AuNPs and c-PSA/XRITC-labeled AuNPs added to sandwich an immunocomplex on the surface of a magnetic bead (2017), AgNPs/ labeled anti-CA153, anti-CA125, anti-CEA/DTNB, 4MBA and 2-naphthalenthiol (2NAT) (Raman reporters)/developed a modified SERS-microfluidic chip (2018)	F-PSA and c-PSA (a marker of prostate cancer) (2017), CA153, CA125, and CEA (2018)	Serum	F-PSA-0.012 ng ml^{-1} and c-PSA and 0.15 ng ml^{-1} (2017), CA153 and CA125 have 0.01 U ml^{-1} while CEA is 1 pg ml^{-1} (2018)	[31, 77]
12.	SERS fabricated LFIA as a SARS-CoV-2 detector	2020	Dual-layer DTNB-modified SiO_2@AgNPs	SARS-CoV-2	Whole blood, serum, plasma	1.0 pg ml^{-1}	[109]
13.	SERS-LFIA	2021	Iodide functionalized inkjet-printed SERS	Narcotics	Heroin, fentanyl, and cocaine as a solution	Heroin (10 ng ml^{-1}) and cocaine (100 ng ml^{-1})	[98]
14.	SERS as a pesticide detector on fruits	2022	Flame aerosol deposited Ag–SiO_2 SERS	Pesticides	Apple	0.04 ppm	[108, 111]

set-ups are often large platforms that cost a lot of money to build. Recent research, however, has revealed that Raman spectra can be produced using a mobile phone camera, highlighting its potential as a reasonably inexpensive point-of-care tool [119].

4.6 The merits of nanotechnology to improve the performance of detection

Noble metal nanoparticles are one of the materials used most commonly to build SERS substrates because of their LSPR properties. These qualities are only applicable to materials at the nanoscale, or dimensions less than 100 nm. Several studies have recently been published on the methodizing and development of metal nanostructures, with a focus on the tailored shapes and dimensions for SERS applications. Colloidal monodisperse metal NPs produce good SERS enhancement due to their controlled size and shape. In a comprehensive study on colloidal Ag nanostructures with a size range of 60–100 nm, it was discovered that the SERS enhancement was dependent on the size and shape of the nanoparticles [120]. In contrast to virtually spherical Ag nanoparticles, cubical nanoparticles with sharp edges produced eco friendly-SERS (EFSERS) in the order of 105. It was discovered that EFSERS improves as nanoparticle size increases from 60 to 100 nm (in the order of 104). When compared to spherical AgNPs, the electric field disperses evenly over the surface, whereas the cubical Ag nanoparticles have directed nonuniform hot spots near the sharp edges. For instance, it has been demonstrated that altering the colloidal nanoparticles' shape from spherical to anisotropic morphologies can change the strength of the hot spots [121]. It was discovered that an anisotropic nanoparticle's EFSERS increased from 104 to 107, making it appropriate for single-molecule detection because a spherical nanoparticle produces a weak hot spot in comparison. Additionally, scientists have shown that adding additional anisotropy or increasing the aspect ratio of these colloidal metal nanoparticles will enhance the EFSERS [122]. By utilizing aggregated colloidal Ag nanoclusters, an improvement factor as high as 1014 was also demonstrated [123, 124].

Numerous researchers have also studied the application of colloidal gold (Au) nanoparticles for SERS. In comparison to silver nanoparticles, gold is more costly and frequently produces moderate EFSERS. However, because of its high bio-compatibility, Au is a good SERS alternative for biological materials. The SERS features of Au nanoparticles with various sizes of about 10–200 nm plus shapes such as triangles, spheres, pentagons, hexagons, etc, have been reported, according to Quester *et al* [122]. A rapid synthesis approach for SERS applications was created by Lu *et al* [125] employing laser irradiation and a variety of shaped colloidal gold nanoparticles using this approach. Using nanospheres of AuNPs has successfully demonstrated the detection of Rhodamine 6G (R6G) dyes at concentration levels as low as 10^{-11} M.

Another significant element enhancing the SERS is the size of the metal nano-particles. The metal nanoparticles should have a size equivalent to or smaller than the wavelength of the incident light for the LSPR effect, as is widely known. The nanoparticles begin to exhibit weak polarization at very tiny sizes, losing their LSPR capabilities and rendering them useless for SERS applications [120]. According to a modern study on the size influence of Ag nanoparticles on SERS, the signal of EFSERS was lowered (on the order of 102) when the size of the nanoparticle was decreased from around 65–35 nm [123].

4.7 Conclusion

Stimulated by the meteoric developments of the past 40 years, great progress in biological and biomedical sensing has been achieved using SERS. In this chapter we described the present-day advances in bio-analytical applications in SERS-based biosensors. The basics of SERS, dealing with the enhancing mechanisms and structures were described briefly with the customary fabrication methods for biosensing in label-free or indirect detection. Modern-day applications dealing with *in vitro* or *ex vivo* fluid associated with SERS-based biosensors were presented with examples. Some practices covered include the detection of biomolecules such as proteins, DNA, etc, and we systematically review the use for cellular properties such as ion concentration, temperature, and pH. SERS-based biosensors are gaining a lot of interest in terms of *in vivo* point-of-care diagnosis, imaging, and therapy, while *ex vivo* remains a challenge for sensing applications. One of the basic drawbacks lies in the improvement of sensitivity detection beyond the innate enhancement delivered by SERS substrates and nanotechnology. Nanotechnology in combination with SERS presents a better performance in terms of reproducibility, high sensitivity, and improved instrumental capabilities. Still, some drawbacks related to the specificity and sensitivity of detection, the degradation from interference from molecules in the matrix apart from photoluminescence it enhances the signal from the substrate. SERS-based biosensing has tremendous potential with some improvements needed to diversify its clinical applications.

Acknowledgments

Thanks to the Department of Biotechnology, Central Research Cell MM(DU), Mullana for their continued support and help.

References

[1] Zong C, Xu M, Xu L J, Wei T, Ma X, Zheng X S, Hu R and Ren B 2018 Surface-enhanced Raman spectroscopy for bio-analysis: reliability and challenges *Chem. Rev.* **118** 4946–80

[2] Moore T J, Moody A S, Payne T D, Sarabia G M, Daniel A R and Sharma B 2018 *In vitro* and *in vivo* SERS biosensing for disease diagnosis *Biosensors* **8** 46

[3] Lane L A, Xue R and Nie S 2018 Emergence of two near-infrared windows for *in vivo* and intraoperative SERS *Curr. Opin. Chem. Biol.* **45** 95–103

[4] Jamieson L E, Asiala S M, Gracie K, Faulds K and Graham D 2017 Bioanalytical measurements enabled by surface-enhanced Raman scattering (SERS) probes *Ann. Rev. Anal. Chem.* **10** 415–37

[5] Henry A I, Sharma B, Cardinal M F, Kurouski D and Van Duyne R P 2016 Surface-enhanced Raman spectroscopy biosensing: *in vivo* diagnostics and multi-modal imaging *Anal. Chem.* **88** 6638–47

[6] Ding S Y, You E M, Tian Z Q and Moskovits M 2017 Electromagnetic theories of surface-enhanced Raman spectroscopy *Chem. Soc. Rev.* **46** 4042–76

[7] Cheng C, Yan B, Wong S M, Li X, Zhou W, Yu T, Shen Z, Yu H and Fan H J 2010 Fabrication and SERS performance of silver-nanoparticle-decorated Si/ZnO nanotrees in ordered arrays *ACS Appl. Mater. Interfaces* **2** 1824–8

[8] Banaei N, Foley A, Houghton J M, Sun Y and Kim B 2017 Multiplex detection of pancreatic cancer biomarkers using a SERS-based immunoassay *Nanotechnology* **28** 455101

[9] Kiefer W 2011 *Surface Enhanced Raman Spectroscopy: Analytical, Biophysical and Life Science Applications* (New York: Wiley)

[10] Mousavi S M, Hashemi S A, Rahmanian V, Kalashgrani M Y, Gholami A, Omidifar N and Chiang W H 2022 Highly sensitive flexible SERS-based sensing platform for detection of COVID-19 *Biosensors* **12** 466

[11] Kneipp K, Dasari R R and Wang Y 1994 Near-infrared surface-enhanced Raman scattering (NIR SERS) on colloidal silver and gold *Appl. Spectrosc.* **48** 951–5

[12] Schütz M and Schlücker S 2015 Molecularly linked 3D plasmonic nanoparticle core/satellite assemblies: SERS nanotags with single-particle Raman sensitivity *Phys. Chem. Chem. Phys.* **17** 24356–60

[13] Romo-Herrera J M, Alvarez-Puebla R A and Liz-Marzán L M 2011 Controlled assembly of plasmonic colloidal nanoparticle clusters *Nanoscale* **3** 1304–15

[14] Hamm L, Gee A and De Silva Indrasekara A S 2019 Recent advancement in the surface-enhanced Raman spectroscopy-based biosensors for infectious disease diagnosis *Appl. Sci.* **9** 1448

[15] Wang J, Koo K M, Wang Y and Trau M 2019 Engineering state-of-the-art plasmonic nanomaterials for SERS-based clinical liquid biopsy applications. *Adv. Sci.* **6** 1900730

[16] Çelik Y and Ayşe K U 2021 Three dimensional porous expanded graphite/silver nano-particles nanocomposite platform as a SERS substrate *Appl. Surf. Sci.* **568** 150946

[17] Guo Q, Xu M, Yuan Y, Gu R and Yao J 2016 Self-assembled large-scale monolayer of Au nanoparticles at the air/water interface used as a SERS substrate *Langmuir* **32** 4530–7

[18] Jiao Y, Ryckman J D, Ciesielski P N, Escobar C A, Jennings G K and Weiss S M 2011 Patterned nanoporous gold as an effective SERS template *Nanotechnology* **22** 295302

[19] Li Z, Leustean L, Inci F, Zheng M, Demirci U and Wang S 2019 Plasmonic-based platforms for diagnosis of infectious diseases at the point-of-care *Biotechnol. Adv.* **37** 107440

[20] Lee H K, Lee Y H, Koh C S, Phan-Quang G C, Han X, Lay C L, Sim H Y, Kao Y C, An Q and Ling X Y 2019 Designing surface-enhanced Raman scattering (SERS) platforms beyond hotspot engineering: emerging opportunities in analyte manipulations and hybrid materials *Chem. Soc. Rev.* **48** 731–56

[21] Cardinal M F, Vander Ende E, Hackler R A, McAnally M O, Stair P C, Schatz G C and Van Duyne R P 2017 Expanding applications of SERS through versatile nanomaterials engineering *Chem. Soc. Rev.* **46** 3886–903

[22] Cialla-May D, Zheng X S, Weber K and Popp J J 2017 Recent progress in surface-enhanced Raman spectroscopy for biological and biomedical applications: from cells to clinics *Chem. Soc. Rev.* **46** 3945–61

[23] Zheng X S, Jahn I J, Weber K, Cialla-May D and Popp J 2018 Label-free SERS in biological and biomedical applications: recent progress, current challenges and opportunities *Spectrochim. Acta* A **197** 56–77

[24] Szlag V M, Rodriguez R S, He J, Hudson-Smith N, Kang H, Le N, Reineke T M and Haynes C L 2018 Molecular affinity agents for intrinsic surface-enhanced Raman scattering (SERS) sensors *ACS Appl. Mater. Interfaces* **10** 31825–44

[25] Kahraman M, Mullen E R, Korkmaz A and Wachsmann-Hogiu S 2017 Fundamentals and applications of SERS-based bio-analytical sensing *Nanophotonics* **6** 831–52

[26] Karadan P, Aggarwal S, Anappara A A, Narayana C and Barshilia H C 2018 Tailored periodic Si nanopillar based architectures as highly sensitive universal SERS biosensing platform *Sensors Actuators* B **254** 264–71

[27] Szekeres G P and Kneipp J 2019 SERS probing of proteins in gold nanoparticle agglomerates *Front. Chem.* **7** 30

[28] Lenzi E, Jimenez de Aberasturi D and Liz-Marzan L M 2019 Surface-enhanced Raman scattering tags for three-dimensional bioimaging and biomarker detection *ACS Sens.* **4** 1126–37

[29] Yang Y, Zhu J, Zhao J, Weng G J, Li J J and Zhao J W 2019 Growth of spherical gold satellites on the surface of Au@Ag@SiO$_2$ core–shell nanostructures used for an ultra-sensitive SERS immunoassay of alpha-fetoprotein *ACS Appl. Mater. Interfaces* **11** 3617–26

[30] Wang Z, Zong S, Wu L, Zhu D and Cui Y 2017 SERS-activated platforms for immunoassay: probes, encoding methods, and applications *Chem. Rev.* **117** 7910–63

[31] Cheng Z, Choi N, Wang R, Lee S, Moon K C, Yoon S Y, Chen L and Choo J 2017 Simultaneous detection of dual prostate specific antigens using surface-enhanced Raman scattering-based immunoassay for accurate diagnosis of prostate cancer *ACS Nano* **11** 4926–33

[32] Chuong T T, Pallaoro A, Chaves C A, Li Z, Lee J, Eisenstein M, Stucky G D, Moskovits M and Soh H T 2017 Dual-reporter SERS-based biomolecular assay with reduced false-positive signals *Proc. Natl Acad. Sci. USA* **114** 9056–61

[33] Garcia-Rico E, Alvarez-Puebla R A and Guerrini L 2018 Direct surface-enhanced Raman scattering (SERS) spectroscopy of nucleic acids: from fundamental studies to real-life applications *Chem. Soc. Rev.* **47** 4909–23

[34] Li X, Yang T, Li C S, Wang D, Song Y and Jin L 2017 Detection of EGFR mutation in plasma using multiplex allele-specific PCR (MAS-PCR) and surface enhanced Raman spectroscopy *Sci. Rep.* **7** 4771

[35] Tian S, Neumann O, McClain M J, Yang X, Zhou L, Zhang C, Nordlander P and Halas N J 2017 Aluminum nanocrystals: a sustainable substrate for quantitative SERS-based DNA detection *Nano Lett.* **17** 5071–7

[36] Chen C, Li Y, Kerman S, Neutens P, Willems K, Cornelissen S, Lagae L, Stakenborg T and Van Dorpe P 2018 High spatial resolution nanoslit SERS for single-molecule nucleobase sensing *Nat. Commun.* **9** 1733

[37] Li Y, Han X, Yan Y, Cao Y, Xiang X, Wang S, Zhao B and Guo X 2018 Label-free detection of tetramolecular i-motifs by surface-enhanced Raman spectroscopy *Anal. Chem.* **90** 2996–3000

[38] Ye S, Li X, Wang M and Tang B 2017 Fluorescence and SERS imaging for the simultaneous absolute quantification of multiple miRNAs in living cells *Anal. Chem.* **89** 5124–30

[39] Sun Y and Li T 2018 Composition-tunable hollow Au/Ag SERS nanoprobes coupled with target-catalyzed hairpin assembly for triple-amplification detection of miRNA *Anal. Chem.* **90** 11614–21

[40] He M Q, Chen S, Yao K, Wang K, Yu Y L and Wang J H 2019 Oriented assembly of gold nanoparticles with freezing-driven surface DNA manipulation and its application in SERS-based microRNA assay *Small Methods* **3** 1900017

[41] Cheng L, Zhang Z, Zuo D, Zhu W, Zhang J, Zeng Q, Yang D, Li M and Zhao Y 2018 Ultrasensitive detection of serum microRNA using branched DNA-based SERS platform combining simultaneous detection of α-fetoprotein for early diagnosis of liver cancer *ACS Appl. Mater. Interfaces* **10** 34869–77

[42] Joseph M M, Narayanan N, Nair J B, Karunakaran V, Ramya A N, Sujai P T, Saranya G, Arya J S, Vijayan V M and Maiti K K 2018 Exploring the margins of SERS in practical domain: an emerging diagnostic modality for modern biomedical applications *Biomaterials* **181** 140–81

[43] Zhang W, Jiang L, Piper J A and Wang Y 2018 SERS nanotags and their applications in biosensing and bioimaging *J. Anal. Test.* **2** 26–44

[44] Wang J, Geng Y, Shen Y, Shi W, Xu W and Xu S 2019 SERS-active fiber tip for intracellular and extracellular pH sensing in living single cells *Sens. Actuators* B **290** 527–34

[45] Zhang Z, Bando K, Mochizuki K, Taguchi A, Fujita K and Kawata S 2019 Quantitative evaluation of surface-enhanced Raman scattering nanoparticles for intracellular pH sensing at a single particle level *Anal. Chem.* **91** 3254–62

[46] Aioub M and El-Sayed M A 2016 A real-time surface enhanced Raman spectroscopy study of plasmonic photothermal cell death using targeted gold nanoparticles *J. Am. Chem. Soc.* **138** 1258–64

[47] Chen J, Sheng Z, Li P, Wu M, Zhang N, Yu X F, Wang Y, Hu D, Zheng H and Wang G P 2017 Indocyanine green-loaded gold nanostars for sensitive SERS imaging and subcellular monitoring of photothermal therapy *Nanoscale* **9** 11888–901

[48] Piotrowski P and Bukowska J 2015 2-mercaptoethanesulfonate (MES) anion-functionalized silver nanoparticles as an efficient SERS-based sensor of metal cations *Sens. Actuators* B **221** 700–7

[49] Tsoutsi D, Montenegro J M, Dommershausen F, Koert U, Liz-Marzan L M, Parak W J and Alvarez-Puebla R A 2011 Quantitative surface-enhanced Raman scattering ultra-detection of atomic inorganic ions: the case of chloride *ACS Nano* **5** 7539–46

[50] Li C, Wang H, Luo Y, Wen G and Jiang Z 2019 A novel gold nanosol SERS quantitative analysis method for trace Na^+ based on carbon dot catalysis *Food Chem.* **289** 531–6

[51] Zheng P, Li M, Jurevic R, Cushing S K, Liu Y and Wu N 2015 A gold nanohole array based surface-enhanced Raman scattering biosensor for detection of silver (I) and mercury (II) in human saliva *Nanoscale* **7** 11005–12

[52] Zhuang H, Wang Z, Zhang X, Hutchison J A, Zhu W, Yao Z, Zhao Y and Li M 2017 A highly sensitive SERS-based platform for Zn(II) detection in cellular media *Chem. Commun.* **53** 1797–800

[53] Pramanik A, Chavva S R, Viraka Nellore B P, May K, Matthew T, Jones S, Vangara A and Ray P C 2017 Development of a SERS probe for selective detection of healthy prostate and malignant prostate cancer cells using ZnII *Chem. Asian J.* **12** 665–72

[54] Smolsky J, Kaur S, Hayashi C, Batra S K and Krasnoslobodtsev A V 2017 Surface-enhanced Raman scattering-based immunoassay technologies for detection of disease biomarkers *Biosensors* **7** 7

[55] Tang S, Liu H, Tian Y, Chen D, Gu C, Wei G, Jiang T and Zhou J 2021 Surface-enhanced Raman scattering-based lateral flow immunoassay mediated by hydrophilic–hydrophobic Ag-modified PMMA substrate *Spectrochim. Acta* A **262** 120092

[56] Bozkurt A G, Buyukgoz G G, Soforoglu M, Tamer U, Suludere Z and Boyaci I H 2018 Alkaline phosphatase labeled SERS active sandwich immunoassay for detection of *Escherichia coli Spectrochim. Acta* A **194** 8–13

[57] Hwang M J, Jang A S and Lim D K 2021 Comparative study of fluorescence and surface-enhanced Raman scattering with magnetic microparticle-based assay for target bacterial DNA detection *Sens. Actuators* B **329** 129134

[58] Yu Z, Chen L, Wang Y, Wang X, Song W, Ruan W, Zhao B and Cong Q A 2014 SERS-active enzymatic product used for the quantification of disease-related molecules *J. Raman Spectrosc.* **45** 75–81

[59] Dong J, Li Y, Zhang M, Yan T and Qian W 2014 Ultrasensitive surface-enhanced Raman scattering detection of alkaline phosphatase *Anal. Methods* **6** 9168–72

[60] Ingram A, Moore B D and Graham D 2009 Simultaneous detection of alkaline phosphatase and β-galactosidase activity using SERRS *Bioorg. Med. Chem. Lett.* **19** 1569–71

[61] Su Y, Wu D, Chen J, Chen G, Hu N, Wang H, Wang P, Han H, Li G and Wu Y 2019 Ratiometric surface enhanced Raman scattering immunosorbent assay of allergenic proteins via covalent organic framework composite material based nanozyme tag triggered Raman signal 'turn-on' and amplification *Anal. Chem.* **91** 11687–95

[62] Neng J, Li Y, Driscoll A J, Wilson W C and Johnson P A 2018 Detection of multiple pathogens in serum using silica-encapsulated nanotags in a surface-enhanced Raman scattering-based immunoassay *J. Agric. Food Chem.* **66** 5707–12

[63] Wang Z, Yang H, Wang M, Petti L, Jiang T, Jia Z, Xie S and Zhou J 2018 SERS-based multiplex immunoassay of tumor markers using double SiO$_2$@Ag immune probes and gold-film hemisphere array immune substrate *Colloids Surf.* A **546** 48–58

[64] Chen R, Liu B, Ni H, Chang N, Luan C, Ge Q, Dong J and Zhao X 2019 Vertical flow assays based on core–shell SERS nanotags for multiplex prostate cancer biomarker detection *Analyst* **144** 4051–9

[65] Zhang W, Tang S, Jin Y, Yang C, He L, Wang J and Chen Y 2020 Multiplex SERS-based lateral flow immunosensor for the detection of major mycotoxins in maize utilizing dual Raman labels and triple test lines *J. Hazard. Mater.* **393** 122348

[66] Chen S *et al* 2021 SERS-based lateral flow immunoassay for sensitive and simultaneous detection of anti-SARS-CoV-2 IgM and IgG antibodies by using gap-enhanced Raman nanotags *Sens. Actuators* B **348** 130706

[67] Chen Y T, Lee Y C, Lai Y H, Lim J C, Huang N T, Lin C T and Huang J J 2020 Review of integrated optical biosensors for point-of-care applications *Biosensors* **10** 209

[68] Gao R, Lv Z, Mao Y, Yu L, Bi X, Xu S, Cui J and Wu Y 2019 SERS-based pump-free microfluidic chip for highly sensitive immunoassay of prostate-specific antigen biomarkers *ACS Sens.* **4** 938–43

[69] Zhang W S, Wang Y N, Wang Y and Xu Z R 2019 Highly reproducible and fast detection of 6-thioguanine in human serum using a droplet-based microfluidic SERS system *Sens. Actuators* B **283** 532–7

[70] Kant K and Abalde-Cela S 2018 Surface-enhanced Raman scattering spectroscopy and microfluidics: towards ultrasensitive label-free sensing *Biosensors* **8** 62

[71] Ackermann K R, Henkel T and Popp J 2007 Quantitative online detection of low-concentrated drugs via a SERS microfluidic system *Chem. Phys. Chem.* **8** 2665–70

[72] Lee D, Lee S, Seong G H, Choo J, Lee E K, Gweon D G and Lee S 2006 Quantitative analysis of methyl parathion pesticides in a polydimethylsiloxane microfluidic channel using confocal surface-enhanced Raman spectroscopy *Appl. Spectrosc.* **60** 373–7

[73] Yazdi S H and White I M 2013 Multiplexed detection of aquaculture fungicides using a pump-free optofluidic SERS microsystem *Analyst* **138** 100–3

[74] Ahi E E, Torul H, Zengin A, Sucularlı F, Yıldırım E, Selbes Y, Suludere Z and Tamer U 2022 A capillary driven microfluidic chip for SERS based hCG detection *Biosens. Bioelectron.* **195** 113660

[75] Wang L, Zhou G, Guan X L and Zhao L 2020 Rapid preparation of surface-enhanced Raman substrate in microfluidic channel for trace detection of amoxicillin *Spectrochim. Acta* A **235** 118262

[76] Chen R, Du X, Cui Y, Zhang X, Ge Q, Dong J and Zhao X 2020 Vertical flow assay for inflammatory biomarkers based on nanofluidic channel array and SERS nanotags *Small* **16** 2002801

[77] Zheng Z, Wu L, Li L, Zong S, Wang Z and Cui Y 2018 Simultaneous and highly sensitive detection of multiple breast cancer biomarkers in real samples using a SERS microfluidic chip *Talanta* **188** 507–15

[78] Gao R, Cheng Z, Wang X, Yu L, Guo Z, Zhao G and Choo J 2018 Simultaneous immunoassays of dual prostate cancer markers using a SERS-based microdroplet channel *Biosens. Bioelectron.* **119** 126–33

[79] Nie Y, Jin C and Zhang J X 2021 Microfluidic *in situ* patterning of silver nanoparticles for surface-enhanced Raman spectroscopic sensing of biomolecules *ACS Sens.* **6** 2584–92

[80] Wang C, Madiyar F, Yu C and Li J 2017 Detection of extremely low concentration waterborne pathogen using a multiplexing self-referencing SERS microfluidic biosensor *J. Biol. Eng.* **11** 9

[81] Zhang Y, Zhao S, Zheng J and He L 2017 Surface-enhanced Raman spectroscopy (SERS) combined techniques for high-performance detection and characterization *TrAC Trends Anal. Chem.* **90** 1–13

[82] Castaño-Guerrero Y, Moreira F T, Sousa-Castillo A, Correa-Duarte M A and Sales M G 2021 SERS and electrochemical impedance spectroscopy immunoassay for carcinoembryonic antigen *Electrochim. Acta.* **366** 137377

[83] Wang J, Zhang R, Ji X, Wang P and Ding C 2021 SERS and fluorescence detection of circulating tumor cells (CTCs) with specific capture-release mode based on multifunctional gold nanomaterials and dual-selective recognition *Anal. Chim. Acta.* **1141** 206–13

[84] Lee H G, Choi W, Yang S Y, Kim D H, Park S G, Lee M Y and Jung H S 2021 PCR-coupled paper-based surface-enhanced Raman scattering (SERS) sensor for rapid and sensitive detection of respiratory bacterial DNA *Sens. Actuators* B **326** 128802

[85] Xu Y, Hassan M M, Zhu A, Li H and Chen Q 2021 Dual-mode of magnetic assisted Au@Ag SERS tags and cationic conjugated UCNPs for qualitative and quantitative analysis of multiple foodborne pathogens *Sens. Actuators* B **344** 130305

[86] Mahmoudi T, de la Guardia M, Shirdel B, Mokhtarzadeh A and Baradaran B 2019 Recent advancements in structural improvements of lateral flow assays towards point-of-care testing *TrAC Trends Anal. Chem.* **116** 13–30

[87] Kim K, Kashefi-Kheyrabadi L, Joung Y, Kim K, Dang H, Chavan S G, Lee M H and Choo J 2021 Recent advances in sensitive surface-enhanced Raman scattering-based lateral flow assay platforms for point-of-care diagnostics of infectious diseases *Sens. Actuators* B **329** 129214

[88] Nguyen V T, Song S, Park S and Joo C 2020 Recent advances in high-sensitivity detection methods for paper-based lateral-flow assay *Biosens. Bioelectron.* **152** 112015

[89] Banerjee R and Jaiswal A 2018 Recent advances in nanoparticle-based lateral flow immunoassay as a point-of-care diagnostic tool for infectious agents and diseases *Analyst* **143** 1970–96

[90] Hwang J, Lee S and Choo J 2016 Application of a SERS-based lateral flow immunoassay strip for the rapid and sensitive detection of *Staphylococcal enterotoxin* B *Nanoscale* **8** 11418–25

[91] Sánchez-Purrà M, Carré-Camps M, de Puig H, Bosch I, Gehrke L and Hamad-Schifferli K 2017 Surface-enhanced Raman spectroscopy-based sandwich immunoassays for multiplexed detection of Zika and Dengue viral biomarkers *ACS Inf. Dis.* **3** 767–76

[92] Fu X, Cheng Z, Yu J, Choo P, Chen L and Choo J 2016 A SERS-based lateral flow assay biosensor for highly sensitive detection of HIV-1 DNA *Biosens. Bioelectron.* **78** 530–7

[93] Shen H, Xie K, Huang L, Wang L, Ye J, Xiao M, Ma L, Jia A and Tang Y 2019 A novel SERS-based lateral flow assay for differential diagnosis of wild-type pseudorabies virus and gE-deleted vaccine *Sens. Actuators* B **282** 152–7

[94] Huang J C, Chang Y F, Chen K H, Su L C, Lee C W, Chen C C, Chen Y M and Chou C 2009 Detection of severe acute respiratory syndrome (SARS) coronavirus nucleocapsid protein in human serum using a localized surface plasmon coupled fluorescence fiber-optic biosensor *Biosens. Bioelectron.* **25** 320–5

[95] Khlebtsov B and Khlebtsov N 2020 Surface-enhanced Raman scattering-based lateral-flow immunoassay *Nanomaterials* **10** 2228

[96] Sánchez-Purrà M, Roig-Solvas B, Versiani A, Rodriguez-Quijada C, De Puig H, Bosch I, Gehrke L and Hamad-Schifferli K 2017 Design of SERS nanotags for multiplexed lateral flow immunoassays *Mol. Syst. Des. Eng.* **2** 401–9

[97] Lin L K and Stanciu L A 2018 Bisphenol A detection using gold nanostars in a SERS improved lateral flow immunochromatographic assay *Sens. Actuators* B **276** 222–9

[98] Maneeprakorn W, Bamrungsap S, Apiwat C and Wiriyachaiporn N 2016 Surface-enhanced Raman scattering based lateral flow immunochromatographic assay for sensitive influenza detection *RSC Adv.* **6** 112079–85

[99] Khlebtsov B N, Bratashov D N, Byzova N A, Dzantiev B B and Khlebtsov N G 2019 SERS-based lateral flow immunoassay of troponin I by using gap-enhanced Raman tags *Nano Res.* **12** 413–20

[100] Fleischmann M, Hendra P J and McQuillan A J Raman spectra of pyridine adsorbed at a silver electrode *Chem. Phys. Lett.* **26** 163–6

[101] Kneipp K, Wang Y, Kneipp H, Perelman L T, Itzkan I, Dasari R R and Feld M S 1997 Single molecule detection using surface-enhanced Raman scattering (SERS) *Phys. Rev. Lett.* **78** 1667

[102] Tian Z Q, Ren B and Wu D Y 2002 Surface-enhanced Raman scattering: from noble to transition metals and from rough surfaces to ordered nanostructures *J. Phys. Chem.* B **106** 37

[103] Stockle R M, Suh Y D, Deckert V and Zenobi R 2000 Nanoscale chemical analysis by tip-enhanced Raman spectroscopy *Chem. Phys. Lett.* **318** 131–6

[104] Zhang X, Shah NC and Van Duyne R 2006 Sensitive and selective chem/bio sensing based on surface-enhanced Raman spectroscopy (SERS) *Vib. Spectrosc.* **42** 2–8

[105] Neng J, Harpster M H, Wilson W C and Johnson P A 2013 Surface-enhanced Raman scattering (SERS) detection of multiple viral antigens using magnetic capture of SERS-active nanoparticles *Biosens. Bioelectron.* **41** 316–21

[106] Ren W, Cho I H, Zhou Z and Irudavaraj J 2016 Ultrasensitive detection of microbial cells using magnetic focus enhanced lateral flow sensors *Chem. Commun.* **52** 4930–3

[107] Saviñon-Flores F, Méndez E, López-Castaños M, Carabarin-Lima A, López-Castaños K A, González-Fuentes M A and Méndez-Albores A 2021 A review on SERS-based detection of human virus infections: influenza and coronavirus *Biosensors* **11** 66

[108] Li H, Merkl P, Sommertune J, Thersleff T and Sotiriou G A 2022 SERS hotspot engineering by aerosol self-assembly of plasmonic Ag nanoaggregates with tunable interparticle distance *Adv. Sci.* **9** 2201133

[109] Yadav S, Sadique M A, Kumar N, Singhal A, Ranjan P, Srivastava A K and Khan R 2021 SERS based lateral flow immunoassay for point-of-care detection of SARS-CoV-2 in clinical samples *ACS Appl. Biol.* **4** 2974–95

[110] Tay Lin L, Poirier S, Ghaemi A, Hulse J and Wang S 2021 Iodide functionalized paper-based SERS sensors for improved detection of narcotics *Front. Chem.* **9** 680556

[111] Li H, Merkl P, Sommertune J, Thersleff T and Sotiriou G A 2022 SERS hotspot engineering by aerosol self-assembly of plasmonic Ag nanoaggregates with tunable interparticle distance *Adv. Sci.* **9** 2201133

[112] Marcu L, Boppart S A, Hutchinson M R, Popp J and Wilson B C 2017 Biophotonics: the big picture *J. Biomed. Opt.* **23** 021103

[113] Beswick D M *et al* 2017 Biomedical device innovation methodology: applications in biophotonics *J. Biomed. Opt.* **23** 021102

[114] Popp J, Matthews D, Martinez-Coll A, Mayerhöfer T and Wilson B C 2018 Challenges in translation: models to promote translation *J. Biomed. Optics* **23** 021101

[115] Kosack C S, Page A L and Klatser P R 2017 A guide to aid the selection of diagnostic tests *Bull. World Health Organ.* **95** 639–45
Langer J *et al* 2020 Present and future of surface-enhanced Raman scattering *ACS Nano* **14** 28–117

[116] Ayas S, Cupallari A, Ekiz O O, Kaya Y and Dana A 2014 Counting molecules with a mobile phone camera using plasmonic enhancement *ACS Photon.* **1** 17–26

[117] McLellan J M, Siekkinen A, Chen J and Xia Y 2006 Comparison of the surface-enhanced Raman scattering on sharp and truncated silver nanocubes *Chem. Phys. Lett.* **427** 122–6

[118] Le Ru E C and Etchegoin P G 2012 Single-molecule surface-enhanced Raman spectroscopy *Ann. Rev. Phys. Chem.* **63** 65–87

[119] Ali A, Nettey-Oppong E E, Effah E, Yu C Y, Muhammad R, Soomro T A, Byun K M and Choi S H 2022 Miniaturized Raman instruments for SERS-based point-of-care testing on respiratory viruses *Biosensors* **12** 590

[120] Nie S and Emory S 1997 Probing single molecules and single nanoparticles by surface-enhanced Raman scattering *Science* **275** 1102–6

[121] Quester K, Avalos-Borja M, Vilchis-Nestor A R, Camacho-López M A and Castro-Longoria E 2013 SERS properties of different sized and shaped gold nanoparticles biosynthesized under different environmental conditions by *Neurospora crassa* extract *PLoS One* **8** e77486

[122] Liu D, Li C, Zhou F, Zhang T, Zhang H, Li X, Duan G, Cai W and Li Y 2015 Rapid synthesis of monodisperse Au nanospheres through a laser irradiation-induced shape conversion, self-assembly and their electromagnetic coupling SERS enhancement *Sci. Rep.* **5** 7686

[123] Ko H, Singamaneni S and Tsukruk V V 2008 Nanostructured surfaces and assemblies as SERS media *Small* **4** 1576–99

[124] He R X, Liang R, Peng P and Norman Zhou Y 2017 Effect of the size of silver nanoparticles on SERS signal enhancement *J. Nanoparticle Res.* **19** 267
Krpetić Ž, Guerrini L, Larmour I A, Reglinski J, Faulds K and Graham D 2012 Importance of nanoparticle size in colorimetric and SERS-based multimodal trace detection of Ni(II) ions with functional gold nanoparticles *Small* **8** 707–14

[125] Lu R, Konzelmann A, Xu F, Gong Y, Liu J, Liu Q, Xin M, Hui R and Wu J Z 2015 High sensitivity surface enhanced Raman spectroscopy of R6G on *in situ* fabricated Au nano-particle/graphene plasmonic substrates *Carbon* **1** 78–85

Chapter 5

Significance, design, and synthesis methods of SERS tags/probes

Ayushi Singhal, Apoorva Shrivastava, Arpana Parihar and Raju Khan

SERS tags are unique entities that have been developed recently within the SERS community, particularly spurred by the need to carrying out experiments within the biomedical and medical fields, wherein the heterogeneity and constant changing of the environment and samples reduce the applicability of direct SERS sensing methods. The components of SERS tags include plasmonic nanoparticle cores, Raman reporters, a coating layer, and the targeting ligands. All the components involved in the design of SERS tags need to be rationally designed and custom-made as per the requirements. Due to the fingerprint-like spectra obtained from SERS nanotags, they can deliver highly specific results. SERS tags have proven to be essential for *in vivo*, *ex vivo*, and *in vitro* imaging and biomarker detection, to improve prognostic and diagnostic outcomes. This chapter introduces the basics of SERS and SERS tags, and their components and applications.

5.1 Introduction

Surface-enhanced Raman spectroscopy (SERS) is a strong vibrational spectroscopy strategy that achieves exceptionally detailed elemental recognition of analytes at low concentrations through the intensification of electromagnetic fields created by the excitation of localized surface plasmons. SERS has advanced from investigations of model frameworks on roughened electrodes to exceptionally modern studies, such as single-particle spectroscopy [1]. SERS combines sub-atomic fingerprint specificity with potential single-particle observation. In this respect, the SERS procedure is an attractive device for detecting molecules at trace levels in various fields such as chemical and biochemical studies [2]. There are two fundamental methodologies involving SERS for biological analyte detection—label-based detection with SERS labels and label-free SERS detection [3]. SERS label-based recognition expects to identify the vibrational spectroscopic fingerprints of biological analytes via indirect interaction, by utilizing a Raman reporter molecule to mark the SERS labels. Label-free SERS detection is a direct methodology; it recognizes and makes images of biological analytes [4–6] after adsorption on the SERS substrates/nanostructures, which frequently brings about superior signal intensity [7]. In the label-based identification scheme, the SERS nanosubstrates contain four main parts: (i) a nano-structured metallic substrate, normally made of gold or silver to further improve the SERS power and action; (ii) a suitable protective shell or layer to improve the solidity and biocompatibility; (iii) a Raman reporter particle layer to enable label-based location with a novel and unique SERS fingerprint; and (iv) target specific detection using bioconjugate. In the label-free detection scheme, the third part is not used [8]. SERS labels have recently received a lot of attention as emerging optical nanoprobes due to their extremely high sensitivity, limited Raman bands for multiplex discovery [9]. However, the design and production of SERS-encoded particles, including their composition, dimensions, and biocompatibility, depend on each specific application. The size of NP-based SERS substrates is much larger than that of the majority of biomolecules, SERS tags cannot identify the intracellular gradient of biomolecule distribution, and the reproducibility of the response is inadequate. SERS labels are therefore unable to detect the intracellular gradient of biomolecule distribution [10]. Despite the great interest of researchers in developing SERS labels/tags, research has been slow in comparison to other nanoprobes. The possible reason behind this may be the need for sophisticated instrument facilities, well-trained personnel, etc. Another reason may be the complex principles of SERS which are not easily understood [11]. Researchers are expected to advance SERS labels with high sensitivity, excellent reproducibility, and small size for single-particle marking or intracellular biomolecule preparation in the future. SERS labels could find an ideal role in the identification of malignant skin growths, which do not need deep tissue access, in determining cancer edges during a medical procedure (for instance in brain tumors), or on the other hand for the endoscopic imaging of sick tissues, where the laser can be coupled to the endoscope, which gives a pathway for the backscattered light to the identifier (e.g. in a colonoscopy). Different applications in which SERS labels can find a significant role involve the *ex vivo* investigation of samples, such as the identification of biomarkers in blood or circulating cancer cells [12]. The different constituents involved in the fabrication of SERS tag are shown in figure 5.1.

5.2 Components of SERS tags

To understand how to best use SERS labels in the clinical field, it is vital to spend some effort in describing the individual parts of a tag and the role they play, recalling that SERS identification and imaging in the clinical field ought to follow the indirect methodology [13]. Ideally, SERS labels should be injected into a subject intravenously, applied during a medical procedure as a type of gel to the area of interest, blended into cell media during *in vitro* examinations, or drop cast onto histopathological samples during *ex vivo* tissue assessment [14]. Considering these conventions, clearly, other than protection from opsonization (as described below), the nanoparticles should be non-cytotoxic, the Raman reporter should be firmly attached to the nanoparticle surface (ideally covalently), and should be protected from the enzymatic cleavage and acidic conditions that are typical

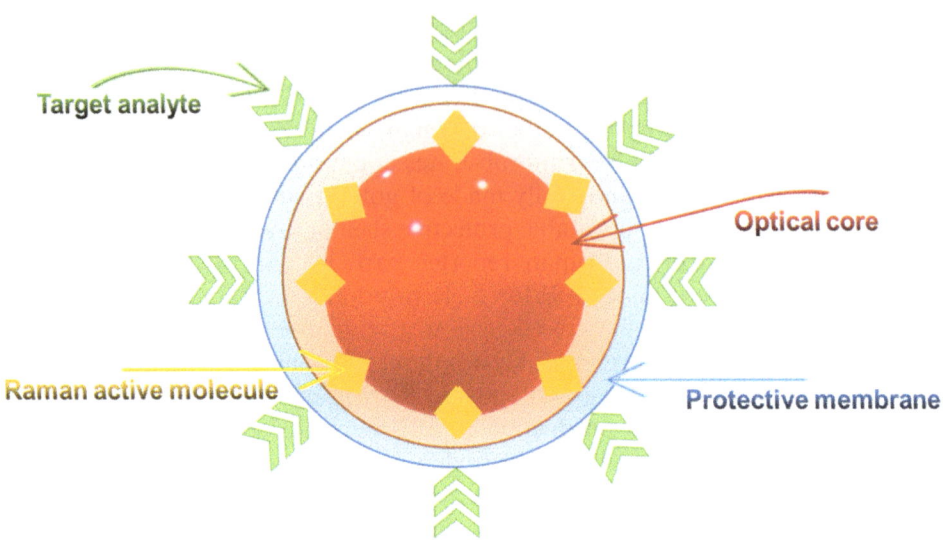

Figure 5.1. Graphical representation of different constituents of SERS tag

of endosomal up-take in cells. In addition, their size should be somewhere in the range of 20 to 200 nm to permit cell up-take and tissue extravasation while decreasing harm, and they need to have underlying hot spots for signal improvement and brightness [15]. For detection purposes, a SERS tag commonly contains a core of plasmonic nanoparticles, a layer of Raman reporter molecules, a coating shell outside the Raman reporters for protection, and also some ligands on the protective shell, as shown in figure 5.2. The plasmonic nanoparticle centers improve the Raman signals, and their composition, structure, and morphology influence the exhibition of SERS labels fundamentally. The increment in the Raman signals on the surface of the plasmonic nanoparticles may quantify the analyte when used for biological analysis. Because of the intricacy of biomolecules, the design in which Raman reporters are connected to the plasmonic center might become unstable; the protective layer seems, by all accounts, to be fundamental. The ligands present on the outer part are expected to supply SERS labels with the capacity to distinguish specific biological molecules [11].

5.2.1 The nanoparticle/plasmonic nanoparticle cores

Metal nanosubstrates act as the underlying framework and Raman signal intensifier for designing tags at the nanoscale [16]. As a rule, their size distribution, amount, elemental composition, and surface science can impact the Raman improvement capacity. As per the surface plasmon resonance (SPR) hypothesis, the SERS power upgrade occurs just when the laser excitation is in oscillation with the plasmon frequency of the NPs. In this manner, choosing a specific nanoparticle that works under the favored laser excitation is significant for designing SERS labels [17].

    i. *Gold and silver nanospheres*:

        Gold and silver are the most extensively used nanosubstrates employed for Raman signal enhancement. Gold and silver have modifiable size, excellent stability, and are also biologically compatible [18].

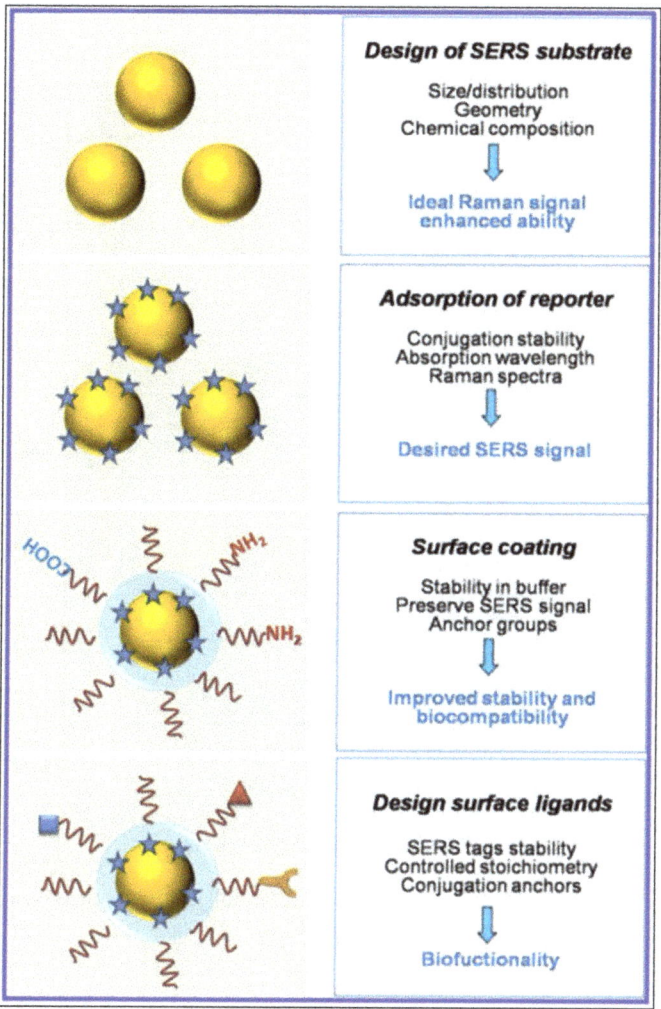

Figure 5.2. Common steps and design strategy in SERS tag engineering. (Reproduced with permission from [11]. Copyright 2013 American Chemical Society.)

ii. *Nanorods*:

In contrast to nanospheres, nanorods have two plasmon resonance groups—the more accessible transverse group in the visible range and the more stronger longitudinal group in the longer wavelength range. The longitudinal plasmon resonance groups can be tuned from the visible to the NIR region by expanding the long axis of the nanorods. This allows a more advanced laser penetration depth of tissue and is necessary for *in vivo* recognition and bioimaging. Thus, gold nanorods can be chosen readily based on the available excitation laser and specific identification conditions. Likewise, plasmon resonance groups shift to longer frequency as the solution's refractive index increases [19, 20].

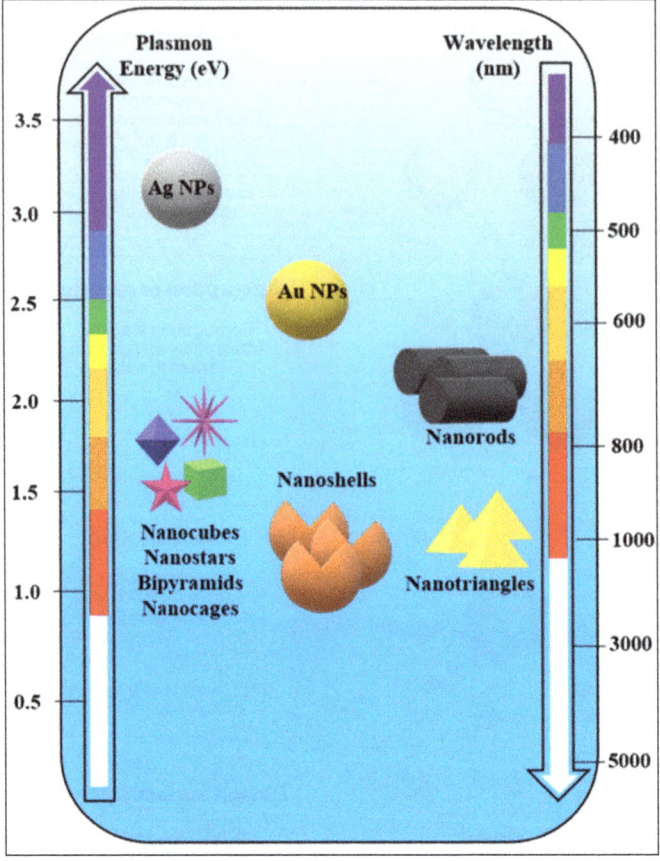

Figure 5.3. Spectral dependence of the plasmon resonance of differently shaped silver (Ag) and gold (Au) nanoparticles (NPs). (Reproduced with permission from [8]. CC BY 3.0.)

   iii. *Nanoshells*:

      These are emerging substrates with a specific core–shell structure comprising two sections: a dielectric core and a shell made up of metal (normally gold or silver). This is particularly critical for *in vivo* imaging because a long frequency laser is more penetrative in tissues, and this excitation additionally limits the tissue auto-fluorescence for better picture contrast [21, 22]. Thus, comparable nanostructures, for example, empty nanoshells and nanocages, are likewise commonly proposed for SERS applications (figure 5.3).

5.2.2 Raman reporters

Raman reporter (RR) molecules are the important basic constituents of SERS tags. The SERS results of the RR provide indirect identification of the target species [11]. The RRs should have a high cross-section to generate a robust response to the signal. They should minimize the number of peaks to avoid any type of overlap and enhance selectivity [23]. They should not be sensitive to the light coming from the laser and should be able to bind with the colloids of the metals [24, 25]. Normally, an RR is a conventional aromatic substance that can absorb physically and chemically onto the surface of the gold and need not be fluorescent. The selection of the RR should be done carefully, to avoid any type of intensification in the background of the SERS spectra, which can occur due to the plasmonic nanoparticles [26]. Some common examples of RRs include mercaptobenzoic acid, thiophenols, naphthalene dithiol, and many others. The RRs are tiny, tough, bind covalently to gold, possess a high cross-section, and show poor florescence properties [27].

5.2.3 The coating layer

The surface coating for labels designed for clinical use is a major component as it removes the unfavorable affects of direct contact with physiological liquids (e.g. blood), which manifest themselves as opsonization and conglomeration [28]. Three types of coatings are generally utilized: (i) biomolecules such as bovine serum albumin (BSA), (ii) polymers, such as PEG, and (3) ceramics, for example, silica [29]. Although one may be tempted to think that coatings of natural origin might be the most appropriate to provide stability while maintaining biocompatibility, it is necessary to ensure that these particles can actually adsorb to the nanoparticle surface forming a protein corona, and be guaranteed to resist enzymatic cleavage, as in this way they would undoubtedly lose their action in a short time [30]. The utilization of a biocompatible polymeric coating, for example, PEG, gives the label great strength with biocompatibility, while simultaneously furnishing it with chemical end groups that make it suitable for surface functionalization, which is significant to emphatically tie moieties of interest to the tag [31–33]. Polar functionalization, for example, has been shown to stabilize SERS labels during cell up-take for more than 24 h, which thus prompts broader SERS action *in vitro* and *in vivo* [34]. Silica coatings were the main coatings to be produced for SERS labels and has at the present time been marketed for quite some opportunity. Silica shells can be developed following the customary Stöber method with thicknesses that can be changed by shifting how much tetraethyl orthosilicate (TEOS) is in the alkali [35].

5.2.4 Attachment of targeting molecules

The water-soluble labels in SERS should be bonded to antibodies, aptamers, or small molecules to deliver it to well-defined natural targets. SERS labels can be functionalized through sulfhydryl-group containing particles [36, 37]. For example, after the incubation of thiolated aptamers, the metal surface arrives at a balance, causing a partial replacement of the underlying coating particles, citrate. Stable covalent bonds can likewise be formed by covering the labels with ortho-pyridyl disulfide-polyethylene glycol-N-succinimidyl propionate (OPSS-PEG-NHS) [38]. The mercapto aggregates can bond to the metal NP's surface, and N-succinimidyl can form stable amide bonds with amines in different biomolecules [39]. Essentially, with the help of coupling reagents such as 1-ethyl-3-(3-dimethylaminopropyl) carbodiimide (EDC) and N-hydroxysuccinimides (NHS), carboxylic acid groups on surface level coating particles (such as BSA) are activated for the response with the amine groups in the antibody [40, 41]. Biotin-modified labels can likewise be utilized for coating since they can definitely be connected to streptavidin-labeled biomolecules. Additionally, electrostatic interactions between the negative polyelectrolyte (e.g. poly (4-styrene sulfonate), PSS)-covered NPs and positive antibodies can likewise provide a simple method for mixing it up of natural functionalities can be promptly joined to SERS labels encapsulated in silica shells by utilizing advanced silane science [42, 43].

5.3 Application of SERS tags

The special features of SERS nanotags offers a fantastic stage for biological sensing purposes. Here, we will talk about the new proposed SERS biosensing applications, from biomarker detection to bioimaging applications [44, 45].

5.3.1 Biomarker detection

For the initial phase of examining various types of malignant developments, *in vitro* testing is crucial. Numerous biomarkers, including nucleic acids and other bio-molecules, have been investigated for the early diagnosis and imaging of disease [46]. The precise examination of these biomarkers will be very beneficial for implement-ing preventative actions [47]. The SERS labels' specificity and recognition enable the precise localization of physiologically relevant analytes in complex organic liquids [48]. The SERS labels are marked with contrasting recognition atoms (such as antibodies and aptamers) to enable precise detection of foci using Raman signals, which are used to separate the biomarkers [49]. With this theory, multitarget location stages with unmatched multiplexing ability and great awareness have also been established with the SERS labels [50, 51].

With its distinctive features of ultra-sensitivity and pattern recognition, SERS technology has received a lot of attention in the field of biomarker detection. For a very sensitive protein such as C-reactive protein (CRP) biomarker detection, a novel aptamer SERS biosensor was developed as shown in figure 5.4. This SERS tag (reporter-labeled Au nano-bridged nanogap particles (AuNNPs)) is accompanied by a metallic substrate biosensor for capturing (Ag-coated Fe_3O_4–AuNPs, AgMNPs). Aptamers against CRP were modified on both the magnetic capture substrate and SERS tag for specific recognition by a AuNNP–CRP–AgMNP sandwich assay. This achieved sensitive detection of CRP with a limit of detection (LOD) of 10 fM (1.14 pg ml^{-1}). Likewise, this strategy can also be used in the detection of other protein biomarkers of clinical importance [52].

5.3.2 *In vitro* imaging

In vitro cell studies can be carried out with the aid of a SERS tags. The brightness of the SERS tags benefits *in vitro* analysis to recognize infected cells in comparison to normal cells [53]. The infected or diseased cells contain specific biomarkers on their

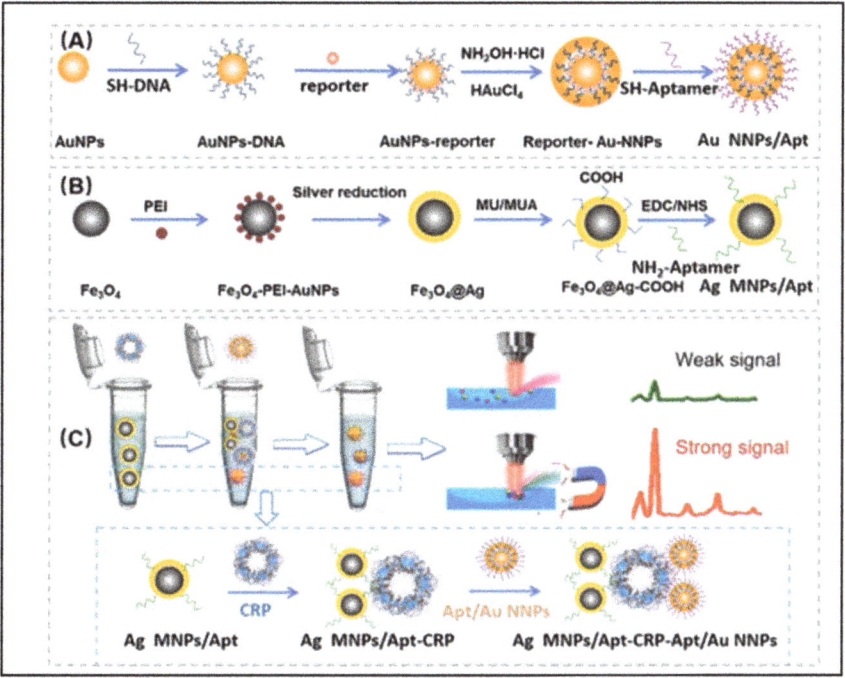

Figure 5.4. (A) Fabrication of a AuNNP SERS tag. (B) Substrate for AgMNP magnetic capture. (C) Protein detection by AgMNP–CRP–AuNNP 'sandwich' structure using SERS. (Reproduced with permission from [52]. Copyright 2021 from Elsevier.)

surfaces that are specific to the disease [54, 55]. By modifying the functional groups present on the surface of the SERS tags concerning the target, images can be taken and targets can be recognized [56]. For instance, for the three cancerous growth markers EGFR, CD44, and TGFβRII, Dinish *et al* synthesized three biologically compatible nanotags [57].

Recently, Liu *et al* developed another folate-designated SERS nanotag for particular bioimaging and determination of FR-overexpressed disease cells. This technique shows high potential to be ideal for bioimaging specialists for advances focusing on therapeutics [58]. With the help of gold nanostars and direct monitoring, the transport and release of the anticancer medication mitoxantrone (MTX) in both healthy and lung cancer (diseased) mouse models as well as single living cells was performed, as shown in figure 5.5. This *in vivo* and *in vitro* SERS detection technique has a lot of potential for application as a non-specific anti-inflammatory or in image-guided cancer treatment [59]

5.3.3 *In vivo* imaging

In vivo imaging using SERS is generally employed to distinguish the occurrence and area of tumors, in this manner directing careful cancer removal, sometimes in combination with correlative imaging methods, consequently prompting

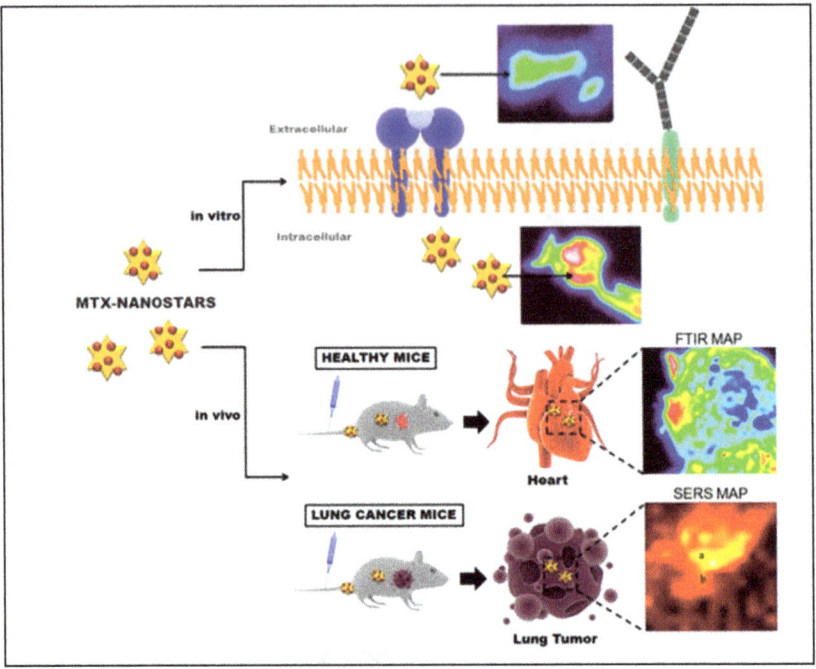

Figure 5.5. *In vivo* and *in vitro* SERS detection combined with Raman imaging. (Reproduced with permission from [59]. Copyright 2016 Elsevier.)

multimodal imaging [60, 61]. Most studies of *in vivo* imaging include the utilization of SERS tags that are infused into the creature and either collect in the cancer because of the improved enhanced penetration and maintenance (EPR) effect or explicitly focus on specific cells or cancers through direct infusion or biologically recognized surface ligands [11]. Once more, the principal constraint is given by the short penetration depth of the excitation laser beam; subsequently, much effort is being committed toward developing new instrumentation for *in vivo* imaging with SERS [62, 63]. In a recent study, multiplexed imaging was performed on a living mouse in an invasive manner. Figure 5.6(A) shows the Raman map of the whole liver of that live mouse after 2 h of the SERS administration at different concentrations [64, 65]. In the figure, the white color represents the maximum Raman intensity whereas black shows the opposite. Figure 5.6(B) shows a graphical representation of the quantitative assessment of the Raman intensity with varying concentrations, which is increasing with increased concentration [66].

5.3.4 Multimodal imaging

One of the preferred methods for obtaining the most data possible for precise disease diagnosis is the combination of mutually compatible imaging techniques [67, 68]. Platforms that enable the employment of many approaches are extremely desirable since each technique has the potential to contribute significant and complementary information [69, 70]. For instance, the presence of both magnetic and plasmonic

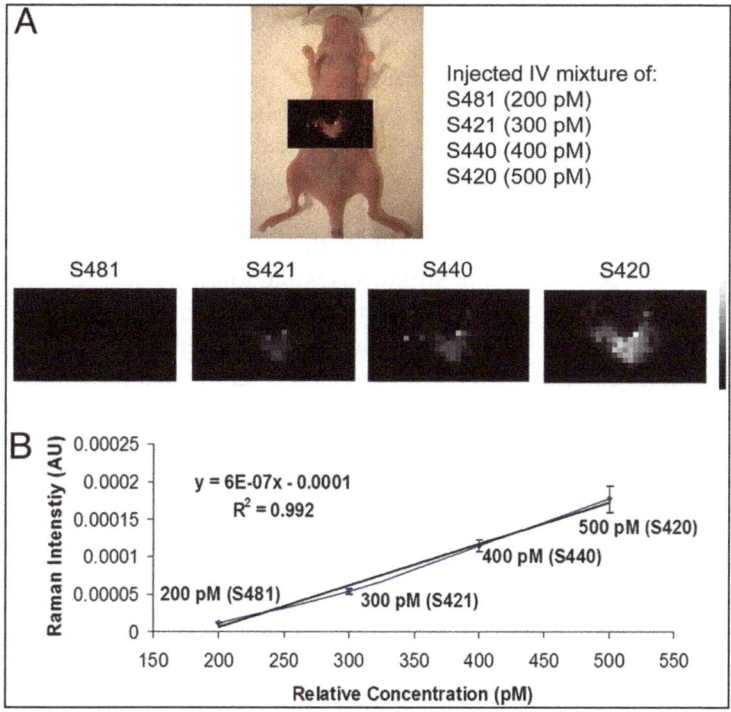

Figure 5.6. (A) Bioimaging with the aid of SERS tags. (B) Graph representing increased Raman intensities with increasing concentration. (Reproduced with permission from [66]. Copyright 2009 PNAS.)

properties in a single nanoscale object should enable the use of magnetic resonance imaging (MRI) through the contrast provided by an iron oxide component, while a plasmonic component, such as RR labeled gold, can be monitored by SERS imaging, offering high sensitivity and spatial resolution [71, 72].

5.4 Conclusion and future perspectives

SERS tags are now a crucial component in SERS-related biomedical applications. This is primarily because of the difficulties experienced during direct SERS sensing in the biological and clinical domains, where the environment is highly varied and frequently changing. In such complicated biological conditions, and particularly for SERS imaging, well-defined SERS-labeled elements with distinct signals that are not altered over time can be utilized as a reference. However, direct SERS would offer supplementary data on analyte changes. Therefore, we suggest that combining the two methods should be quite advantageous. In this regard, recent advancements in the controlled and repeatable synthesis of anisotropic metal nanoparticles, along with encoding, protecting, and targeting technologies, are leading to extremely complex systems that may be designed 'à la carte' for each unique situation. A lot of the recent developments in the field of tag-based SERS imaging are centered on improvements in spatial and temporal resolutions. The use of ultrafast lasers, coupled imaging approaches, and high spatial resolution techniques such as TERS are pushing the boundaries to achieve nanoscale resolutions and femtosecond time scales. To accomplish these goals, multivariate data analysis and the application of precise 3D cell and tissue models are crucial tools. As a result, we expect a rapid increase in new developments in ultrafast and extremely accurate SERS imaging shortly. *In vivo* biomarker detection, which requires open surgery, is another area where SERS tags have a lot to offer. Endoscopic SERS probes can supplement the analysis and identification of tumor cells in this application. Due to the improved sensitivity that may be acquired in situations when analytes such as cell biomarkers are present at extremely low concentrations, the development of SERS-based point-of-care testing (POCT) is increasing. The incorporation of SERS within micro-fluidics devices enables one to generate more consistent measurement circumstances, leading to reliable quantitative results, even though reproducibility is still the key issue. As a result, we can expect new clinical applications based on SERS as well as continued advancements in portable devices for *in situ* studies, such as reduced dimensions, automated analysis, and more sophisticated components. Although SERS tags have been used successfully for liquid biopsies, POCT has not yet adopted them broadly. The lack of inexpensive, high-sensitivity equipment and detection techniques are the key constraints. In recent years, some portable instruments have been made available. However, when compared the larger devices, their laser power and adjustability are substantially lower. Future efforts should focus on creating novel testing platforms for quick *in vitro* diagnostics in addition to building sophisticated instruments. The quick examination of bio-logical samples will benefit greatly from the integration of SERS tags with advanced POCT devices. One method of multiplexing detection is the fabrication of non-overlapping SERS tags. The majority of the works discussed in this review use this methodology. There is growing popularity for multiplex detection and bioimaging of different biomolecules utilizing SERS technology. Nevertheless, it appears that most applications fall far short of demonstrating the clinical usefulness of SERS technology, despite the early success of some clinical studies based on this technology. Therefore, it is important to support ongoing research into SERS-based biomedicine to maximize its potential for practical applications. Practical and clinical applications of SERS nanotechnology must be accepted and evaluated based on their assay time and cost, sensitivity, and accuracy of quantitative detection to replace conventional fluorescence-based diagnostics. Therefore, any significant advancement in the structural reproducibility of SERS-active nano-structure production will inevitably lead to a new era of SERS-based diagnostics as an alternative to traditional systems in nanobiotechnology and nanomedicine. As, even with small detection areas, current SERS technology requires a long spectral collection time, limiting its potential application to high-throughput screening and *in vitro* or *in vivo* bioimaging, there is a need to shorten the SERS signal acquisition time when scanning large areas or whole animal bodies. As was done in the case of MRI and fluorescence scanning, rapid promotion of the development of SERS instrumentation and spectroscopy capable of giving a fast and sensitive read-out of signals from large scanning regions is therefore required. However, by combining all of the benefits of SERS nanotechnology with sophisticated SERS spectroscopy, all of the concerns identified in this review might be resolved, which would significantly advance the fields of nano-bioscience and nano-biomedicine.

References

[1] Sharma B, Frontiera R R, Henry A I, Ringe E and Van Duyne R P 2012 SERS: materials, applications, and the future *Mater. Today* **15** 16–25

[2] Cialla D, März A, Böhme R, Theil F, Weber K, Schmitt M and Popp J 2012 Surface-enhanced Raman spectroscopy (SERS): progress and trends *Anal. Bioanal. Chem.* **403** 27–54

[3] Liu Y, Zhou H, Hu Z, Yu G, Yang D and Zhao J 2017 Label and label-free based surface-enhanced Raman scattering for pathogen bacteria detection: a review *Biosens. Bioelectron.* **94** 131–40

[4] van Lierop D, Faulds K and Graham D 2011 Separation free DNA detection using surface enhanced Raman scattering *Anal. Chem.* **83** 5817–21

[5] van Lierop D, Krpetić Ž, Guerrini L, Larmour I A, Dougan J A, Faulds K and Graham D 2012 Positively charged silver nanoparticles and their effect on surface-enhanced Raman scattering of dye-labelled oligonucleotides *Chem. Commun.* **48** 8192–4

[6] Gracie K, Moores M, Smith W E, Harding K, Girolami M, Graham D and Faulds K 2016 Preferential attachment of specific fluorescent dyes and dye labeled DNA sequences in a surface enhanced Raman scattering multiplex *Anal. Chem.* **88** 1147–53

[7] Wang H N, Fales A M and Vo-Dinh T 2015 Plasmonics-based SERS nanobiosensor for homogeneous nucleic acid detection *Nanomed. Nanotechnol. Biol. Med.* **11** 811–4

[8] Tahir M A, Dina N E, Cheng H, Valev V K and Zhang L 2021 Surface-enhanced Raman spectroscopy for bioanalysis and diagnosis *Nanoscale* **13** 11593–634

[9] Han X X, Rodriguez R S, Haynes C L, Ozaki Y and Zhao B 2022 Surface-enhanced Raman spectroscopy *Nat. Rev. Methods Primers* **1** 87

[10] Plou J, Valera P S, García I, de Albuquerque C D, Carracedo A and Liz-Marzán L M 2022 Prospects of surface-enhanced Raman spectroscopy for biomarker monitoring toward precision medicine *ACS Photonics* **9** 333–50

[11] Wang Y, Yan B and Chen L 2013 SERS tags: novel optical nanoprobes for bioanalysis *Chem. Rev.* **113** 1391–428

[12] Wu Z, Wang Z, Xie H, Wang Y, He H, Nie S, Ye J and Lin L 2022 Raman-guided bronchoscopy: feasibility and detection depth studies using *ex vivo* lung tissues and SERS nanoparticle tags *Photonics* **9** 429

[13] Lin J, Akakuru O U and Wu A 2021 Advances in surface-enhanced Raman scattering bioprobes for cancer imaging *View* **2** 20200146

[14] Langer J *et al* 2019 Present and future of surface-enhanced Raman scattering *ACS Nano* **14** 28–117

[15] Liu H, Gao X, Xu C and Liu D 2022 SERS tags for biomedical detection and bioimaging *Theranostics* **12** 1870

[16] Xie J, Zhang Q, Lee J Y and Wang D I 2008 The synthesis of SERS-active gold nanoflower tags for *in vivo* applications *ACS Nano* **2** 2473–80

[17] Liang X, Li N, Zhang R, Yin P, Zhang C, Yang N, Liang K and Kong B 2021 Carbon-based SERS biosensor: from substrate design to sensing and bioapplication *NPG Asia Mater.* **13** 8

[18] Amaravathi K Y 2015 Green synthesis of gold nanoparticles formulated with natural Indian medicine to perform cancer theranostic study *Doctoral Dissertation* Texas A&M University–Kingsville, TX

[19] Pérez-Juste J, Pastoriza-Santos I, Liz-Marzán L M and Mulvaney P 2005 Gold nanorods: synthesis, characterization and applications *Coord. Chem. Rev.* **249** 1870–901

[20] Chen H, Shao L, Li Q and Wang J 2013 Gold nanorods and their plasmonic properties *Chem. Soc. Rev.* **42** 2679–724

[21] Hirsch L R, Gobin A M, Lowery A R, Tam F, Drezek R A, Halas N J and West J L 2006 Metal nanoshells *Ann. Biomed. Eng.* **34** 15–22

[22] Jackson J B and Halas N J 2001 Silver nanoshells: variations in morphologies and optical properties *J. Phys. Chem.* B **105** 2743–6

[23] Li M, Cushing S K and Wu N 2015 Plasmon-enhanced optical sensors: a review *Analyst* **140** 386–406

[24] Hirsch L R, Stafford R J, Bankson J A, Sershen S R, Rivera B, Price R E, Hazle J D, Halas N J and West J L 2003 Nanoshell-mediated near-infrared thermal therapy of tumors under magnetic resonance guidance *Proc. Natl Acad. Sci. USA* **100** 13549–54

[25] Fabris L 2016 SERS tags: the next promising tool for personalized cancer detection? *ChemNanoMat* **2** 249–58

[26] Samanta A *et al* 2011 Ultrasensitive near-infrared Raman reporters for SERS-based *in vivo* cancer detection *Angew. Chem.* **123** 6213–6

[27] Fabris L, Schierhorn M, Moskovits M and Bazan G C 2010 Aptatag-based multiplexed assay for protein detection by surface-enhanced Raman spectroscopy *Small* **6** 1550–7

[28] Ranganathan R, Madanmohan S, Kesavan A, Baskar G, Krishnamoorthy Y R, Santosham R, Ponraju D, Rayala S K and Venkatraman G 2012 Nanomedicine: towards development of patient-friendly drug-delivery systems for oncological applications *Int. J. Nanomed.* **7** 1043

[29] Pallaoro A, Braun G B and Moskovits M 2015 Biotags based on surface-enhanced Raman can be as bright as fluorescence tags *Nano Lett.* **15** 6745–50

[30] Chien Y H, Chan K K, Anderson T, Kong K V, Ng B K and Yong K T 2019 Advanced near-infrared light-responsive nanomaterials as therapeutic platforms for cancer therapy *Adv. Ther.* **2** 1800090

[31] Khullar P, Singh V, Mahal A, Dave P N, Thakur S, Kaur G, Singh J, Singh Kamboj S and Singh Bakshi M 2012 Bovine serum albumin bioconjugated gold nanoparticles: synthesis, hemolysis, and cytotoxicity toward cancer cell lines *J. Phys. Chem.* C **116** 8834–43

[32] Doering W E and Nie S 2003 Spectroscopic tags using dye-embedded nanoparticles and surface-enhanced Raman scattering *Anal. Chem.* **75** 6171–6

[33] Mulvaney S P, Musick M D, Keating C D and Natan M J 2003 Glass-coated, analyte-tagged nanoparticles: a new tagging system based on detection with surface-enhanced Raman scattering *Langmuir* **19** 4784–90

[34] Indrasekara A D, Meyers S, Shubeita S, Feldman L C, Gustafsson T and Fabris L 2014 Gold nanostar substrates for SERS-based chemical sensing in the femtomolar regime *Nanoscale* **6** 8891–9

[35] Stöber W, Fink A and Bohn E 1968 Controlled growth of monodisperse silica spheres in the micron size range *J. Colloid Interface Sci.* **26** 62–9

[36] Nie S and Emory S R 1997 Probing single molecules and single nanoparticles by surface-enhanced Raman scattering *Science* **275** 1102–6

[37] Fang Y, Seong N H and Dlott D D 2008 Measurement of the distribution of site enhancements in surface-enhanced Raman scattering *Science* **321** 388–92

[38] Tian S, Neumann O, McClain M J, Yang X, Zhou L, Zhang C, Nordlander P and Halas N J 2017 Aluminum nanocrystals: a sustainable substrate for quantitative SERS-based DNA detection *Nano Lett.* **17** 5071–7

[39] Moskovits M 1985 Surface-enhanced spectroscopy *Rev. Mod. Phys.* **57** 783

[40] Kneipp K, Wang Y, Kneipp H, Perelman L T, Itzkan I, Dasari R R and Feld M S 1997 Single molecule detection using surface-enhanced Raman scattering (SERS) *Phys. Rev. Lett.* **78** 1667

[41] Wu S, Shen Y and Jin C 2019 Surface-enhanced Raman scattering induced by the coupling of the guided mode with localized surface plasmon resonances *Nanoscale* **11** 14164–73

[42] Park S G, Mun C, Xiao X, Braun A, Kim S, Giannini V, Maier S A and Kim D H 2017 Surface energy-controlled SERS substrates for molecular concentration at plasmonic nano-gaps *Adv. Funct. Mater.* **27** 1703376

[43] Chirumamilla M, Chirumamilla A, Roberts A S, Zaccaria R P, De Angelis F, Kjær Kristensen P, Krahne R, Bozhevolnyi S I, Pedersen K and Toma A 2017 Hot-spot engineering in 3D multi-branched nanostructures: ultrasensitive substrates for surface-enhanced Raman spectroscopy *Adv. Opt. Mater.* **5** 1600836

[44] Wang L, Vendrell-Dones M O, Deriu C, Doğruer S, Harrington P D and McCord B 2021 Multivariate analysis aided surface-enhanced Raman spectroscopy (MVA-SERS) multiplex quantitative detection of trace fentanyl in illicit drug mixtures using a handheld Raman spectrometer *Appl. Spectrosc.* **75** 1225–36

[45] Yadav S, Sadique M A, Ranjan P, Kumar N, Singhal A, Srivastava A K and Khan R 2021 SERS based lateral flow immunoassay for point-of-care detection of SARS-CoV-2 in clinical samples *ACS Appl. Biomater.* **4** 2974–95

[46] Küstner B, Gellner M, Schütz M, Schöppler F, Marx A, Ströbel P, Adam P, Schmuck C and Schlücker S 2009 SERS labels for red laser excitation: silica-encapsulated SAMs on tunable gold/silver nanoshells *Angew. Chem. Int. Ed.* **48** 1950–3

[47] Murphy C J, Sau T K, Gole A M, Orendorff C J, Gao J, Gou L, Hunyadi S E and Li T 2005 Anisotropic metal nanoparticles: synthesis, assembly, and optical applications *J. Phys. Chem.* B **109** 13857–70

[48] Hu Q, Tay L L, Noestheden M and Pezacki J P 2007 Mammalian cell surface imaging with nitrile-functionalized nanoprobes: biophysical characterization of aggregation and polarization anisotropy in SERS imaging *J. Am. Chem. Soc.* **129** 14–5

[49] Xu L, Yan W, Ma W, Kuang H, Wu X, Liu L, Zhao Y, Wang L and Xu C 2015 SERS encoded silver pyramids for attomolar detection of multiplexed disease biomarkers *Adv. Mater.* **27** 1706–11

[50] Lutz B, Dentinger C, Sun L, Nguyen L, Zhang J, Chmura A J, Allen A, Chan S and Knudsen B 2008 Raman nanoparticle probes for antibody-based protein detection in tissues *J. Histochem. Cytochem.* **56** 371–9

[51] Michalet X, Pinaud F F, Bentolila L A, Tsay J M, Doose S J, Li J J, Sundaresan G, Wu A M, Gambhir S S and Weiss S 2005 Quantum dots for live cells, *in vivo* imaging, and diagnostics *Science* **307** 538–44

[52] Hu Z *et al* 2021 Aptamer-based novel Ag-coated magnetic recognition and SERS nanotags with interior nanogap biosensor for ultrasensitive detection of protein biomarker *Sensors Actuators* B **334** 129640

[53] Huang X, El-Sayed I H, Qian W and El-Sayed M A 2006 Cancer cell imaging and photothermal therapy in the near-infrared region by using gold nanorods *J. Am. Chem. Soc.* **128** 2115–20

[54] Du Z, Qi Y, He J, Zhong D and Zhou M 2021 Recent advances in applications of nanoparticles in SERS *in vivo* imaging *Wiley Interdiscip. Rev. Nanomed. Nanobiotechnol.* **13** e1672

[55] Bock S *et al* 2022 Highly sensitive near-infrared SERS nanoprobes for *in vivo* imaging using gold-assembled silica nanoparticles with controllable nanogaps *J. Nanobiotechnol.* **20** 130

[56] Fabris L 2015 Gold-based SERS tags for biomedical imaging *J. Opt.* **17** 114002

[57] Dinish U S, Balasundaram G, Chang Y T and Olivo M 2014 Actively targeted *in vivo* multiplex detection of intrinsic cancer biomarkers using biocompatible SERS nanotags *Sci. Rep.* **4** 4075

[58] Liu R, Zhao J, Han G, Zhao T, Zhang R, Liu B, Liu Z, Zhang C, Yang L and Zhang Z 2017 Click-functionalized SERS nanoprobes with improved labeling efficiency and capability for cancer cell imaging *ACS Appl. Mater. Interfaces* **9** 38222–9

[59] Tian F, Conde J, Bao C, Chen Y, Curtin J and Cui D 2016 Gold nanostars for efficient *in vitro* and *in vivo* real-time SERS detection and drug delivery via plasmonic-tunable Raman/FTIR imaging *Biomaterials* **106** 87–97

[60] Li J F *et al* 2010 Shell-isolated nanoparticle-enhanced Raman spectroscopy *Nature* **464** 392–5

[61] Du Z, Qi Y, He J, Zhong D and Zhou M 2021 Recent advances in applications of nanoparticles in SERS *in vivo* imaging *Wiley Interdiscip. Rev. Nanomed. Nanobiotechnol.* **13** e1672

[62] Abramczyk H and Brozek-Pluska B 2013 Raman imaging in biochemical and biomedical applications. Diagnosis and treatment of breast cancer *Chem. Rev.* **113** 5766–81

[63] Fang J, Du S, Lebedkin S, Li Z, Kruk R, Kappes M and Hahn H 2010 Gold mesostructures with tailored surface topography and their self-assembly arrays for surface-enhanced Raman spectroscopy *Nano Lett.* **10** 5006–13

[64] Zhang R *et al* 2013 Chemical mapping of a single molecule by plasmon-enhanced Raman scattering *Nature* **498** 82–6

[65] Andreou C, Gregoriou Y, Ali A and Pal S 2022 *In vivo* imaging with SERS nanoprobes *SERS for Point-of-Care and Clinical Applications* (New York: Elsevier) p 199–235

[66] Zavaleta C L, Smith B R, Walton I, Doering W, Davis G, Shojaei B, Natan M J and Gambhir S S 2009 Multiplexed imaging of surface enhanced Raman scattering nanotags in living mice using noninvasive Raman spectroscopy *Proc. Natl Acad. Sci.* **106** 13511–6

[67] Lim D K, Jeon K S, Hwang J H, Kim H, Kwon S, Suh Y D and Nam J M 2011 Highly uniform and reproducible surface-enhanced Raman scattering from DNA-tailorable nano-particles with 1-nm interior gap *Nat. Nanotechnol.* **6** 452–60

[68] Iakab S A, Baquer G, Lafuente M, Pina M P, Ramírez J L, Ràfols P, Correig-Blanchar X and García-Altares M 2022 SALDI-MS and SERS multimodal imaging: one nanostructured substrate to rule them both *Anal. Chem.* **94** 2785–93

[69] Camden J P, Dieringer J A, Wang Y, Masiello D J, Marks L D, Schatz G C and Van Duyne R P 2008 Probing the structure of single-molecule surface-enhanced Raman scattering hot spots *J. Am. Chem. Soc.* **130** 12616–7

[70] Diebold E D, Mack N H, Doorn S K and Mazur E 2009 Femtosecond laser-nanostructured substrates for surface-enhanced Raman scattering *Langmuir* **25** 1790–4

[71] Lenzi E, Jimenez de Aberasturi D and Liz-Marzan L M 2019 Surface-enhanced Raman scattering tags for three-dimensional bioimaging and biomarker detection *ACS Sens.* **4** 1126–37

[72] Zhang X, Zheng Y, Liu X, Lu W, Dai J, Lei D Y and MacFarlane D R 2015 Hierarchical porous plasmonic metamaterials for reproducible ultrasensitive surface-enhanced Raman spectroscopy *Adv. Mater.* **27** 1090–6

Chapter 6

SERS integrated detection techniques for clinical samples: overcoming challenges

**Pushpesh Ranjan, Lal Singh Banjara, Shalu Yadav,
Mohd Abubakar Sadique and Raju Khan**

Surface-enhanced Raman spectroscopy (SERS)-based biosensing techniques exhibit promise in the detection of infectious diseases, pathogenic bacteria, and protein biomarkers. SERS technology is a high sensitivity, rapid, and multiplex diagnostic platform. Coupled efficiently with analytical diagnostic methods such as electrochemical, optical, microfluidic, machine learning, and artificial intelligence approaches, the SERS technique can be advanced further as a point-of-care detection platform. The integration of the SERS technique enables an advanced diagnostic platform that improves the sensitivity enormously and achieves ultra-low detection limits even up to single cell detection. In addition, it overcomes the issues with single detection techniques that require a high sample volume, a time-consuming process, and detection at a mass scale. In this chapter, we discuss the recent advances in the development of the SERS integrated detection technique platform for highly sensitive and selective detection of pathogenic bacteria and infectious diseases such as viruses. Lastly, we address the challenges associated with the integration of the SERS technique and the possible solutions to overcome this issue to further improve their function and their future prospects.

6.1 Introduction

In the current challenging diagnostic landscape, sensitive, rapid, selective, and accurate sensing analytical tools are in demand. This concerns the healthcare issue of the detection of highly pathogenic particles. In recent years, various detection techniques have been validated for the qualitative or quantitative estimation of disease-associated antibodies and protein biomarkers of pathogenic bacteria, viruses, cancer, cardiac conditions, and other diseases, which identify major health problems allowing timely treatment. In this respect, the most common gold-standard analytical techniques, such as polymerase chain reaction (PCR), reverse transcription-quantitative polymerase chain reaction (RT-qPCR), and enzyme-linked immunosorbent assay (ELISA), are employed on a large scale for the detection of disease-specific biomarkers. However, they still struggle with several limitations such as a costly set-up, limited testing, and time-consuming process, including sample preparation and washing steps which significantly constrain performing point-of-care (POC) rapid sensing of infectious diseases in large-scale testing. On the other hand, several POC diagnostic platforms such as electrochemical, optical, lateral flow immunoassay (LFIA), microfluidic, and microscopic imaging have been reported for the detection of such infectious disease-causing particles in a rapid fashion. They are highly sensitive, cost-effective, rapid, and can detect multiple biomarkers with a single testing kit. Moreover, their easy fabrication methods, portability, disposability, and on-site testing have made them highly attractive for biosensing applications [1–6]. The prominent spectroscopic technique known as surface-enhanced Raman spectroscopy (SERS) is extensively utilized in biosensor platforms owing to several advantages, such as fingerprint recognition ability, high sensitivity, non-invasiveness, label-free detection, and extremely good detection capacity up to the single molecule level [2]. Furthermore, the integration of SERS with other analytic detection techniques improves the biosensor performance with ultra-low detection efficiency and resolves the issues associated with individual detection techniques [7].

Some of the most promising diagnostics are electrochemical technique-based biosensors, in which the working electrodes are fabricated using highly conductive and functional nanostructured materials which possess a large surface area and high stability. Further, they are modified by the immobilization of target-specific biomolecules, i.e. antigens, antibodies, or aptamers, on the modified surface that specifically capture and detect the analyte of interest with high selectivity [8–10]. Electrochemical biosensors allow rapid, sensitive, and label-free detection. However, their cross-reactivity, limited shelf life, and environmental sensitivity are the major weakness of these sensing techniques.

Optical biosensors are analytical sensing devices that include an optical transducer such as fluorescence, luminescence, surface plasmon resonance (SPR), Raman, and fiber optics integrated with biorecognition elements that produce a high-throughput measurable result of the target analyte concentration based on the produced optical signal after the binding of the analyte on the sensing surface. In optical biosensors, plasmonic nanomaterials are essential for the fabrication of immunoassays, where the signal intensity of the light after capturing analytes has been used for the detection and estimation of the biomarker. An optical biosensor is sensitive, however, their complex surface modification steps and the requirement for bulky instruments has restricted their mass-scale applicability [11, 12].

Similarly, the LFIA platform has been the most applicable diagnostic kit for virus sensing and is cost-effective, rapid, and easy to use for end-users, and provides a reliable result. In LFIA strips, the result is analysed based on a colorimetric signal that appears on the test and control lines, which can be observed by either the naked eye or by a simple camera. Since the sensing operation and result interpretation are quite easy, it has been in high demand for biosensing of infectious diseases such as SARS-CoV-2. However, the limited sensitivity, cross-reactivity, false-positive and -negative results, and qualitative results are major concerns in LFIA and limit their applicability. However, the integration of the SERS technique with the LFIA platform overcomes these issues and enables quantitative and sensitive results [13–15].

Emerging microfluidic-based biosensing is the most promising POC diagnostic platform which deals with the detection of target analytes in a low-volume sample ($\leqslant \mu l$). They offer numerous advantages, such as ease for integration with quantitative analytical techniques, multiplex detection, low-cost devices, disposability, rapidity, and reliable results. However, they could not have their sensing where the integration of analytical techniques is necessary for the quantification of the analyte. Therefore, SERS integration with a microfluidic device makes them appropriate for the detection of infectious diseases [16–18]. This chapter presents the advantages of SERS and its integration with current existing diagnostic methods for infectious diseases in POC settings.

6.2 SERS integrated detection techniques

6.2.1 SERS integrated lateral flow immunoassay

The LFIA is a diagnostic tool utilized for the detection of various target analytes. They are employed extensively for the detection of antibodies or antigens specific to infectious diseases such as influenza virus, severe acute respiratory syndrome coronavirus (SARS-CoV)-1, SARS-CoV-2, bacterial infections, cancerous protein biomarkers, and toxic environmental chemicals. The LFIA consists of a sample pad, conjugate pad, test line, control line, and absorption pad, which are fabricated on a porous nitrocellulose membrane paper. The conjugate pad of the LFIA is modified using selective antibody/antigen conjugated metal nanoparticles (AuNPs, AgNPs, etc). The test line is modified using a target-specific capture antibody or antigen and the control line using the respective target anti-IgM or anti-IgG antibody. When the target analyte containing the clinical sample is dropped on the sample pad, it flows on the porous paper substrate due to the capillary force and binds to the functionalized metal nanoparticles on the conjugation pad. Further, it moves and binds to biospecies immobilized on the test line to make a sandwich-type assay. In this process, the colors that appear in both the test and control lines confirm the presence of the target analyte. Therefore, LFIA-based detection is easy to interpret using visual observation, and at the same time it offers high-throughput qualitative results. It offers several advantages such as ease-of-use, long-term stability, cost-effectiveness, and rapid, multiplex detection [13–15]. However, the limited sensitivity and false results of LFIAs are the foremost issues of concern. These may occur because a very low concentration of analyte in the clinical sample can affect the true result and it is sometimes difficult to accept the diagnostic accuracy. Combination with the SERS technique overcomes these issues of conventional LFIAs. In the case of SERS-LFIA, Raman nanotag-labeled metal nanoparticles are employed for modification of the conjugate pad of the LFIA strip, and an appropriate laser light is directed on the test line which delivers highly sensitive, quantitative, and reliable results [19, 20]. In a recent study, Liu *et al* reported a SERS integrated LFIA for quick detection of IgM and IgG antibodies for SARS-CoV-2 simultaneously in serum. Herein, the authors prepared the conjugate pad of the test strip using SiO_2@Ag nanoparticles modified with dual layers of Raman tag and further functionalized with the S-protein of SARS-CoV-2. The two test lines and one control line of the strip were modified by goat anti-human IgM, goat anti-human IgG, and SARS-CoV-2 S-protein antibody, respectively. A laser was focused on the colorimetric signal of the test line when it appeared after selectively capturing IgM and IgG antibodies for the quantitative estimation of antibodies. This immunoassay offers a highly sensitive result, which has 800-fold higher sensitivity compared to AuNP-based LFIA. The ultra-low detection ability can benefit early detection of SARS-CoV-2 before the onset of COVID-19 symptoms. In addition, they tested 19 positive and 49 negative serum samples for the validation of clinical applicability [21]. In another study, Xiao *et al* reported a similar SERS-based platform for the detection of avian influenza H7N9 virus. For this assay the authors employed a 4-aminothiophenol (4-ATP) Raman reporter functionalized with AuAg@AgNPs conjugated with a specific antibody for the modification of the test line. AuNPs and AgNPs have a plasmonic property and high surface area which improves the SERS intensity, as a result they are promising candidates for sensitive and rapid testing in a real sample. In this test, the color of the test line can be observed visually, where the color intensity is related directly to the concentration of the viral antigen. The quantitative estimation was performed using a portable Raman instrument [22]. Recently, Wang *et al* reported a Fe_3O_4@Ag magnetic nanoparticle as a SERS tag modified LFIA for quantification of influenza A (H1N1) and human adenovirus (HAdV) simultaneously. The LFIA strip was fabricated by the modification of two test lines using an H1N1 antibody and HAdV antibody followed by a control line of goat anti-mouse IgG. The Fe_3O_4@Ag SERS tag was placed in a clinical sample containing virus particles as they bind selectively, and were separated magnetically. The advantage of the utilization of magnetic nanoparticles (MNPs) is that they facilitate a high degree of capturing of biomolecules and can be separated magnetically in a single step which reduces the time-consuming washing and separation process. After that, the functionalized MNP solution flowed on the test strip and were captured specifically by their respective antibody-modified test line which appeared as a colorimetric signal. A laser of 785 nm was irradiated on the test line to estimate the virus particles at much lower concentrations of 50 and 10 PFU ml^{-1} for H1N1 and HAdV, respectively. The authors also found that the assay had 2000-times higher sensitivity compared to the gold nanoparticle-based LFIA. Additionally, in this assay there is no need to sample pre-treatment for the detection process [23]. To extend this work, Zhou *et al* developed an aptamer-conjugated Fe_3O_4@Au magnetic nanoparticle-based SERS-LFIA for pathogen enrichment and a staphylococcus protein modified-SERS tags (Au@DTNB@PA) for simultaneous detection of *Escherichia coli* (*E. coli*), *Listeria monocytogenes* (*L. mono*), and *Salmonella typhimurium* (*S. typhi*) bacteria in food samples [24]. Similarly, Li *et al*

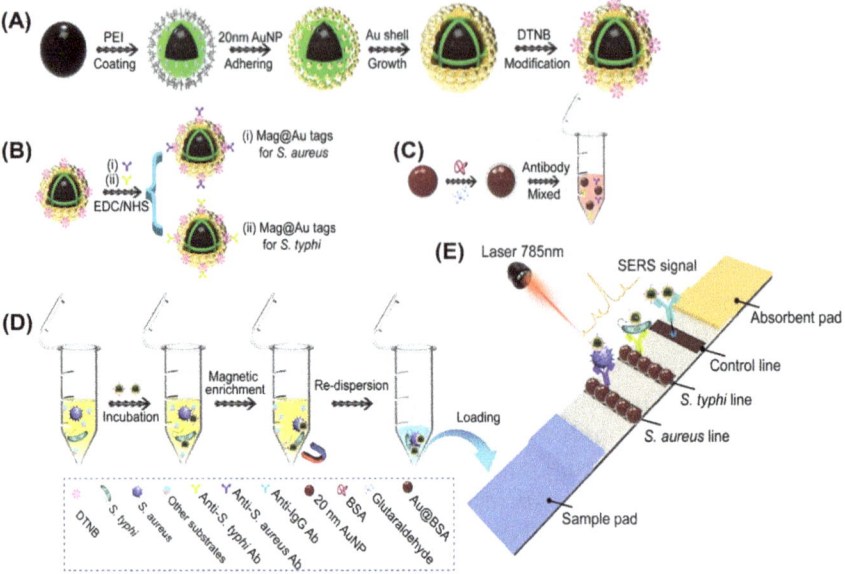

Figure 6.1. (A) Synthesis of the SERS tag labeled magnetic nanoparticles, (B) and (C) its antibody-modification, and (D) magnetic separation of modified nanoparticles. (E) Representation of the magnetic SERS-based LFIA for the multiplex detection of foodborne bacteria. (Reproduced with permission from [25]. Copyright 2022 American Chemical Society.)

developed a similar LFIA strip using Fe_3O_4@AuNPs for rapid detection of multiple bacteria such as *Staphylococcus aureus* (*S. aureus*) and *S. typhi*. The test lines of this assay were fabricated by the immobilization of detection antibody functionalized bovine serum albumin (BSA)-coated gold nanoparticles. This assay was rapid and required less than 30 min for the detection of both bacteria having a low LOD of 12 and 9 cells/ml. A schematic representation of the synthesis and antibody function-alization of magnetic nanoparticles, their separation, and detection of bacteria on SERS-LFIA are illustrated in figure 6.1 [25].

In another study, the *Yersinia pestis* (*Y. pestis*), *Francisella tularensis* (*F. tularensis*), and *Bacillus anthracis* (*B. anthracis*) pathogenic bacteria were detected by Wang *et al* using a malachite green isothiocyanate-labeled AuNP functionalized detection antibody-based SERS-LFIA strip. Herein, gold nanoparticles with a size of 40 nm were used which were further treated with polyvinylpyrrolidone (PVP) and 10G surfactant that stabilized the SERS tag as well as improved the hydrophobic property which maximized the capturing of antibodies immobilized on the test line, resulting in improved sensitivity of the immunoassay. A schematic representation of the SERS-based LFIA sensing platform for *Y. pestis*, *F. tularensis*, and *B. anthracis* is shown in figure 6.2 [26]. Recently, Wang *et al* detected the four bacteria *S. aureus*, *S. typhi*, *L. mono*, and *E. coli* on two test lines of a bi-channel LFIA strip. The test lines were made by DTNM and MBA Raman tag modified GO@Au/AgNPs labeled with the target antibodies. The high surface area and oxygen functionalities of the

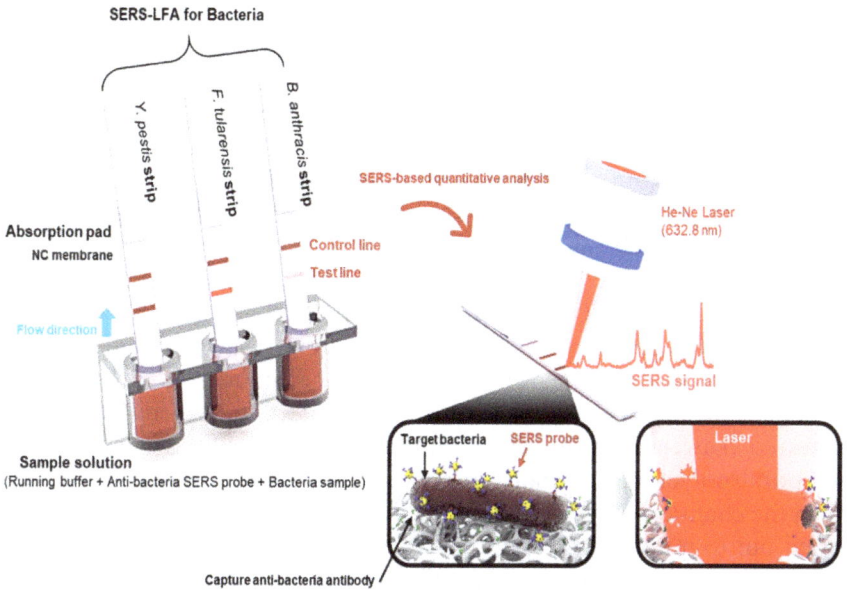

Figure 6.2. Schematic of the SERS-based LFIA sensing platform for *Y. pestis*, *F. tularensis*, and *B. anthracis*. (Reproduced with permission from [26]. Copyright 2016 Elsevier.)

nanocomposites offer high degrees of capturing of bacteria and fast detection within 20 min at a very low LOD of 9 cells/ml. This assay expresses a great affinity for multiplex detection of pathogens; therefore, it can also be utilized successfully for other infectious diseases [27]. SERS-LFIAs display excellent detection capability even the multiplex sensing which has better than single biomarker detection and generates reproducible results. However, further research will be required to explore their detection ability beyond the protein and antibody biomarkers.

6.2.2 SERS integrated microfluidic device

The microfluidic device is an emergent platform for the analysis of numerous biomarkers from proteins to cells. The fabrication of the microfluidic chip is performed through the construction of microchannels on glass or silicon plate surfaces and molded using polydimethylsiloxane (PDMS) polymer. PDMS polymer is employed widely because of its low cost and non-reactive behavior with the sample solution which can otherwise cause interference in the result. Furthermore, the microchannels are modified using nanomaterials followed by biomolecules specific to the target analyte, where they capture the selective analytes and exhibit a measurable signal. Microfluidic devices offer several advantages, including rapid detection, ease-of-use, portability, disposability, cost-effectiveness, a low required sample volume, multiplex detection, controlled sample injection, and an ultra-low detection limit. An analytical technique needs to be coupled with the microfluidic assay to produce the quantitative results throughout the detection process, and the integration of the SERS technique with microfluidic assays enables quantitative results as well as improved sensitivity. In a SERS integrated microfluidic chip, the microchannels are modified using SERS tag labeled nanomaterials and capture antibodies or antigens. The analyte sample is injected into the sample inlet where the sample flows in the channel through the capillary force, is separated and captured on the modified surface, and is detected using the SERS technique. Since the SERS integration improves the sensitivity and quantitative results as well as improving the detection efficacy of the microfluidic device, they are utilized widely for the estimation of biomarkers [28–32]. In a recent study, a SERS integrated microfluidics platform was developed by Choi *et al* for the detection of fraction 1 (F1) antigen in *Y. pestis* with a low LOD of 59.6 pg ml^{-1}. Herein, they fabricated microfluidic devices of PDMS through the soft lithography technique to construct a micro-channel. The sandwich method was utilized to detect the F1 antigen, where they were captured between a monoclonal antibody functionalized carboxylated magnetic bead and polyclonal antibody functionalized AuNPs labeled with the SERS nanotag in the channels of the microfluidic assay. Subsequently, magnetic separation was carried out to remove the functionalized magnetic bead, and then the recorded Raman intensity was measured to determine the F1 antigen quantitatively. The proposed immunoassay was twice as sensitive as the conventional ELISA as well being rapid (<10 min) and fully automated which reduces the overall detection time. A representation of the composition of the SERS integrated microfluidic device and its detection process for F1 antigens is shown in figure 6.3 [33].

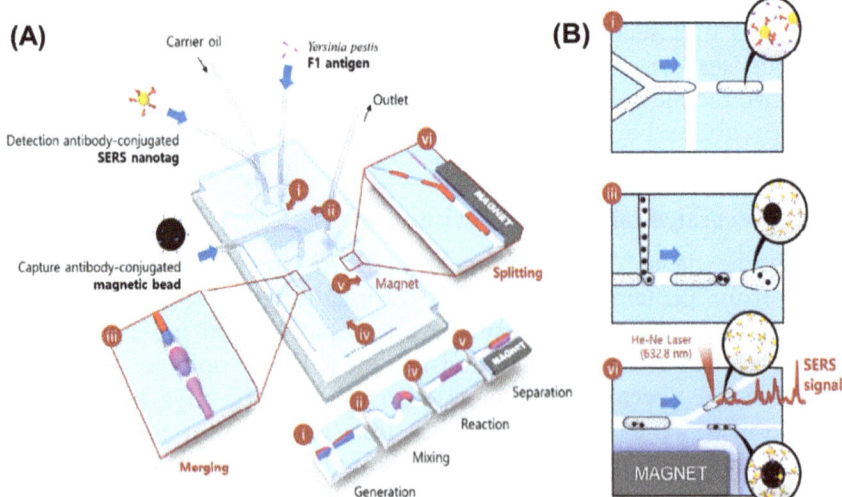

Figure 6.3. (A) Schematic of a SERS integrated microfluidic channel composed of six microdroplet compartments: (i) droplet generation, (ii) droplet mixing, (iii) droplet merging, (iv) droplet mixing, (v) droplet splitting, and (vi) Raman detection of unbound SERS nanotags. (B) Detailed images for (i) droplet generation, (iii) droplet merging, and (vi) droplet splitting. (Reproduced with permission from [33]. Copyright 2017 American Chemical Society.)

In another study, the detection of *L. monocytogenes* was achieved within 100 s on a microfluidic chip. This immunostrip was developed by Rodríguez-Lorenzo *et al* using SERS tag labeled gold nanostars coated with silica nanoparticles. This integrated system provided a controlled sampling and automated detection strategy with excellent reproducibility. Gold nanostars have a high plasmonic nature that improves the signal intensity and their high surface area increases the high immobilization of antibodies which improves the sensitivity of the assay. In addition, gold nanostars affect the binding chemistry of the antibody–antigen which impacts the binding efficacy of the conjugate antibody compared to the free antibody which can deviate from the original result [34]. A similar sensing approach using Ag nanoclusters has been proposed by Dina and co-workers for the rapid detection of bacteria. Herein, they grew the Ag nanoclusters *in situ* in the microfluidic channel through the passage of silver nitrate salt and citrate reducing agent. The four bacteria were captured in separate channels where they exhibited similar Raman signals at 725 cm^{-1}, 1089 cm^{-1}, and 1316 cm^{-1} at different intensities [35]. Similarly, Kraft *et al* applied colloidal AgNP solution with 60–70 nm NP size and a concentration of 0.1–4.0 mg ml^{-1} for identifying *E. coli* and *Pseudomonas taiwanensis* (*P. taiwanensis*) bacteria in water. They studied the effect of varying the concentrations of the AgNPs, and the maximum SERS intensity was achieved for 1.0 mg ml^{-1} of AgNPs, which showed a high surface enhancement effect, resulting in the effective sensing of both bacteria at lower detection concentrations [36]. Another work was reported by Zhuang *et al* using a recombinase polymerase amplification (CRISPR/Cas)-combined SERS microfluidic device to detect *S. typhimurium* in meat and milk samples. This study shows the effects of the concentration of bacteria

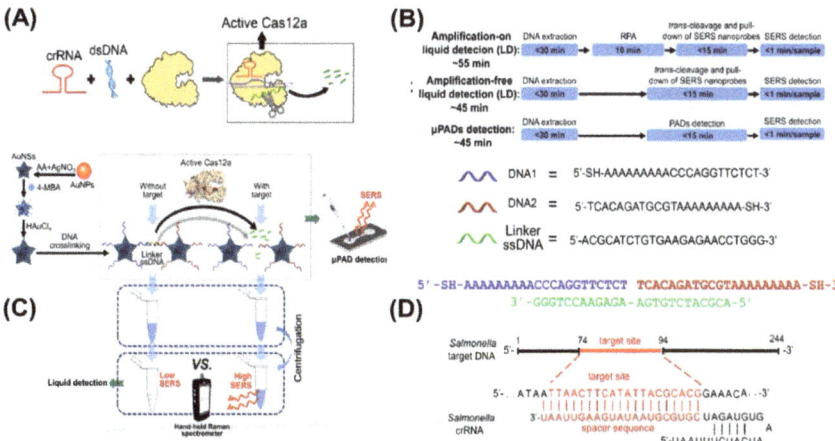

Figure 6.4. The Raman-based CRISPR/Cas biosensor for detection of pathogenic bacteria. (A) The activation of CRISPR/Cas12a for trans-cleavage. The green ribbon represents single-stranded DNA subject to trans-cleavage. (B) The preparation of AuNS@4-MBA@Au and their utility in combination with CRISPR/Cas12a for SERS-based bacterial detection for both in-tube and *μ*PAD detection. (C) The schematics of the biosensing processes with the estimated assay time for each step. (D) The nucleic acid sequences required for the proposed biosensor and the hybridization of linker ssDNA with DNA1 and DNA2. (Reproduced with permission from [37]. Copyright 2022 Elsevier.)

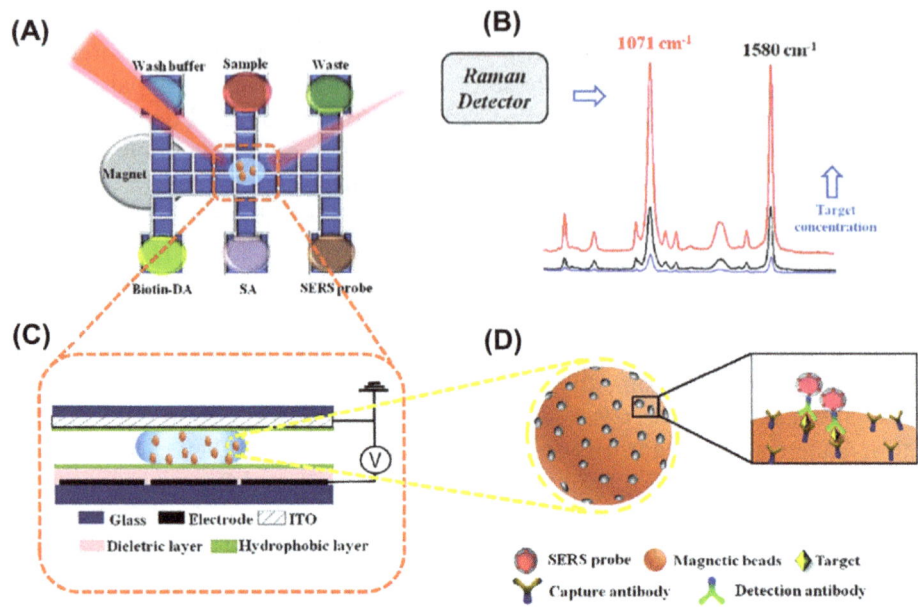

Figure 6.5. Schematic of the SERS-based immunoassay with digital microfluidics (DMF). (A) DMF-SERS method and bottom plate of the DMF chip. (B) Two characteristic Raman peaks of 4-MBA. (C) Side view of the DMF chip containing a droplet with magnetic beads. (D) Immunocomplex functionalized with SERS tags on magnetic beads. (Reproduced with permission from [38]. Copyright 2018 American Chemical Society.)

on the agglomeration of SERS probes which were estimated on the microfluidic paper device through Raman spectrum measurements (figure 6.4) [37].

A study by Wang *et al* proposed an ultrasensitive sandwich assay of a SERS integrated programmed digital microfluidic device for detection of the avian influenza H5N1 virus in the serum sample. Herein, the Raman reporter 4-mercaptobenzoic acid (4-MBA) was labeled on the Au@Ag core–shell nanostructure to prepare the SERS tag. Since AgNPs display a high enhancement factor compared to AuNPs, therefore the authors chose the AgNPs for the coating. Furthermore, the SERS tag was modified through the detection antibody coated with magnetic beads that selectively target the H5N1 antigen. It has been found that the reported device detected the H5N1 antigen within 1 h in as low as ~30 μl of the clinical sample having a low LOD of 74 pg ml^{-1}. Since the assay is fully automated and digitalized, it could be potentially utilized for other viral and pathogenic bacterial detection. A schematic representation of the SERS-based immunoassay with digital microfluidics for the detection of the influenza virus is shown in figure 6.5 [38].

A loop-mediated isothermal amplification (LAMP)-based SERS microfluidic device was proposed by Teixeira *et al* for the detection of *L. monocytogenes*. Thiolated polyethylene glycol (PEG) was functionalized on AuNPs labeled with glutathione as a chelating agent and a 1-naphthalenethiol Raman reporter. The *L. monocytogenes* was quantified through the examination of Raman intensity of the reporter molecule which was associated with the agglomeration of AuNPs. The nanoparticle agglomeration was triggered by the formation of pyrophosphate in the LAMP reaction during the DNA amplification process causing stable complex formation which improves the Raman intensity [39]. In another report, Witkowska *et al* developed a SERS-magnetomicrofluidic platform for the detection of two pathogens, *Porphyromonas gingivalis* and *Aggregatibacter actino-mycetemcomitans* bacteria, in human saliva samples, which cause a gum disease related to Alzheimer's disease. The bacteria were mixed with silver coated magnetic nanoparticles (Fe_3O_4@AgNPs), where bacteria were absorbed, separated magnetically, and detected on the microfluidic device. However, the assay was coupled with the Si/Ag SERS platform to achieve the enhanced Raman signal, which significantly improved the sensitivity of the device. In addition to this, the authors successfully separated *P. gingivalis* with 89% accuracy from the *A. actinomycetemcomitans* strain in the saliva sample through principal component analysis (PCA). Thus, the SERS-PCA technique provides a selective, sensitive, and cost-effective detection strategy and could also be used to detect bacteria in cerebrospinal fluid and blood samples [40].

6.2.3 SERS integrated electrochemical biosensor

The electrochemical (EC) technique appears to be a highly significant biosensor platform for the detection of infectious diseases owing to several advantages, including quantitative results, high sensitivity, selectivity, portability, ease of fabrication and operation, disposability, cost-effectiveness, and very small sample volumes (a drop of the sample) for the whole detection process. Electrochemical biosensors are classified based on the technique applied for the quantitative estimation, which can be voltammetric, amperometric, or impedimetric [41, 42]. The materials for the fabrication of the electrochemical working electrodes need to be easy to synthesize or commercially available. The frequently utilized nano-materials are metal nanoparticles (AuNPs, AgNPs, CuNPs, etc), metal oxides (ZnO, CeO_2, TiO_2, ZrO_2, etc), conductive polymeric materials, carbon-based materials (graphene oxide, reduced graphene oxide, quantum dots, carbon nanotubes), and their hybrid nanocomposites. The nanomaterials are immobilized on either a glassy carbon electrode (GCE), screen printed electrode (SPE), indium tin oxide (ITO), or fluorine-doped tin oxide (FTO) surface to fabricate the working electrode followed by surface modification using a target-specific antibody that selectively captures the target antigen to generate a quantifiable result. EC biosensors offer label-free detection and avoid the sample pre-treatment process which benefit the rapid detection of biomolecules and hazardous chemicals. In addition, they can transform into wearable and flexible devices which provide a low-cost POC diagnostic platform for on-site healthcare applications [43, 44]. The right combination of two techniques, such as electrochemical with SERS, provides a superior sensing platform for quantitative detection of infectious diseases. The integration of both technologies in a single sensing strategy overcomes the drawbacks of single-technique-based detection as well as providing a dual sensing platform.

Researchers found that the SERS signal intensity is affected greatly by potential dependent electromagnetic enhancement, which is associated with the characteristics of surface plasmon resonance. However, potential applied through the electro-chemical technique improves the electromagnetic field through a change in elec-tronic distribution, surface orientation, and electric field, which attract the molecules near the electromagnetic field and improves their electromagnetic effect. Therefore, EC integration improved the above phenomena effectively, resulting in a high sensitivity of biosensors [45–47]. For instance, Lynk et al, for the first time, used a SERS coupled EC biosensor to identify and detect bacteria. Herein, they coated three layers of 24 nm sized AgNPs on SPE to produce uniform coverage of the electrode surface. Furthermore, it was treated with 0.5 M KCl to remove the citrate ions attached to the AgNPs. The removal of citrate ions improves the intensity of the SERS signal considerably, which improves the sensitivity for bacterial detection [48]. Similar work was reported by McLeod et al based on SERS-EC electrodes using the deposition of three layered AgNPs on SPE for the detection of either *Bacillus megaterium* or *E. coli* bacteria. Herein, they fabricated the electrodes and immersed them in *B. megaterium* or *E. coli* bacteria solution which was dried under ambient conditions, and then a potential was applied on the electrode surface that appeared with characteristic Raman signals for both different bacteria. The developed method is highly sensitive and reliable and can also be employed for screening other pathogens [49]. Very recently, Lee et al utilized a similar platform for quantification of *Enterococcus faecium* (*E. faecium*) and *S. aureus* bacteria. Before the detection, they performed the electrodeposition of gold nanopillars which were functionalized by the complementary DNA that selectively targeted both bacteria [50]. Very recently, Hendricks-Leukes et al proposed a SERS-EC platform for *Mycobacterium tuberculosis* (*M. tuberculosis*) detection. In this study, a uniform layer of AgNPs on the electrode surface was immobilized through the Tollens' based synthesis process. This biosensor was able to detect and differentiate between three strains of tuber-culosis, TB-H37Rv, TB-CDC1551, and TB-HN878. Therefore, it improved the ability to identify the exact disease-causing bacteria. A schematic of a SERS integrated electrochemical biosensor for the detection of mycobacteria is shown in figure 6.6 [51].

6.2.4 SERS integrated machine learning device

Machine learning is a statistics-based advanced algorithm technique that assumes the property of target species without calculating their electronic assembly. It predicts the energy of the surface, band gap, bond energy, and so forth. On this basis, researchers can determine the materials and molecules precisely [52–56]. A machine-learning-based detection approach combined with the SERS technique has been demonstrated by Rahman et al for selective detection of the *E. coli* 8739 strain. In this method, the SERS sensor was made using AuNPs modified with lectin functionalized bacterial cellulose nanocrystals. This sensor showed an excellent accuracy of 87.7% and an LOD of 10^3 CFU ml^{-1} and could efficiently distinguish the 19 bacterial strains which were investigated using a support vector machine [57].

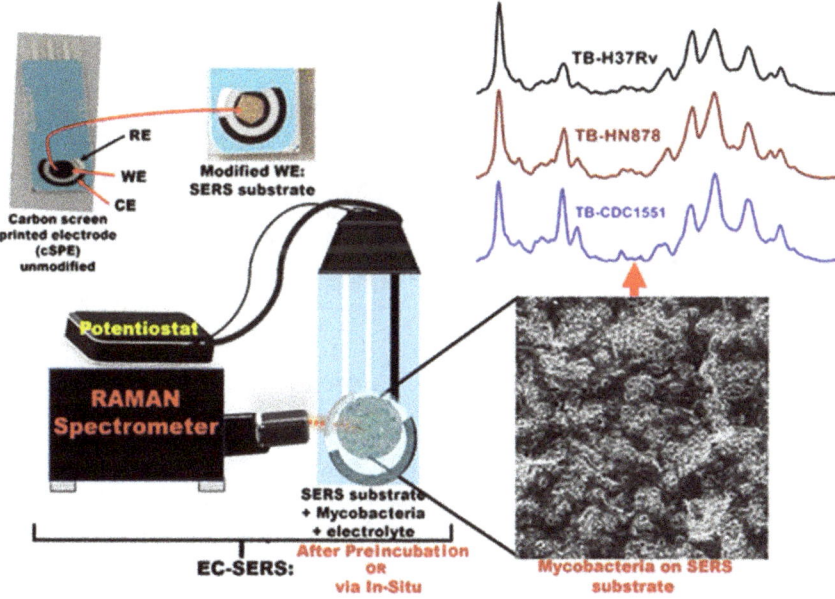

Figure 6.6. Schematic of a SERS integrated electrochemical biosensor for detection of mycobacteria. (Reproduced with permission from [51]. Copyright 2022 American Chemical Society.)

Very recently, Torun *et al* reported an aptamer-based SERS sensor for the detection of SARS-CoV-2 as well as its alpha and beta variants. The machine learning statistics showed a high sensitivity of 95.2% and good selectivity after testing of 33 negative and 36 positive samples, which is confirmed by PCR technique [58]. However, much research remains in this field to advance the algorithmic- or statistic-based real-time prediction for the rapid detection of infectious diseases.

6.2.5 Other SERS integrated devices

Numerous other SERS integrated detection platforms have been reported for the detection of infectious diseases. For example, Gao *et al* developed a SERS integrated platform for the detection and photothermal killing of *S. aureus* bacteria in a whole blood sample. The authors used a sandwich assay where one part was the vancomycin-modified gold core and Prussian blue shell nanoparticles which represented the SERS tag, while the second part was 4-mercaptophenyl boronic acid modified plasmonic gold film and 4-mercaptobenzonitrile as the SERS substrate. When the bacteria are captured between both substrates, a characteristic Raman signal appeared. An 808 nm laser was used to kill the bacteria through the photothermal effect. Therefore, this method offers a promising platform for the detection and killing of bacteria. The process of the preparation of nanomaterials, their modifications and the detection of bacteria is depicted in figure 6.7 [59]. Paul *et al* reported a bioconjugated gold nanoparticle-based SERS platform for the detection of mosquito-borne viruses such as dengue and West Nile virus. The gold

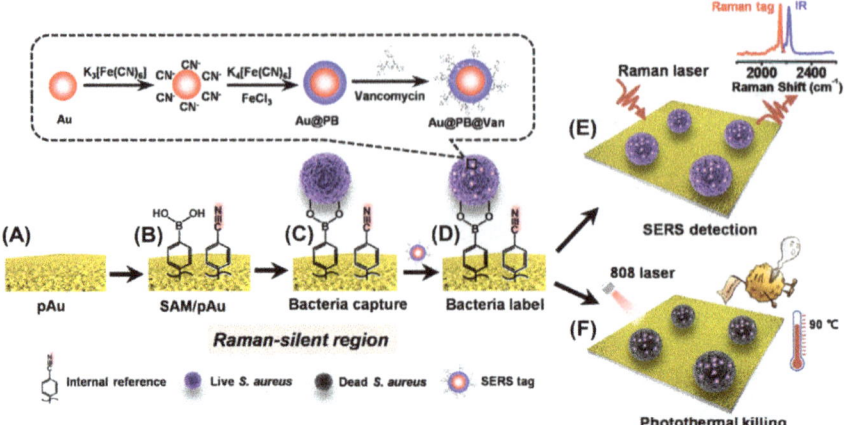

Figure 6.7. (A) and (B) The procedure for the preparation of SAM/pAu. (C) Bacteria capture and (D) their labeling process. (E) Bacteria determination is based on the sandwich SERS platform. (F) *In situ* elimination of bacteria due to the synergistic photothermal effect. (Reproduced with permission from [59]. Copyright 2020 American Chemical Society.)

nanoparticles functionalized to the 4G2 antibody which selectively captured the dengue and West Nile viruses that exhibited Raman signatures, with an LOD of 10 PFU ml^{-1}. Moreover, this assay showed a 10^4-fold Raman enhancement effect due to the assembled structure causing strong electric field enhancement [60]. To extend this work, the gold nanoparticle coated silicon dioxide (Au@SiO$_2$)-based SERS substrate chip was demonstrated by Boardman *et al* for rapid quantification of two bacteria, *S. aureus* and *E. coli*, in as little as a microliter of the whole blood sample. The developed platform detected these two bacteria within 7 h with 88% and 97% sensitivity and specificity, respectively [61].

In another study, a SERS platform was developed using gold nanorods (GNRs) by Tadesse *et al* for the estimation of gram-positive and -negative bacteria in a water sample. A varied concentration ratio of GNRs and bacteria samples were mixed where the positively charged GNRs bound to the negatively charged bacteria; as they appear to have specific SERS signal with enhanced intensities. The enhancement of the SERS signal is related to the higher surface charge density of bacteria, in which gram-positive bacteria exhibit high signal enhancement compared to gram-negative bacteria that are used to distinguish the gram-positive and -negative bacteria (figure 6.8) [62].

In another study, Kukushkin *et al* developed a sandwich-type SERS-based aptasensor for the detection of the influenza virus. The authors prepared RHA0385 aptamers functionalized via the thiol group of silver nanoparticles as a Raman substrate and Raman dye-labeled with a secondary aptamer. The virus particles capture both aptamers and generate Raman signals in the fingerprint region. The developed biosensor is rapid and detected the virus within 12 min, with an LOD of 10^4 particle/sample. In addition to this, the aptasensor is capable of detecting different strains such as H1, H3, and H5 of the influenza virus sensitively.

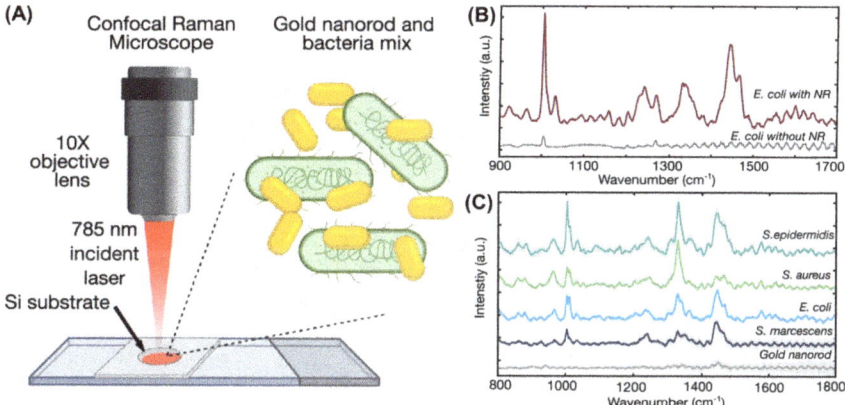

Figure 6.8. Overview of the liquid-SERS chamber and plasmonic nanoparticles employed. (A) Liquid well imaging set-up with bacteria and gold nanorods. (B) Comparison of *E. coli* Raman spectra with and without the 670 nm nanorods. (C) Liquid-SERS spectra of the four bacterial species mixed with the 670 nm nanorods. (Reproduced with permission from [62]. Copyright 2020 American Chemical Society.)

Hence, the high efficacy of the biosensors offers the detection of a wide range of infection-causing particles [63]. Similarly, Chen *et al* detected the SARS-CoV-2 in nasopharyngeal swabs using the SERS-based aptasensor. In this aptasensor, the receptor was a Cy3 Raman reporter conjugated spike protein deoxyribonucleic acid aptamer and the SERS detection component of 4-MBA was an internal standard reporter modified gold nanopopcorn. They observed that the DNA aptamer moved away from the surface of the gold nanopopcorn when the binding of the spike protein increased and, as a result, the peak intensity of the Cy3 was reduced which estimated the quantification of SARS-COV-2 at an LOD of 10 PFU ml^{-1}. The resulting aptasensor has two-fold higher sensitivity than the commercially available kit which makes it a more promising sensor for SARS-CoV-2 detection (table 6.1). A schematic of the quantitative estimation of SARS-CoV-2 through a SERS-based aptasensor is illustrated in figure 6.9 [64].

6.3 Challenges and outlook

SERS is a most fascinating technique which offers highly sensitive diagnostic applications for a wide range of analytes, including pathogenic bacteria, viruses, cancer biomarkers, and toxic chemicals. SERS provides significant Raman signals in the fingerprint region which make the detection process easier. Their ultra-low detection limits make them promising candidates in healthcare applications. The SERS technique can be coupled readily with other analytical techniques that improve the sensitivity and detection limit of the biosensor [7, 65]. Further research is required to enhance the wide-ranging applicability SERS before achieving full implementation. Despite its several advantages, SERS suffers from several challenges in the diagnostic field. One of the drawbacks of the SERS technique is the requirement for plasmonic nanomaterials and further labeling with the Raman

Table 6.1. SERS integrated detection techniques for the quantification of infectious diseases.

Nanomaterial	Detection method	Target analyte	LOD	Clinical sample	Time	Reference
SiO$_2$@Ag	LFIA	Anti-SARS-CoV-2 IgM/IgG	1.0 pg ml^{-1}	Serum	25 min	[21]
AuAg4-ATP@AgNPs	LFIA	Influenza virus	0.0018 HAU	Swab	20 min	[22]
Fe$_3$O$_4$@AgNPs	LFIA	Influenza A H1N1 and HAdV virus	50 and 10 PFU ml^{-1}	Blood, serum, and sputum	30 min	[23]
Fe$_3$O$_4$@Au/ Au@DTNB@PA	Aptasensor	E. coli, L. mono, and S. typhimurium	10–25 cells/ml	Food	—	[24]
Fe$_3$O$_4$@Au/Au@BSA	LFIA	S. typhimurium and S. aureus	12 and 9 cells ml^{-1}	Food	30 min	[25]
AuNPs	LFIA	Y. pestis, F. tularensis, and B. anthracis	43.4 CFU ml^{-1}, 45.8 CFU ml^{-1}, and 357 CFU ml^{-1}	—	15 min	[26]
GO@Au/Ag	LFIA	S. aureus, S. typhi, L. mono, and E. coli	9 cells/ml	—	20 min	[27]
Carboxylated magnetic bead and AuNPs	Microfluidic	Antigen fraction 1	59.6 pg ml^{-1}	—	<10 min	[33]
Gold nanostars	Microfluidic	L. monocytogenes	1 × 10^5 CFU ml^{-1}	Food	100 sec	[34]
AgNPs	Microfluidic	E. coli TOP10, P. aeruginosa, S. aureus, and E. faecalis	—	Tap water	15 min	[35]
AgNPs	Microfluidic	E. coli and P. taiwanesis	—	Water	—	[36]
—	Microfluidic	S. typhimurium	3–4 CFU ml^{-1}	Milk and meat	45 min	[37]
Au@AgNPs	Microfluidic	Avian influenza H5N1 virus	74 pg ml^{-1}	Serum	< 1 h	[38]
AuNPs	LAMP	L. monocytogenes	—	Food, milk	—	[39]
Fe$_2$O$_3$@AgNPs	Microfluidic	P. gingivalis and A. actinomycetemcomitans	10^3 CFU ml^{-1}	Saliva	—	[40]
AgNPs/GCE	EC	B. megaterium or E. coli	—	—	—	[49]
AuNPs-DNA	EC	E. faecium and S. aureus	~0.035 nM	Blood	10 min	[50]

(*Continued*)

Table 6.1. (*Continued*)

Nanomaterial	Detection method	Target analyte	LOD	Clinical sample	Time	Reference
Polyelectrolyte wrapping of AgNPs	EC	*Mycobacterium tuberculosis*	—	Sputum and urine	—	[51]
Lectin-modified bacterial cellulose nanocrystals-AuNPs	Machine Learning	*E. coli*	10^3 CFU ml^{-1}	—	—	[57]
AuNPs	—	Dengue virus (DENV) and West Nile virus (WNV)	10 PFU ml^{-1}	Blood	30 min	[60]
—	—	*Staphylococcus aureus* and *E. coli*	—	Blood	—	[61]
Gold nanorod	—	*E. coli, S. marcescens, S. aureus*, and *S. epidermidis*	—	Water	—	[62]
AgNPs	Aptasensor	Influenza virus	1×10^{-4} HAU/probe	—	12 min	[63]
Au nanopopcorn	Aptasensor	SARS-CoV-2	10 CFU ml^{-1}	Nasopharyngeal swab	15 min	[64]

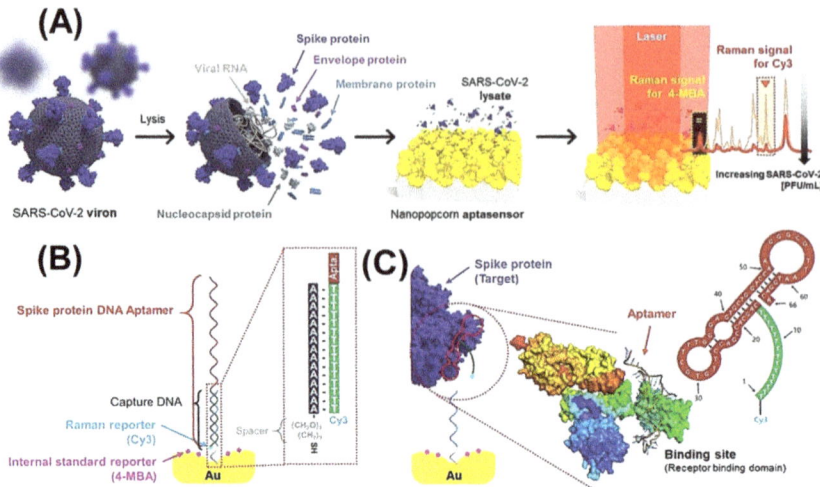

Figure 6.9. Schematic of the quantitative estimation of SARS-CoV-2 using a SERS-based aptasensor. (A) After SARS-CoV-2 lysates release the target spike proteins. (B) Cy3-tagged aptamer DNAs are hybridized with capture DNAs on the Au nanopopcorn substrate. (C) Recognition of the spike protein of SARS-CoV-2 induces a conformational change of aptamer DNAs, enabling the aptamer DNAs to bind with the receptor-binding domain (RBD) on the spike protein. (Reproduced with permission from [64]. Copyright 2021 American Chemical Society.)

reporter to enhance the signal intensity. Since the nanomaterials are less efficient, they possess low optical signal intensity for the target molecule. In addition, the plasmonic nanomaterials have limited stability in a solution. Specific Raman reporters and their selection for the labeling of molecules are needed urgently to improve the enhancement factor. In addition to this, the signal consistency and reproducibility over the large batch of sample detection concerns the reliability of the results. However, costly and bulkier instrumentation can further restrict the full employment of SERS-based diagnostics for POC home sensing [66]. The integrated SERS techniques also suffer from some challenging issues. One of the foremost problems of the SERS integrated electrochemical technique is to avoid the distortion of the solvent layer and the adsorption of the analyte on the electrode surface. The potential dependent multiple electrochemical scans and degradation of the reactive surface can affect the optical signal [2, 46, 67]. The LFIA strip offers a simple qualitative detection process through the visual analysis of the colors which appear on the test and control lines. SERS integration with LFIA strips overcomes their limited sensitivity and qualitative results, as well as improving the detection ability even in the presence of a low concentration of infectious biomarkers. Similarly, electrochemical and automated microfluidic devices coupled with SERS enhance the high-throughput results [2, 19, 67]. Thus far, machine learning and artificial intelligence (AI)-based statistical results offer a new direction in the diagnostic field. The advantages, challenges, and prospects of SERS-based assays in bioanalysis and diagnosis are shown in figure 6.10 [2]. Beyond the challenges, SERS has huge

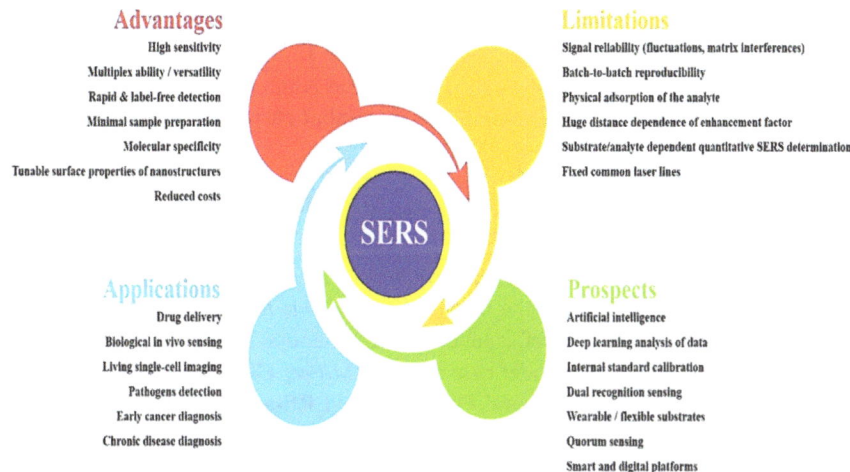

Figure 6.10. Prospects and challenges of SERS-based assays in bioanalysis and diagnosis. (Reproduced with permission from [2]. CC BY 3.0.)

potential in the biosensor-based diagnostic platform. Furthermore, SERS integration with sensitive analytical techniques can resolve the limitations of single-technique-based diagnosis which significantly improves the detection efficiency, reproducibility, and accuracy of the biosensor.

6.4 Summary

A concise review of SERS and its integration with sensitive analytical techniques for the detection of infectious diseases including viruses and pathogenic bacteria have been discussed in this chapter. In addition, the fabrication of the different types of biosensors, and their working and detection processes are discussed. Then, we cover briefly the limitations and future advancements in SERS integrated techniques for the detection of infectious particles.

Conflicts of interest

The authors declare no conflict of interest.

Acknowledgments

The authors thank sincerely Director, CSIR-AMPRI for their encouragement in this work. PR and SY are grateful to CSIR, India, for SRF and JRF, respectively. MAS is grateful to DST-SERB for JRF. RK would like to acknowledge CSIR for providing funds in the form of the IPA/2020/000130 project.

References

[1] Yadav S *et al* 2021 SERS based lateral flow immunoassay for point-of-care detection of SARS-CoV-2 in clinical samples *ACS Appl. Bio Mater.* **4** 2974–95

[2] Tahir M A, Dina N E, Cheng H, Valev V K and Zhang L 2021 Surface-enhanced Raman spectroscopy for bioanalysis and diagnosis *Nanoscale* **13** 11593–634

[3] Parihar A, Ranjan P, Sanghi S K, Srivastava A K and Khan R 2020 Point-of-care biosensor-based diagnosis of COVID-19 holds promise to combat current and future pandemics *ACS Appl. Bio Mater.* **3** 7326–43

[4] Sadique M A, Yadav S, Ranjan P, Akram Khan M, Kumar A and Khan R 2021 Rapid detection of SARS-CoV-2 using graphene-based IoT integrated advanced electrochemical biosensor *Mater. Lett.* **305** 130824

[5] Ranjan P *et al* 2021 Rapid diagnosis of SARS-CoV-2 using potential point-of-care electro-chemical immunosensor: toward the future prospects *Int. Rev. Immunol.* **40** 126–42

[6] Sadique M A *et al* 2021 High-performance antiviral nano-systems as a shield to inhibit viral infections: SARS-CoV-2 as a model case study *J. Mater. Chem.* B **9** 4620–42

[7] Wang Z, Zong S, Wu L, Zhu D and Cui Y 2017 SERS-activated platforms for immuno-assay: probes, encoding methods, and applications *Chem. Rev.* **117** 7910–63

[8] Zhou X, Schuh D A, Castle L M and Furst A L 2022 Recent advances in signal amplification to improve electrochemical biosensing for infectious diseases *Front. Chem.* **10** 1–8

[9] Sadique M A, Ranjan P, Yadav S and Khan R 2022 Advanced high-throughput biosensor-based diagnostic approaches for detection of severe acute respiratory syndrome-coronavirus-2 *Computational Approaches for Novel Therapeutic and Diagnostic Designing to Mitigate SARS-CoV-2 Infection* (New York: Academic) pp 147–69

[10] Ranjan P, Sadique M A, Yadav S and Khan R 2022 Approaches for fabrication of point-of-care biosensors for viral infection *Advanced Biosensors for Virus Detection: Smart Diagnostics to Combat SARS-CoV-2* (New York: Academic) pp 353–71

[11] Yoo S M and Lee S Y 2016 Optical biosensors for the detection of pathogenic micro-organisms *Trends Biotechnol.* **34** 7–25

[12] Sharma A *et al* 2021 Optical biosensors for diagnostics of infectious viral disease: a recent update *Diagnostics* **11** 2083

[13] Liu Y, Zhan L, Qin Z, Sackrison J and Bischof J C 2021 Ultrasensitive and highly specific lateral flow assays for point-of-care diagnosis *ACS Nano* **15** 3593–611

[14] Sohrabi H, Majidi M R, Fakhraei M, Jahanban-Esfahlan A, Hejazi M, Oroojalian F, Baradaran B, Tohidast M, de la Guardia M and Mokhtarzadeh A 2022 Lateral flow assays (LFA) for detection of pathogenic bacteria: a small point-of-care platform for diagnosis of human infectious diseases *Talanta* **243** 123330

[15] Ince B and Sezgintürk M K 2022 Lateral flow assays for viruses diagnosis: up-to-date technology and future prospects *TrAC Trends Anal. Chem.* **157** 116725

[16] Jagannath A, Cong H, Hassan J, Gonzalez G, Gilchrist M D and Zhang N 2022 Pathogen detection on microfluidic platforms: recent advances, challenges, and prospects *Biosens. Bioelectron.* X **10** 100134

[17] Su W, Gao X, Jiang L and Qin J 2015 Microfluidic platform towards point-of-care diagnostics in infectious diseases *J. Chromatogr.* A **1377** 13–26

[18] Tay A, Pavesi A, Yazdi S R, Lim C T and Warkiani M E 2016 Advances in microfluidics in combating infectious diseases *Biotechnol. Adv.* **34** 404–21

[19] Kim K *et al* 2021 Recent advances in sensitive surface-enhanced Raman scattering-based lateral flow assay platforms for point-of-care diagnostics of infectious diseases *Sens. Actuators* B **329** 129214

[20] Ranjan P, Sadique M A, Yadav S, Parihar A and Khan R 2022 Miniaturized analytical system for point-of-care coronavirus infection diagnostics *Advanced Biosensors for Virus Detection: Smart Diagnostics to Combat SARS-CoV-2* (New York: Academic) pp 305–40

[21] Liu H *et al* 2021 Development of a SERS-based lateral flow immunoassay for rapid and ultra-sensitive detection of anti-SARS-CoV-2 IgM/IgG in clinical samples *Sens. Actuators* B **329** 129196

[22] Xiao M *et al* 2019 Ultrasensitive detection of avian influenza A (H7N9) virus using surface-enhanced Raman scattering-based lateral flow immunoassay strips *Anal. Chim. Acta.* **1053** 139–47

[23] Wang C *et al* 2019 Magnetic SERS strip for sensitive and simultaneous detection of respiratory viruses *ACS Appl. Mater. Interfaces* **11** 19495–505

[24] Zhou Z *et al* 2021 A universal SERS-label immunoassay for pathogen bacteria detection based on Fe3O4@Au-aptamer separation and antibody–protein A orientation recognition *Anal. Chim. Acta.* **1160** 338421

[25] Li J *et al* 2022 Nanogapped Fe_3O_4@Au surface-enhanced Raman scattering tags for the multiplex detection of bacteria on an immunochromatographic strip *ACS Appl. Nano Mater.* **5** 6–11

[26] Wang R *et al* 2018 Highly sensitive detection of high-risk bacterial pathogens using SERS-based lateral flow assay strips *Sens. Actuators* B **270** 72–9

[27] Wang C, Wang C, Li J, Tu Z, Gu B and Wang S 2022 Ultrasensitive and multiplex detection of four pathogenic bacteria on a bi-channel lateral flow immunoassay strip with three-dimensional membrane-like SERS nanostickers *Biosens. Bioelectron.* **214** 3–5

[28] Yue S, Fang J and Xu Z 2022 Advances in droplet microfluidics for SERS and Raman analysis *Biosens. Bioelectron.* **198** 113822

[29] Chen H *et al* 2020 Recent advances in surface-enhanced Raman scattering-based microdevices for point-of-care diagnosis of viruses and bacteria *Nanoscale* **12** 21560–70

[30] Guo J, Zeng F, Guo J and Ma X 2020 Preparation and application of microfluidic SERS substrate: challenges and future perspectives *J. Mater. Sci. Technol.* **37** 96–103

[31] Khan R, Dhand C, Sanghi S K, Salammal S T and Mishra A B P 2022 *Commercialization of Microfluidic Point-of-Care Diagnostic Devices* 1st edn (Boca Raton, FL: CRC Press)

[32] Parihar A, Parihar D S, Ranjan P and Khan R 2022 *Role of Microfluidics-Based Point-of-Care Testing (POCT) for Clinical Applications* 1st edn (Boca Raton, FL: CRC Press)

[33] Choi N *et al* 2017 Integrated SERS-based microdroplet platform for the automated immunoassay of F1 antigens in *Yersinia pestis Anal. Chem.* **89** 8413–20

[34] Rodríguez-Lorenzo L *et al* 2019 Gold nanostars for the detection of foodborne pathogens via surface-enhanced Raman scattering combined with microfluidics *ACS Appl. Nano Mater.* **2** 6081–6

[35] Dina N E, Colniță A, Marconi D and Gherman A M R 2020 Microfluidic portable device for pathogens' rapid SERS detection *Proceedings* **60** 2

[36] Krafft B, Tycova A, Urban R D, Dusny C and Belder D 2021 Microfluidic device for concentration and SERS-based detection of bacteria in drinking water *Electrophoresis* **42** 86–94

[37] Zhuang J *et al* 2022 SERS-based CRISPR/Cas assay on microfluidic paper analytical devices for supersensitive detection of pathogenic bacteria in foods *Biosens. Bioelectron.* **207** 114167

[38] Wang Y *et al* 2018 Highly sensitive and automated surface enhanced Raman scattering-based immunoassay for H5N1 detection with digital microfluidics *Anal. Chem.* **90** 5224–31

[39] Teixeira A *et al* 2020 Multifunctional gold nanoparticles for the SERS detection of pathogens combined with a LAMP-in-microdroplets approach *Materials* **13** 1934

[40] Witkowska E, Łasica A M, Niciński K, Potempa J and Kamińska A 2021 In search of spectroscopic signatures of periodontitis: a SERS-based magnetomicrofluidic sensor for detection of *Porphyromonas gingivalis* and *Aggregatibacter actinomycetemcomitans ACS Sens.* **6** 1621–35

[41] Kaushik A K *et al* 2020 Electrochemical SARS-CoV-2 sensing at point-of-care and artificial intelligence for intelligent COVID-19 management *ACS Appl. Bio Mater.* **3** 7306–25

[42] Castle L M, Schuh D A, Reynolds E E and Furst A L 2021 Electrochemical sensors to detect bacterial foodborne pathogens *ACS Sens.* **6** 1717–30

[43] Zhu C, Yang G, Li H, Du D and Lin Y 2015 Electrochemical sensors and biosensors based on nanomaterials and nanostructures *Anal. Chem.* **87** 230–49

[44] Yang A and Yan F 2021 Flexible electrochemical biosensors for health monitoring *ACS Appl. Electron. Mater.* **3** 53–67

[45] Sundaresan V, Do H, Shrout J D and Bohn P W 2022 Electrochemical and spectroelectrochemical characterization of bacteria and bacterial systems *Analyst* **147** 22–34

[46] Moldovan R *et al* 2022 Review on combining surface-enhanced Raman spectroscopy and electrochemistry for analytical applications *Anal. Chim. Acta.* **1209** 339250

[47] Wu D Y, Li J F, Ren B and Tian Z Q 2008 Electrochemical surface-enhanced Raman spectroscopy of nanostructures *Chem. Soc. Rev.* **37** 1025–41

[48] Lynk T P, Sit C S and Brosseau C L 2018 Electrochemical surface-enhanced Raman spectroscopy as a platform for bacterial detection and identification *Anal. Chem.* **90** 12639–46

[49] McLeod K E R, Lynk T P, Sit C S and Brosseau C L 2019 On the origin of electrochemical surface-enhanced Raman spectroscopy (EC-SERS) signals for bacterial samples: the importance of filtered control studies in the development of new bacterial screening platforms *Anal. Methods* **11** 924–9

[50] Lee S H *et al* 2022 Organometallic hotspot engineering for ultrasensitive EC-SERS detection of pathogenic bacteria-derived DNAs *Biosens. Bioelectron.* **210** 114325

[51] Hendricks-Leukes N R, Jonas M R, Mlamla Z C, Smith M and Blackburn J M 2022 Dual-approach electrochemical surface-enhanced Raman scattering detection of *Mycobacterium tuberculosis* in patient-derived biological specimens: proof of concept for a generalizable method to detect and identify bacterial pathogens *ACS Sens.* **7** 1403–18

[52] Hu W *et al* 2019 Machine learning protocol for surface-enhanced Raman spectroscopy *J. Phys. Chem. Lett.* **10** 6026–31

[53] Prezhdo O V 2020 Advancing physical chemistry with machine learning *J. Phys. Chem. Lett.* **11** 9656–8

[54] Leong Y X *et al* 2022 Where nanosensors meet machine learning: prospects and challenges in detecting disease X *ACS Nano* **16** 13279–93

[55] Rojalin T, Antonio D, Kulkarni A and Carney R P 2022 Machine learning-assisted sampling of surface-enhanced Raman scattering (SERS) substrates improve data collection efficiency *Appl. Spectrosc.* **76** 485–95

[56] Pan L, Zhang P, Daengngam C, Peng S and Chongcheawchamnan M 2022 A review of artificial intelligence methods combined with Raman spectroscopy to identify the composition of substances *J. Raman Spectrosc.* **53** 6–19

[57] Rahman A, Kang S, Wang W, Huang Q, Kim I and Vikesland P J 2022 Lectin-modified bacterial cellulose nanocrystals decorated with Au nanoparticles for selective detection of bacteria using surface-enhanced Raman scattering coupled with machine learning *ACS Appl. Nano Mater.* **5** 259–68

[58] Torun H *et al* 2021 Machine learning detects SARS-CoV-2 and variants rapidly on DNA aptamer metasurfaces *MedRxiv*

[59] Gao X *et al* 2021 Integrated SERS platform for reliable detection and photothermal elimination of bacteria in whole blood samples *Anal. Chem.* **93** 1569–77

[60] Paul A M *et al* 2015 Bioconjugated gold nanoparticle based SERS probe for ultrasensitive identification of mosquito-borne viruses using Raman fingerprinting *J. Phys. Chem.* C **119** 23669–75

[61] Boardman A K *et al* 2016 Rapid detection of bacteria from blood with surface-enhanced Raman spectroscopy *Anal. Chem.* **88** 8026–35

[62] Tadesse L F *et al* 2020 Plasmonic and electrostatic interactions enable uniformly enhanced liquid bacterial surface-enhanced Raman scattering (SERS) *Nano Lett.* **20** 7655–61

[63] Kukushkin V I, Ivanov N M, Novoseltseva A A, Gambaryan A S, Yaminsky I V, Kopylov A M and Zavyalova E G 2019 Highly sensitive detection of influenza virus with SERS aptasensor *PLoS One* **14** e0216247

[64] Chen H *et al* 2021 Sensitive detection of SARS-CoV-2 using a SERS-based aptasensor *ACS Sens.* **6** 2378–85

[65] Wang L *et al* 2021 SERS-based test strips: principles, designs and applications *Biosens. Bioelectron.* **189** 113360

[66] Driscoll A J, Harpster M H and Johnson P A 2013 The development of surface-enhanced Raman scattering as a detection modality for portable *in vitro* diagnostics: progress and challenges *Phys. Chem. Chem. Phys.* **15** 20415–33

[67] Zong C *et al* 2018 Surface-enhanced Raman spectroscopy for bioanalysis: reliability and challenges *Chem. Rev.* **118** 4946–80

Chapter 7

SERS based conventional diagnostics for the diagnosis of SARS-CoV-2

Anwesha Kanungo and Sarbari Acharya[1]

The COVID-19 pandemic, caused by the severe acute respiratory syndrome coronavirus-2 (SARS-CoV-2), has been spreading continuously for several years and remains a worldwide menace. To design an accurate mode of treatment for this contagious and refractory disease, early and rapid diagnosis is essential. The current diagnostic techniques implemented for SARS-CoV-2, such as RT-PCR and ELISA, although effective, are often plagued by many defects. Thus, a simple, fast, easy-to-use, and portable diagnostic technique for mass screening is the need of the hour. In this context, an innovative method of Raman fingerprinting, using surface-enhanced Raman spectroscopy (SERS) techniques, has been proposed recently to detect SARS-CoV-2 at an early stage of infection. This analysis technique removes the requirement for sample processing time, giving instantaneous results. These SERS-based point-of-care devices use dedicated artificial intelligence (AI) algorithms and may emerge as a new platform for mass screening for the virus.

7.1 Introduction

Severe acute respiratory syndrome (SARS), initiated by a zoonosis, is a virus-related respiratory illness. SARS-associated coronavirus-1 (SARS-CoV-1) primarily occurred in China, in 2002, and quickly spread to over 30 countries. The first case of pneumonia-like SARS-associated coronavirus-2 (SARS-CoV-2) was recognized in Wuhan, China, in late December 2019. From then on SARS-CoV-2 has reached all the countries of the world. WHO proclaimed COVID-19 a pandemic on 11 March 2020, due to the global morbidity and mortality with increasing socio-economic consequence and severe health issue [1]. The reason for the concern regarding SARS-CoV-2 was that it is transferred easily from an infected person to a

---

[1] Both the authors have contributed equally.

non-infected person due to its extraordinarily infectious nature, and can spread quickly through physical interaction [1]. Thus, curtailing its spread was the most critical issue that healthcare personnel faced throughout the world.

The most important aspect of the management of any disease is its identification and diagnosis, specifically the stage of infection, because this determines the course and outcome of treatment. The most-used screening method during the early and late stages of SARS-CoV-2 viral infection is reverse transcription polymerase chain reaction (RT-PCR) [2]. The technique is highly specific for the virus and is done by altering the viral mRNA into DNA for amplification and detection through PCR. For the timely diagnosis of COVID-19, chest computed tomography (CT) plays an important role and involves taking numerous x-ray images from different angles all over the chest to generate tomographic images of the lungs [3]. In this context, surface-enhanced Raman scattering (SERS) may serve as an answer to surmount all the pitfalls of conventional diagnostic agents implemented for the identification of SARS-CoV-2. In addition being a time-consuming process, CT scans lack distinction between patients infected with COVID-19 or pneumonia making it unreliable, which provides impetus to find a more rapid, reliable, and sensitive diagnostic method for accurate disease detection.

SERS has experience a wide range of developments since its first discovery in 1928 (figure 7.1).

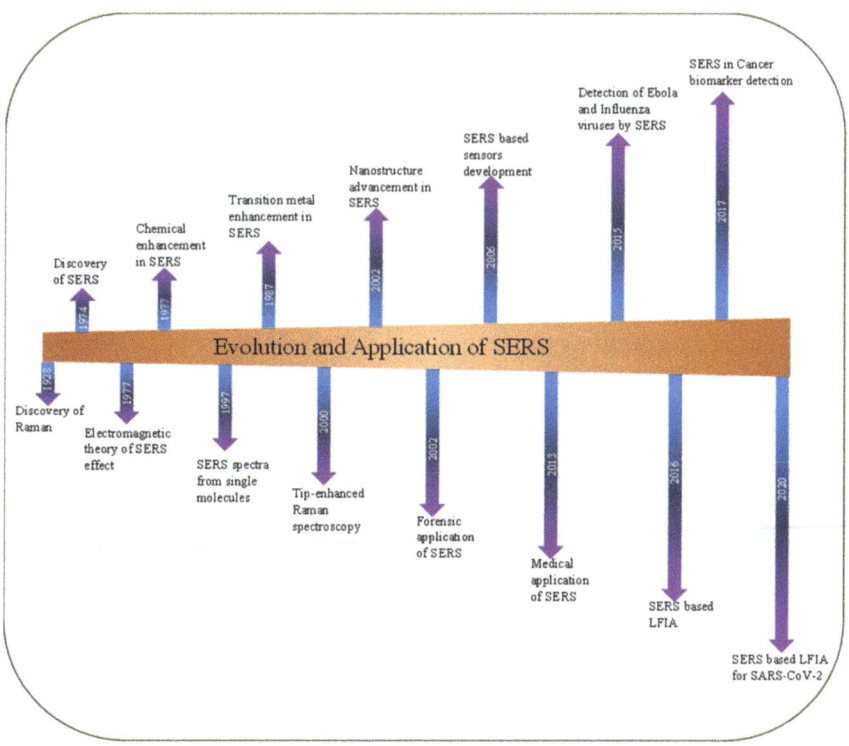

Figure 7.1. The evolution and applications of SERS.

SERS was inadvertently discovered by Fleischmann and co-workers during experiments on the Raman scattering of pyridine on rough silver electrodes in 1974. It is an analytical technique for the accurate diagnosis of viruses by analyte interaction with surface plasmons of metals such as Ag, Au, and Cu, which results in intensification of the Raman response [4, 5]. Commonly the SERS technique comprises two principles: (i) the electromagnetic mechanism (EM) and (ii) the chemical mechanism (CM) effects [6]. With advancing technology, a cheap and effective strip-based test technique is accepted for SARS-CoV-2 virus detection [7]. The traces of IgM/IgG in the serum of COVID-19 patients confirms the occurrence of SARS-CoV-2. When compared with a traditional lateral flow assay (LFA), the SERS-based LFA emerged as more sensitive for the detection of the SARS-CoV-2 virus. SERS has been confirmed to be a rapid, accurate, economical, and sensitive technique for the discovery of several strains of influenza A (H1N1), influenza A (H7N9), and different subtypes of coronavirus SARS-CoV-2 [4]. This chapter is an attempt to understand the principles and uses of SERS for SARS-CoV-2 detection, which may become a gold standard for virus detection in the near future.

7.2 SARS-CoV-2 and the emergence of the pandemic

SARS-CoV is a large single-stranded positive-sense RNA (ssRNA) enveloped virus in the family Coronaviridae. One infected patient possesses the capability to infect three or more healthy people thus making SARS-CoV-2 spread rapidly [3, 8]. In addition to SARS-CoV-1 in 2002, another outbreak occurred in Saudi Arabia in 2012, transmitted from Arabian camels to humans, called middle-east respiratory syndrome coronavirus (MERS-CoV) which spread to over 27 countries. As mentioned above, from the first case of pneumonia-like SARS-CoV-2 in late December 2019, in Wuhan, China, the disease has reached all the countries of the world and was proclaimed a pandemic by the WHO on 11 March 2020 [1]. COVID-19 is highly infection and spreads easily from person to person. Common symptoms found in patients are mostly flu-like symptoms and they may show cough, anosmia, breathlessness, diarrhea, fever, runny nose, and muscular pain. The initial days after contracting SARS-CoV-2 are recognized as the incubation period which lasts 2–7 days and in this stage the patient does not show any signs or symptoms, i.e. they are asymptomatic but highly infectious. Almost 45% of the cases reported are asymptomatic, which is a challenge for tracking and monitoring infected individuals [1].

According to reports, the SARS-CoV-2 virus has four chief structural proteins: S (spike protein), N (nucleocapsid protein), E (envelope protein), and M (membrane protein) [9]. The S and N protein antigens are used as biomarkers for the detection of COVID-19. For the assembly of the virus, M and E proteins are essential. The S protein is essential for its penetration into the target cell where the S protein with a receptor-binding domain (RBD) facilitates the interaction with angiotensin-converting enzyme 2 (ACE2) [3, 10]. For the prevention of SARS-CoV-2, timely diagnosis and screening are currently being pursued to stop the spreading of the virus through direct routes. The most used screening method during the early and late stages of the viral infection is RT-PCR. RT-PCR is highly specific for SARS-

CoV-2 and acts by changing the viral mRNA into DNA for amplification and detection through PCR. However, this technique has the drawback that variations can be observed in PCR results due to faulty sample collection from nasal or throat swabs, and mishandling, which compromise the accuracy by giving improper results, thus leading to false-positive or false-negative results. The life-threatening effect of the virus was reduced due to the rapid distribution of vaccines. It is advised to take two doses of the vaccine followed by a precautionary dose administered nine months after the second dose [2, 11]. Vaccinations that are accepted in different parts of the the world include the Covaxin, Covishield, Sputnik V, Sputnik Light, Zydus Cadila, Moderna, Pfizer, Johnson & Johnson, Novavax, and Corbevax vaccines. With the emerging COVID-19 cases and variants such as Beta, Delta, Lambda, and lately Omicron, the whole globe faced a lack in availability of vaccines and an alarming increase in cases. This pandemic on only had negative effects on health, but also affected the economy and brought about a drastic change in lifestyles in nations all over the globe. Even though the vaccines proved to be excellently effectual, new data raised concerns about the Delta and Omicron variants because they tend to be more contagious [11, 12].

7.3 Conventional methods of SARS-CoV-2 diagnosis

Early and precise infectious disease diagnosis is paramount to enhance the effectiveness of treatments and ward off future complications in infected patients. In addition, patients not being aware of being infected contributes to the transmission of the disease and they can become 'super-spreaders'. Different diagnostic modalities have been used for the diagnosis of SARS-CoV-2, which were considered agile, fast, and flexible (figure 7.2). However, over time, each of the techniques exhibited its drawbacks. Some of the methods used for virus detection are as follows:

i. *Molecular analysis by RT-PCR.*

The first step in RT-PCR is sample collection from nasal or throat swabs, and the procedure is easy, rapid, and harmless. The collected viral sample can be preserved in a viral transport medium (VTM), saline water, Amies transport medium at 2 °C for at least 72 h after the sample is collected. If the sample needs to be further tested after a longer duration, it must be stored at −70 °C or below [13]. The second step in RT-PCR is RNA extraction and purification. The extremely infectious viral sample must be handled in a biosafety cabinet in biosecurity level 2 (BSL-2). This follows the purification and extraction of viral RNA using a lysis buffer which degrades and ruptures the outer protective covering of the virus, releasing the viral RNA which is eluted out with the help of an elution buffer. The third step in RT-PCR is reverse transcription, amplification, and quantification. Once the RNA is extracted it is mixed with a master mix comprising a buffer, nucleotides (dNTPs), reverse transcriptase (RT) enzyme, forward primers, reverse primers, probes, and DNA polymerase. The well-blended mixture is further loaded into a PCR plate and placed in a thermal cycler for further steps to take place. First, the reverse transcriptase forms RNA/DNA

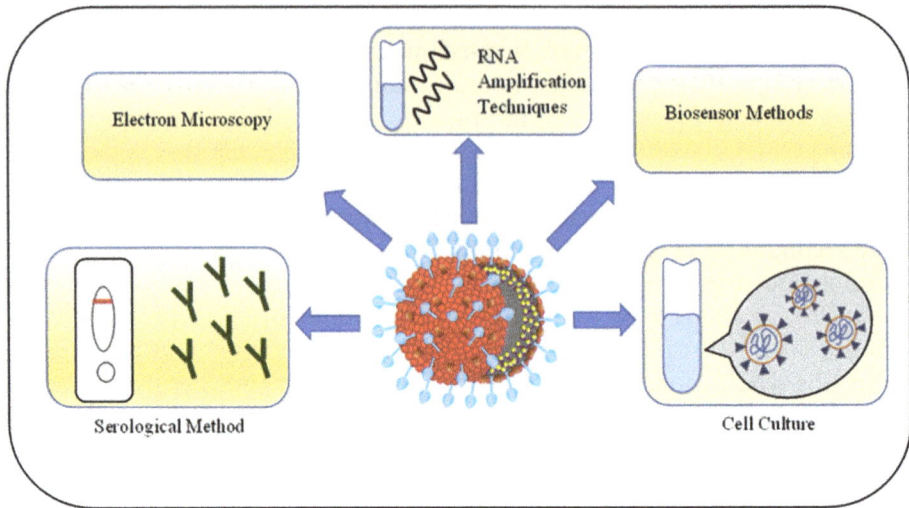

Figure 7.2. Different conventional diagnostic techniques used for SARS-CoV-2 detection.

hybrids followed by denaturation of the hybrids using high temperatures (95 °C) which inactivates the reverse transcriptase, followed by annealing at 60 °C with forward and reverse primers. Finally, a new complementary strand is synthesized by the process of extension. After the extension step, a new double-stranded DNA is achieved [14].

ii. *Diagnosis by chest imaging.*

Chest computed tomography (CT) plays a vital role in the early diagnosis of COVID-19 by taking numerous x-ray images from different angles all over the chest which generates tomographic images of the lungs. CT shows slight changes and lesions in the lungs which are not visible in x-rays and vary according to their number, pattern, and density [3].

iii. *CRISPR/Cas12a-NER.*

CRISPR/Cas12a-NER is a suitable and reliable on-site testing method for local hospitals or community testing centers. It is confirmed that this assay is rapid with a naked eye readout (NER) and can detect up to ten virus gene copies within 45 min exclusive of any instrument. This technique emits a fluorescence signal that is used as a control to confirm the positive result. This technique proved to be trouble-free, sensitive, portable, and specific in the identification of COVID-19 [3, 6].

iv. *Loop-mediated isothermal amplification (LAMP).*

LAMP is a budding molecular detection technique capable of replacing traditional PCR. LAMP comprises two sets of enzymes, where one enzyme helps in converting a viral RNA to DNA and the other helps in copying this DNA. Furthermore, an array of six primers is needed which specify the viral genome sequence. The LAMP technique has the same diagnostic accuracy

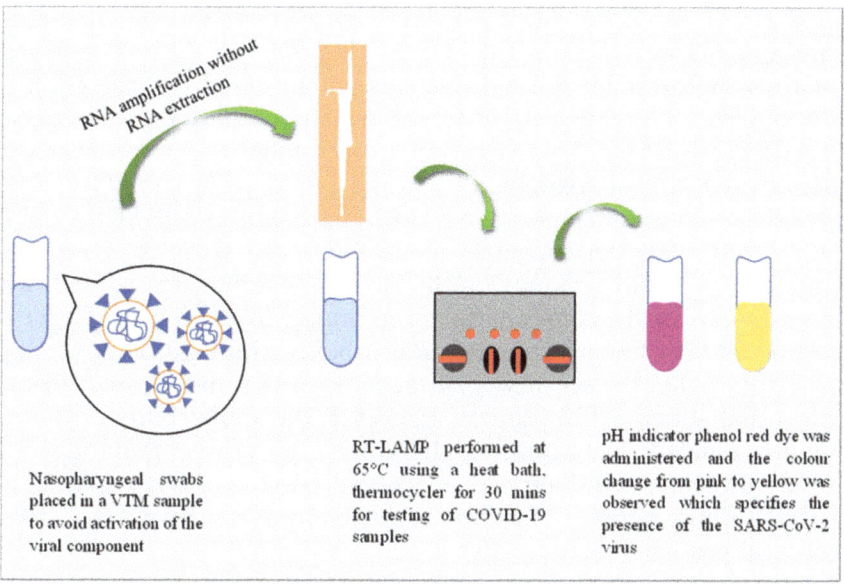

Figure 7.3. SARS-Cov-2 detection using RT-LAMP.

as RT-PCR, and LAMP gained its name due to the formation of looped structures of newly copied DNA strands which are further amplified more effectively when compared to RT-PCR. In contrast, this technique accurately runs a large number of samples at once while exhibiting low precision while working with a small number of samples. RT-LAMP involves the use of a hot plate to maintain the proper temperature as this technique functions at a temperature of 60 °C–65 °C [15] (figure 7.3).

Recently, for SARS-CoV-2 detection in 248 infected people, the LAMP technique detected the presence of the infection in about 90% of the samples, although this technique was found to be less accurate due to cross-contamination [15, 16]. Additional research found a reverse transcription-loop mediated isothermal amplification (RT-LAMP) technique for SARS-CoV-2 detection. This technique was found to work at a constant temperature and be less expensive and laborious. Another benefit of this technique is that the results are observed through color changes and are visible to the naked eye as they are dependent on the pH change which is produced during the amplification process. In this process, the pH of the reaction solution becomes low due to the production of protons, which requires an appropriate pH indicator to identify positive or negative results by changing the color of the solution which can be spotted by the naked eye. The detection sensitivity of this method is 80 copies/ml of the viral RNA in the crude sample [17].

Another similar procedure reported that the nucleocapsid gene detection of SARS-CoV-2 through RT-LAMP can be observed by the naked eye within 30 min of the experiment by using direct RNA amplification without RNA extraction [18]. Herein, the color change was observed when the pH indicator phenol red dye was administered and the color change from pink to yellow was observed which specifies the existence of the SARS-CoV-2 virus. This experiment was found to be more specific against the viral RNA of SARS-CoV-2 when tested with a mixture of HCoV, MERS-CoV, and influenza virus [19]. The diagnosis of SARS-CoV-2 using RT-LAMP was performed by collecting swab samples. To this sample mixture, a small amount of fluorescent calcein was added which is responsible for the color change from orange to green if the target analyte is present. For the colorimetric and turbidity examination of the sample it was found that the sensitivity of the assay was 1 and 2 copies/reaction for the orflab-4 and S-123 primers. However, the applicability of this assay is limited due to fluctuating results caused by primer mutation. Another study presented the diagnosis of SARS-CoV-2 by the RT-LAMP method from a saliva sample. The limit of detection of this assay was ~10^2 copies of viral genome/reaction [20]

v. *Optical-based high-throughput biosensor diagnostics.*

This open-ended threat of SARS-CoV-2 places elevated demands for promising high-throughput biosensor devices. On this front, fluorescence (FL) detection of biomarkers is confirmed to have suitability in biosensing. High-throughput meta-surface fluorescence biosensors are ultra-sensitive and are an appropriate detection method for target analytes such as nucleic acids. In addition, all the dielectric meta-surface biosensors comprise a silicon-on-insulator nanorod arrangement and exhibit out-standing fluorescence emission enhanced by potential electromagnetic resonances. Due to the direct detection procedure, the meta-surface fluorescence biosensors exhibit enhanced performance. For a better under-standing of the practicality of meta-surface biosensors, fluorescence detection of single-stranded oligo DNAs that are similar to SARS-CoV-2 RNA was carried out. It showed the detection of a nucleic acid target to be highly efficient at low concentrations, i.e. 100 amol/ml. Fulfilling the heavy requirements for this test, pre-treatment of meta-surfaces is per-formed with biotin trappings identical to anti-biotin Abs coatings in microplates in immunoassay kits. Then the FL probes are introduced into the RNA sequence, for which an antigen kit of SARS-CoV-2 is used for rapid screening to match the RNA targets in meta-surface nucleic-acid sensors. In addition, these biosensors are capable of detecting unidentified new viral infections rapidly, without the fabrication of required antibodies. A high-throughput surface plasmon resonance (SPR) detection for SARS-CoV-2 spike protein was performed for POC which delivered high accuracy and the limit of detection (LOD) of the spike protein was found to be 0.2 μg ml^{-1}. Hence, this technique was found to be a promising screening method for COVID-19 [53].

vi. *Point-of-care electrochemical immunosensor.*

Previously, for the detection of target analytes, various biosensors were used, of which electrochemical biosensors were found to possess unique properties. Electrochemical biosensors can immobilize the detection of target analytes with the introduction of disease-specific antibodies/antigens as the electrode surfaces of this biosensor are composed of conductive materials. The sensor surface can be assembled with nanocomposites composed of novel metal nanoparticles, nanowires, nanorods, quantum dots, and metal oxides/sulfides [34]. Nanocomposites are characterized as promising materials for the fabrication of biosensors due to their high conductivity, stability, cost-effectiveness, and biocompatibility [35].

Accordingly, the biosensor probe when bound to the target analyte generates electrical signals in response to a small current and exhibits chemistry while antibody–antigen binding. These electrical signals are transformed into a transducer displaying disease growth stages and delivering quantitative results [36]. Eventually, in the case of SARS-CoV-2, electrochemical immunosensors play a key role in its diagnosis and are highly specific, sensitive, rapid, and accurate, and the samples do not require any pre-treatment before the testing and are capable of distinguishing the target analyte at exceptionally low concentration, i.e. femtomolar to attomolar [37, 38]. Some of the advantages of electrochemical biosensors which make them a favorable choice for POC biosensor applications are their effectiveness, ease of incorporating with other devices such as microfluidics, ease of handling, cost-effectiveness, and miniaturization [39]. Moreover, when compared with mass spectrometric methods, PCR, and RT-PCR, electrochemical biosensors do not need any skilled personnel or expensive facilities for the results to be elucidated [40, 41].

7.4 Drawbacks of conventional diagnostic agents

Conventional diagnostic agents typically use serological tests, phenotypic tests, culturing, and biochemical methods, and morphological examination which assists in the identification of diseases. However, these conventional methods do not always provide the correct results and consequently create complications. For example, PCR is a widely accepted detection technique for SARS-CoV-2 due to its sensitivity and selectivity, but this sophisticated technique has anomalies, yielding false-positive and -negative results which has led to an increase in mortality [3]. PCR is also one of the most time-consuming and costly methods. It also requires multistep handling and uses expensive reagents, and requires skilled personnel to deal with the instruments [21]. Another emerging technique for SARS-CoV-2 virus detection is CRISPR-based diagnostics. Although it is one of the most promising and sensitive techniques it still is at its early stages and requires excess time and reagents. It also produces false-positive results because it depends upon amplification, i.e. PCR [3, 21, 22]. One of the easily operated and sensitive techniques for COVID-19 detection is the rapid antigen test

(RAT), but it has its pitfalls. Being sensitive is one of the major disadvantages, and it changes the result if the proportion or the composition of the reagents used in the RATs test vary, which presents the result as false-positive [23].

For the detection of pneumonia-associated diseases, one of the broadly accepted techniques is chest CT [24]. It has proven to be 70 times more effective and sensitive than x-rays and is globally accepted for lung anomalies such as influenza, SARS, and MERS. However, chest CT shows false-positives in the case of SARS, MERS, and influenza due to their similar physical properties, which leads to overlap of infections. A new study suggests that for COVID-19, for 75% of the negative cases shown in RT-PCR, 48% were found to be positive when diagnosed with a CT scan [25, 26]. All these drawbacks led to the elimination of certain diagnostic techniques as they provided perplexing results which led to a worldwide increase in mortality. Thus, finding a new kind of diagnostic technique was the need of the hour and the prime target for all researchers [27].

7.5 SERS as a diagnostic agent

SERS was inadvertently discovered by Fleischmann and co-workers during experimenting on the Raman scattering of pyridine on rough silver electrodes in 1974. It is an analytical technique for the accurate diagnosis of viruses by analyte interaction with surface plasmons of metals such as Ag, Au, and Cu which results in intensification of the Raman response [4, 5]. The entrance of an infectious agent such as a virus can cause an infectious disease, for example influenza (flu) and coronavirus (CoV) which infect millions globally and lead at least hundreds of thousands of mortalities. When an infected individual coughs or sneezes, the tiny infected viral particles are suspended in the air and later on settle on a surface, which are transferred from one person to another by touching the contaminated surface and then touching the nose, mouth, or eyes of a healthy individual [28].

This section focuses on a brief description of the detection and principles of the SERS technique, with quantification and identification of SERS strategies for zoonotic infectious diseases such as influenza and coronavirus.

7.5.1 Principles of SERS

Commonly the SERS technique comprises two working principles: (i) the electro-magnetic mechanism (EM) and (ii) the chemical mechanism (CM) effects. The first principle (EM) is widely understood making it the most used one. The mechanism of EM is quite straightforward, it is generated from the substrate and initiated by the laser exposure of a free-electron-like metal whose frequency pulsates with the frequency developed due to the collective oscillation of the conduction band electron. This aspect is termed surface plasmon resonance (SPR) [29]. In CM, in contrast, the presence of incident light results in alteration of the molecular polarizability when the inherent properties of the adsorbate and the resulting properties of the combined adsorbate–metal nanostructure complex merge with the light (figure 7.4).

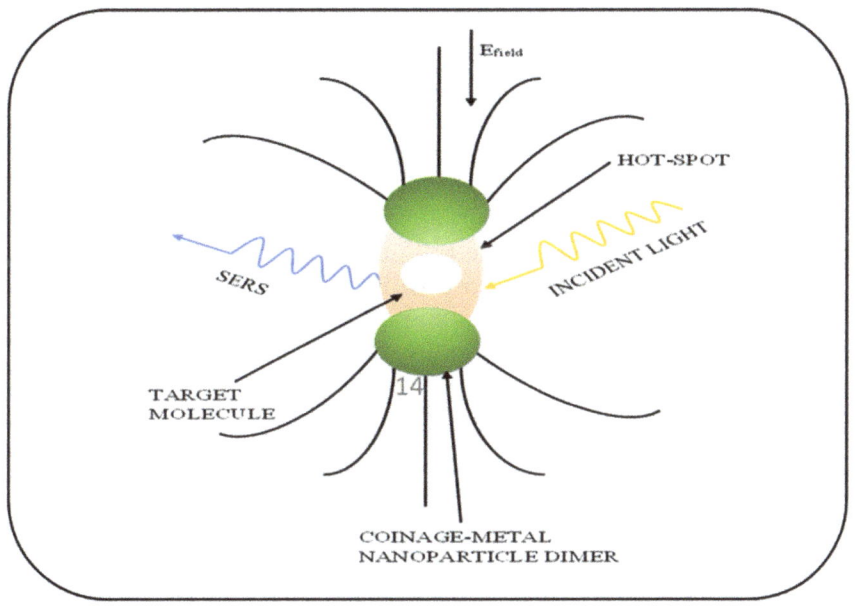

Figure 7.4. Mechanism of SERS.

7.6 SERS-based diagnostic agents and their implication for infectious diseases

7.6.1 SERS detection of influenza A (H1N1) virus

Influenza A (H1N1), commonly known as swine flu, started in pigs and is one of the leading human respiratory infections, having similar symptoms to common flu. H1N1 can be detected through rapid antigen tests, direct immune fluorescence (DFA), viral cultures, and RT-PCR. In addition to these leading detection techniques for the identification and quantification of H1N1, SERS has been proved to be a promising method. For identification, SERS cannot characterize the whole H1N1 virus because of pleomorphism and its large size (150–400 nm), hence a small fragment is used to obtain the Raman shift pattern coming out from the small segment of the viral lipid envelope of the strain [29].

7.6.2 SERS detection of H7N9

Normally H7N9 can be detected through PCR or real-time PCR as well as through the available rapid influenza diagnostic test (RIDT) kits, but these kits are not always accurate, are less sensitive, and cannot differentiate between subtypes. Although PCR is fast, accurate, and sensitive, it is not capable of preventing false-positives, resulting in the search for alternative techniques, such as fluorescence and enzyme-induced metallization.

SERS utilizes a well-organized strip-based test with surface-enhanced Raman scattering-based lateral flow immunoassay strips (SERS-LFIAS) to detect inactive

H7N9 virus. SERS tags comprise anti-H7N9 monoclonal antibodies (H7N9-mAb) with modified AuAg4_ATP@Ag core–shell nanoparticles and 4-aminothioplenol (4-ATP) as a reporter molecule. H7N9-mAb is immobilized in the external layer of silver, whereas 4-ATP remains immobilized between the two layers of silver covering the gold core [29]. LFIA strips were prepared with goat anti-mouse IgG antibody and H7N9-mAb at the control and test lines, respectively (figure 7.3). For the positive sample, iH7N9-mAb-AuAg4_ATP@AgNps immunocomplexes are formed in conjugation and migrate toward the test line through capillary action where is it captured and the Raman signal is recorded. For the negative sample, the excess of mAb–AuAg4_ATP@AgNps complexes migrates towards the control line where it is captured by the goat anti-mouse IgG antibodies [29].

7.6.3 SERS-based diagnostics for SARS-CoV-2

In the brutal COVID-19 pandemic, for the identification of the SARS-CoV-2 virus one of the most accurate, feasible, and fast diagnostic methods is SERS [30]. SERS diagnosis does not require calibration or other reagents because it uses a SERS-active substrate and Raman spectrometer to detect the biochemicals present on the virus envelope. Raman spectroscopy is used to detect analytes through the scattering of incident light [31, 32]. With the advancing technology, a cheap and effective strip-based test technique has been accepted for SARS-CoV-2 virus detection. Lateral flow immunoassay (LFIA) is an advanced characterization technique [7]. The SARS-CoV-2 virus affects humans and leaves them with further health consequences, and is one of the largest single-stranded RNAs, i.e. 26–32 kbp. Essential membrane proteins present on the coronavirus consist of the hemagglutinin esterase (HE), spike (S), nucleocapsid (N), membrane (M), and envelope (E) among which spike plays an important role in virus–host adherence [5, 33]. Currently, identification of the SARS-CoV-2 virus in respiratory samples such as nasal swabs and oral swabs is recommended which further go through real-time PCR for the detection of positive and negative results.

Several tests have been carried out to determine that SERS has the capability of detecting COVID-19 with SERS-based biosensors. It has also been found that development of SERS techniques speeds up SARS-CoV-2 diagnosis. To detect the presence of SARS-CoV-2 in COVID-19 patients, IgM/IgG in serum must be identified. When compared with a traditional lateral flow assay (LFA), SERS-based LFA emerged as more sensitive toward the detection of the SARS-CoV-2 virus. In addition to high sensitivity, the SERS scanner exhibits a greater magnitude with an LOD of about ca. 100 fg/ml. It was also found that the cellular receptor angiotensin-converting enzyme 2 (ACE2) facilitated screening and interrogating the viral components with an RBD for entering human cells when expressed to a silver nanorod SERS array and revealed its potential as a rapid detection method [4].

7.6.4 Lateral flow immunoassay (LFIA)

LFIA is used exclusively as a recognition element; here it is the identification of the SARS-CoV-2 antibody. LFIA, being a fast, cost-effective, and portable technique, is deemed to be an eligible POC diagnostic tool [42, 43]. In LFIA, upon the introduction of the liquid sample on the strip, if SARS-CoV-2 Ab is present then it reacts with the labeled Ab (tag gold colloidal) and binds with the immobilized Ag present on the surface of the nitrocellulose membrane [44]. This immobilized antibody–detection antibody complex results in the formation of a colored band due to the accumulation of colloidal gold. As a result of this in less than 15 min IgM and IgG can be detected in the blood sample [45]. When compared to other antibody detection tests, LFIA proved to show less sensitivity [43, 46].

For viral infection detection of SARS-CoV, MERS-CoV, Ebola, influenza, and swine flu numerous electrochemical biosensors were used [47–49]. It was reported that for the detection of MERS-CoV and human coronavirus (HCoV) an electro-chemical biosensor with a modified carbon electrode was used with high sensitivity. The electrode surface was formed by immobilization of cysteamine on gold nano-particles/carbon electrodes and the detection was performed by square wave voltammetry (SWV) which provided the result in 20 min and had a low LOD of 1.0 pg ml^{-1} and 0.4 pg ml^{-1} for MERS-CoV and HCoV [3].

LFIA is a one-step assay, so any inaccuracy in the volume of the sample can affect the result's precision. However, one major disadvantage of LFIA is that it requires pre-treatment of the non-fluid samples. The response of this assay cannot be enhanced by enzyme reaction in addition the time of the assay depends on the nature of the sample, i.e. viscosity. This assay cannot be done recklessly; it needs good antigen preparation and the total volume in the test brings restrictions to its sensitivity [15] (figure 7.5).

The gold nanoparticle in conjugation with the Au–S bond is attached to a reporter molecule 4-amino thiophenol, which blocks virus–host cell binding, prevents the spreading of viral infection, as well as destroying the viral lipid membrane by attaching to the spike protein. Further peptides were used to catch viral proteins and an ACE2 peptide mimics SERS-based sensor with higher effectiveness and enhanced detection limit was produced, i.e. 300 nM in the presence of bovine serum albumin with higher concentration. Likewise, a functioning diagnostic technique based on SERS combined with a microfluidic system was demonstrated that comprised carbon nanotubes and disposable electrospinning nanofilms/microfilters.

7.6.5 Mass spectrometry diagnostic approaches

Mass spectrometry (MS) uses collected saliva or gargle samples for the identification of SARS-CoV-2 by calculating the mass fragmentation ion intensity of the virus [50]. However, this technique requires effective instrumentation maintenance, and is high-cost, laborious, and slow (~3 h) [51, 52].

7.7 Future perspectives and conclusion

With the alarming rate of spread of COVID-19 infections and escalation in mortality, there is a desperate need to find a cure to eradicate this infectious SARS-CoV-2 virus from the world. The SARS-CoV-2 virus has become a brutal

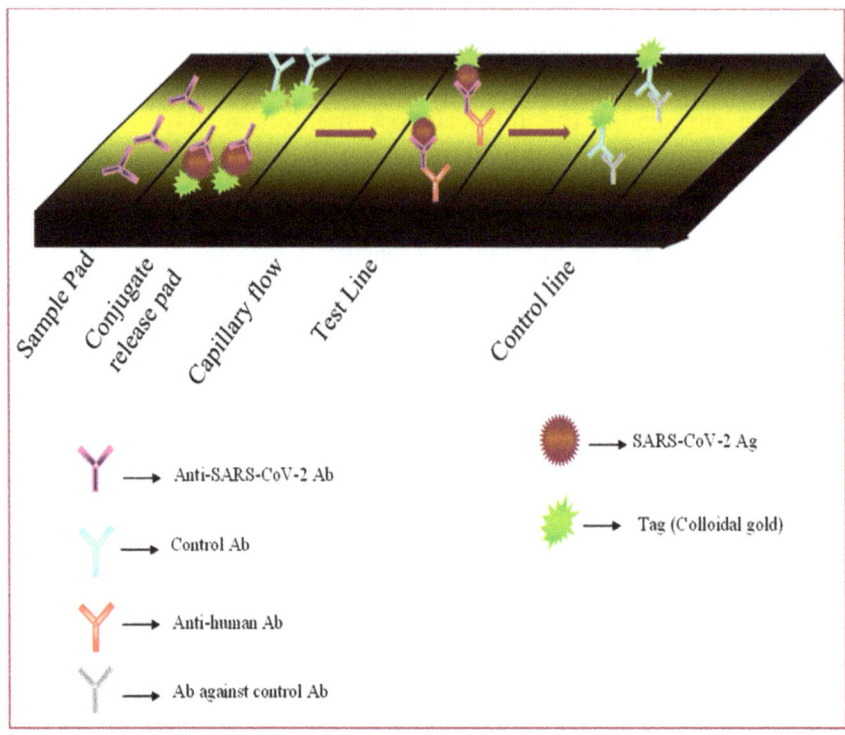

Figure 7.5. Schematic diagram of the LFIA for SARS-CoV-2 IgM/IgG antibodies.

infectious agent which necessitates the development of a new analysis technique for its accurate diagnosis. In this burdensome situation the reliable techniques used for the detection of SARS are real-time PCR (RT-PCR), chest computed tomography (CT scans), CRISPR/Cas12a-NER, and antigen testing. Due to drawbacks in RT-PCR which produces false-positives, one technique emerged as reliable, i.e. surface-enhanced Raman spectroscopy (SERS). SERS has been confirmed to be a rapid, accurate, cost-effective, and sensitive technique for the detection of several strains of influenza A H1N1, influenza A H7N9, and different subtypes of coronavirus SARS-CoV-2. It was shown that this technique lacks some specificity and needs pre-treatment of the samples to avoid pleomorphism while detection. Other than its negligible drawbacks, SERS is believed to be one of the leading effective conventional detection techniques for the detection of viruses [29]. In this chapter, we have mentioned the SERS-based lateral flow immunoassay (LFIA) which proved to be an admirable choice for the detection of SARS-CoV-2 spike RBD protein. SERS-based LFIA utilizes Raman intensities to measure the captured SERS nanotag hence determining the RBD in 20 min. This proved SERS-based LFIA to be an alternative approach for COVID-19 detection due to its rapid, accurate, and on-site diagnosis [7]. One of the surprising approaches of this technique is that it can detect even a single molecule even in low concentrations. When examined for medical and biological diagnosis, SERS was proved to diagnose the disease in a non-destructive manner and with ultra-sensitive detection of viruses. when signal enhancers for Raman scattering, of gold, copper, and silver, were added. In conclusion SERS is one of the leading detection and diagnosis applications for viral diseases such as influenza and COVID-19, making it capable of preventing epidemics or pandemics in the future [14]. This chapter showed SERS to be a promising alternative for the diagnosis and detection of SARS-CoV-2 in medical, biochemical, and biological analyses. This technique is further considered to be a versatile, viable, and long-term alternative for accountable diagnosis of SARS-CoV-2 to contain future outbreaks of a viral pandemic.

Acknowledgments

AK is grateful to KIIT for a fellowship. SA is grateful to KIIT for the opportunity.

References

[1] Yadav S *et al* 2021 SERS based lateral flow immunoassay for point-of-care detection of SARS-CoV-2 in clinical samples *ACS Appl. Bio Mater.* **4** 2974–95

[2] Bistaffa M J, Camacho S A, Pazin W M, Constantino C J L, Oliveira O N Jr and Aoki P H B 2022 Immunoassay platform with surface-enhanced resonance Raman scattering for detecting trace levels of SARS-CoV-2 spike protein *Talanta* **244** 123381

[3] Martin J, Tena N and Asuero A G 2021 Current state of diagnostic, screening and surveillance testing methods for COVID-19 from an analytical chemistry point of view *Microchem. J.* **167** 106305

[4] Eskandari V, Sahbafar H, Zeinalizad L and Hadi A 2022 A review of applications of surface-enhanced Raman spectroscopy laser for detection of biomaterials and a quick glance into its advances for COVID-19 investigations *ISSS J. Micro Smart Syst.* **11** 363–82

[5] Jadhav S A *et al* 2021 Development of integrated microfluidic platform coupled with surface-enhanced Raman spectroscopy for diagnosis of COVID-19 *Med. Hypotheses* **146** 110356

[6] Liang J *et al* 2021 Application of the amplification-free SERS-based CRISPR/Cas12a platform in the identification of SARS-CoV-2 from clinical samples *J Nanobiotechnol.* **19** 273

[7] Serebrennikova K V *et al* 2021 Lateral flow immunoassay of SARS-CoV-2 antigen with SERS-based registration: development and comparison with traditional immunoassays *Biosensors* **11** 510

[8] Huang J *et al* 2021 On-site detection of SARS-CoV-2 antigen by deep learning-based surface-enhanced Raman spectroscopy and its biochemical foundations *Anal. Chem.* **93** 9174–82

[9] Awada C, Abdullah M M B, Traboulsi H, Dab C and Alshoaibi A 2021 SARS-CoV-2 receptor binding domain as a stable-potential target for SARS-CoV-2 detection by surface-enhanced Raman spectroscopy *Sensors* **21** 4617

[10] Zhang D *et al* 2021 Ultra-fast and onsite interrogation of Severe Acute Respiratory Syndrome Coronavirus 2 (SARS-CoV-2) in waters via surface enhanced Raman scattering (SERS) *Water Res.* **200** 117243

[11] Sitjar J *et al* 2022 Synergistic surface-enhanced Raman scattering effect to distinguish live SARS-CoV-2 S pseudovirus *Anal. Chim. Acta.* **1193** 339406

[12] Moitra P *et al* 2022 Probing the mutation independent interaction of DNA probes with SARS-CoV-2 variants through a combination of surface-enhanced Raman scattering and machine learning *Biosens. Bioelectron.* **208** 114200

[13] Cha H *et al* 2022 Surface-enhanced Raman scattering-based immunoassay for severe acute respiratory syndrome coronavirus 2 *Biosens. Bioelectron.* **202** 114008

[14] Sur U K and Santra C 2022 Spectroscopy: a versatile sensing tool for cost-effective and rapid detection of novel coronavirus (COVID-19) *Emerg. Mater.* **5** 249–60

[15] Parihar A, Ranjan P, Sanghi S K, Srivastava A K and Khan R 2020 Point-of-care biosensor-based diagnosis of COVID-19 holds promise to combat current and future pandemics *ACS Appl. Bio Mater.* **3** 7326–43

[16] Yu L *et al* 2020 Rapid detection of COVID-19 coronavirus using a reverse transcriptional loop-mediated isothermal amplification (RT-LAMP) diagnostic platform *Clin. Chem.* **66** 975–7

[17] Huang W E *et al* 2020 RT-LAMP for rapid diagnosis of coronavirus SARS-CoV-2 *Microb. Biotechnol.* **13** 950–61

[18] Mauriz E 2020 Recent progress in plasmonic biosensing schemes for virus detection *Sensors* **20** 4745

[19] Baek Y H *et al* 2020 Development of a reverse transcription-loop-mediated isothermal amplification as a rapid early-detection method for novel SARS-CoV-2 *Emerg. Microbes Infect.* **9** 998–1007

[20] Yan C *et al* 2020 Rapid and visual detection of 2019 novel coronavirus (SARS-CoV-2) by a reverse transcription loop-mediated isothermal amplification assay *Clin. Microbiol. Infect.* **26** 773–9

[21] Choi J H *et al* 2021 Clustered regularly interspaced short palindromic repeats-mediated amplification-free detection of viral DNAs using surface-enhanced Raman spectroscopy-active nanoarray *ACS Nano* **15** 13475–85

[22] Sanchez J E *et al* 2021 Detection of SARS-CoV-2 and its S and N proteins using surface enhanced Raman spectroscopy *RSC Adv.* **11** 25788–94

[23] Yamayoshi S *et al* 2020 Comparison of rapid antigen tests for COVID-19 *Viruses* **12** 1420

[24] Ye Z, Zhang Y, Wang Y, Huang Z and Song B 2020 Chest CT manifestations of new coronavirus disease 2019 (COVID-19): a pictorial review *Eur. Radiol.* **30** 4381–9

[25] Rai P, Kumar B K, Deekshit V K, Karunasagar I and Karunasagar I 2021 Detection technologies and recent developments in the diagnosis of COVID-19 infection *Appl. Microbiol. Biotechnol.* **105** 441–55

[26] Long C *et al* 2020 Diagnosis of the Coronavirus disease (COVID-19): rRT-PCR or CT? *Eur. J. Radiol.* **126** 108961

[27] Liu G and Rusling J F 2021 COVID-19 antibody tests and their limitations *ACS Sens.* **6** 593–612

[28] Sitjar J, Liao J D, Lee H, Tsai H P, Wang J R and Liu P Y 2021 Challenges of SERS technology as a non-nucleic acid or -antigen detection method for SARS-CoV-2 virus and its variants *Biosens. Bioelectron.* **181** 113153

[29] Savinon-Flores F *et al* 2021 A review on SERS-based detection of human virus infections: influenza and coronavirus *Biosensors* **11** 66

[30] Chen H *et al* 2021 Sensitive detection of SARS-CoV-2 using a SERS-based aptasensor *ACS Sens.* **6** 2378–85

[31] Kim G *et al* 2022 Fabrication of MERS-nanovesicle biosensor composed of multi-functional DNA aptamer/graphene–MoS$_2$ nanocomposite based on electrochemical and surface-enhanced Raman spectroscopy *Sens. Actuators* B **352** 131060

[32] Vermisoglou E *et al* 2020 Human virus detection with graphene-based materials *Biosens. Bioelectron.* **166** 112436

[33] Zhai P, Ding Y, Wu X, Long J, Zhong Y and Li Y 2020 The epidemiology, diagnosis and treatment of COVID-19 *Int. J. Antimicrob. Agents* **55** 105955

[34] Lim R R X and Bonanni A 2020 The potential of electrochemistry for the detection of coronavirus-induced infections *TrAC Trends Anal. Chem.* **133** 116081

[35] Huang A T *et al* 2020 A systematic review of antibody mediated immunity to coronaviruses: kinetics, correlates of protection, and association with severity *Nat. Commun.* **11** 4704

[36] Pan Y *et al* 2020 Serological immunochromatographic approach in diagnosis with SARS-CoV-2 infected COVID-19 patients *J. Infect.* **81** e28–32

[37] Ravina M H, Gill P S and Kumar A 2019 Hemagglutinin gene based biosensor for early detection of swine flu (H1N1) infection in human *Int. J. Biol. Macromol.* **130** 720–6

[38] Maity A *et al* 2018 Resonance-frequency modulation for rapid, point-of-care Ebola-glycoprotein diagnosis with a graphene-based field-effect biotransistor *Anal. Chem.* **90** 14230–8

[39] Goral V N, Zaytseva N V and Baeumner A J 2006 Electrochemical microfluidic biosensor for the detection of nucleic acid sequences *Lab Chip* **6** 414–21

[40] Kaushik A K *et al* 2020 Electrochemical SARS-CoV-2 sensing at point-of-care and artificial intelligence for intelligent COVID-19 management *ACS Appl. Bio Mater.* **3** 7306–25

[41] Pashchenko O, Shelby T, Banerjee T and Santra S 2018 A comparison of optical, electro-chemical, magnetic, and colorimetric point-of-care biosensors for infectious disease diagnosis *ACS Infect. Dis.* **4** 1162–78

[42] Xu M *et al* 2020 COVID-19 diagnostic testing: technology perspective *Clin. Transl. Med.* **10** e158

[43] Kontou P I, Braliou G G, Dimou N L, Nikolopoulos G and Bagos P G 2020 Antibody tests in detecting SARS-CoV-2 infection: a meta-analysis *Diagnostics* **10** 319

[44] Koczula K M and Gallotta A 2016 Lateral flow assays *Essays Biochem.* **60** 111–20

[45] Cui F and Zhou H S 2020 Diagnostic methods and potential portable biosensors for coronavirus disease 2019 *Biosens. Bioelectron.* **165** 112349

[46] Carter L J *et al* 2020 Assay techniques and test development for COVID-19 diagnosis *ACS Cent. Sci.* **6** 591–605

[47] Layqah L A and Eissa S 2019 An electrochemical immunosensor for the corona virus associated with the Middle East respiratory syndrome using an array of gold nanoparticle-modified carbon electrodes *Mikrochim. Acta.* **186** 224

[48] Nidzworski D *et al* 2017 A rapid-response ultrasensitive biosensor for influenza virus detection using antibody modified boron-doped diamond *Sci. Rep.* **7** 15707

[49] Dou T, Li Z, Zhang J, Evilevitch A and Kurouski D 2020 Nanoscale structural characterization of individual viral particles using atomic force microscopy infrared spectroscopy (AFM-IR) and tip-enhanced Raman spectroscopy (TERS) *Anal. Chem.* **92** 11297–304

[50] Ranjan P *et al* 2021 Rapid diagnosis of SARS-CoV-2 using potential point-of-care electro-chemical immunosensor: toward the future prospects *Int. Rev. Immunol.* **40** 126–42

[51] Nikolaev E N *et al* 2020 Mass-spectrometric detection of SARS-CoV-2 virus in scrapings of the epithelium of the nasopharynx of infected patients via nucleocapsid N protein *J. Proteome Res.* **19** 4393–7

[52] Gouveia D *et al* 2020 Proteotyping SARS-CoV-2 virus from nasopharyngeal swabs: a proof-of-concept focused on a 3 min mass spectrometry window *J. Proteome Res.* **19** 4407–16

[53] Sadique M A, Ranjan P, Yadav S and Khan R 2022 Advanced high-throughput biosensor-based diagnostic approaches for detection of SARS-CoV-2 *Revolutionary Strategies to Combat Pandemics* (Amsterdam: Elsevier) ch 8 147–69

Chapter 8

SERS-based lateral flow immunoassay for viral infections

Shalu Yadav, Mohd Abubakar Sadique, Pushpesh Ranjan, Neeraj Kumar and Raju Khan

Among recent developments in the field of biosensing, a significant trend has been towards the integration of quantitative and qualitative approaches to diagnose disease more efficiently. Subsequently, to overcome the limitations of current diagnostic techniques, the integration of surface-enhanced Raman spectroscopy (SERS) as a quantitative method with lateral flow immunoassay (LFIA) has shifted the focus of researchers around the globe. The systematic combination of SERS and LFIA has provided more sensitive, rapid, simple, and accurate results for the diagnosis of infectious diseases. The advantages of SERS-based LFIA for viral infections surpass other conventional methods pertinent to commercial and accurate high-throughput clinical testing. This chapter describes the necessity of such integrations, their utilizations, and further improvements achieved for SERS-based LFIA diagnostics. Currently, this field has been little investigated for commercialization, nonetheless, the studies suggest a promising outcome with significant benefits for the diagnostics of viral infections.

8.1 Introduction

Infectious diseases affect human health, with life-threatening pandemics on a global scale. Several well-known viruses, such as human immunodeficiency virus (HIV) and hepatitis are major causes of death. New and brutal viruses are spreading chaos by becoming pandemics and significant outbreaks. The most recent is the coronavirus disease-2019 (COVID-19) pandemic caused by the spread of severe acute respiratory syndrome (SARS-CoV-2), affecting the whole world [1]. Previously, the Ebola outbreak in 2014 and influenza A (H1N1) in 2009 killed thousands in Africa. In 2012 the Middle East respiratory syndrome (MERS-CoV) infected many in Saudi Arabia.

Before that, in 2002 SARS-CoV was responsible a viral outbreak [2]. For the detection of such viruses, plenty of research has been carried out in the biomedical domain. Some therapeutics are also available for past viral infections, but there is still a lack of adequate drugs and vaccinations with an effective treatment that would have better efficacy towards different variants of respiratory illness or recently encountered viruses [3]. Biosensors aid the treatment of such infectious diseases through their rapid diagnostic characteristics. The advancements in recently developed biosensing techniques may lead in a beneficial direction towards the treatment of morbific illness [4].

The conversion of biochemical reactions into some readable output using any analytical tool is the basic mechanism behind biosensors. Immobilization of various biomaterials such as antibodies, enzymes, cell-receptors, microorganisms, and other biorecognition elements on a transducing material governs the biochemical reactions with the target analyte in the test sample [5]. The resultant biochemical activity is then converted into a readable quantity using the transducer. Further, digitization of the signal is performed by a digital signal processing unit that displays the results. Consequently, the versatility of optical sensors is demonstrated by their multiplexing abilities using a single tool for analytical applications. After the transducer detects any interaction with the recognition element, the optical properties and characteristics are studied by such optical devices [6].

Innovative sensor systems in optical sensors include surface-enhanced Raman spectroscopy (SERS) which is an advanced form of Raman spectroscopy. The optical and chemical properties exhibited by plasmonic particles have been utilized along with Raman for analytical purposes and molecular analysis, mainly in biomedical diagnostics [7]. The fundamentals of Raman scattering are used in the detection of biomolecules that give weak peak intensities. This can be enhanced with the help of the SERS technique using SERS nanotags and plasmonic nanomaterials [8]. The radiation intensity of a metallic nanoparticle is enhanced when it interacts with the incident light and generates hotspots. Such hotspots enhance local fields at the surface of the metal creating an oscillating dipole. The basic representation of the EM effect is shown in figure 8.1 [9].

The benefits and suitability of the SERS technique have been covered in-depth in previous chapters. However, there are some limitations associated with SERS that need attention to develop and improve the design, fabrication, and assembly approaches for commercialization [10]. Considering the COVID-19 pandemic, there is a need for accurate, precise, and sensitive diagnostic tools. SERS-based diagnostics have the advantages of high sensitivity, stability, accuracy, etc, that provide a better alternative to replace conventional techniques [11]. The fabrication process of SERS substrates is a complex process when they are to be utilized in the biomedical domain. The tedious methodology, costly metals, and sophisticated instruments limit and restrict the cost-effective and mass-production of such advanced techniques. There is a need to develop advance methods to translate laboratory protocols to point-of-care clinical settings [12].

A paper-based technique rapidly increasing in popularity in the detection of target bioanalytes for clinical set-ups is the lateral flow immunoassay (LFIA).

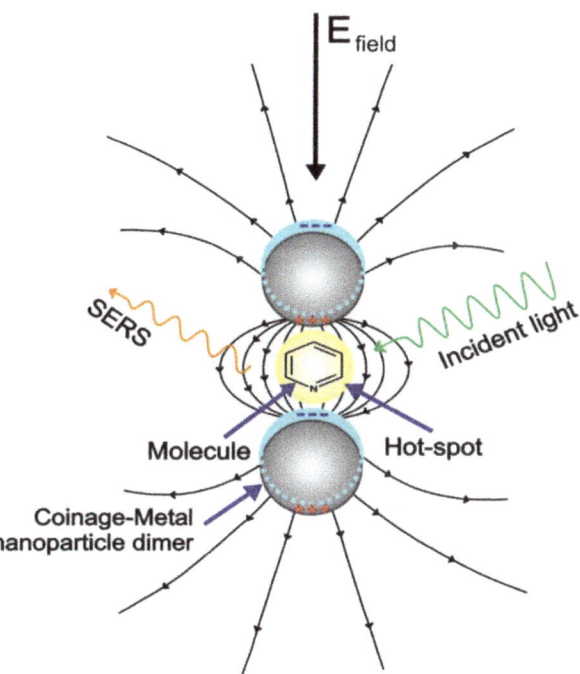

Figure 8.1. Pictorial representation of SERS from the electromagnetic (EM) effect. (Reproduced with permission from [9]. CC BY 4.0.)

The advantages associated with LFIAs include easy usage, eco-friendly production, and rapid, large-scale production. Based on a particular application of the LFIA kit, a specific fabrication process is carried out [13]. Many low-income areas can easily make use of cheap LFIA kits for the diagnosis of infectious diseases even in times of high demand. Further, LFIA requires very little sample volume and has easy processing steps, stable storage, and quick results compared to other available techniques such as reverse-transcriptase polymerase chain reactions (RT-PCR), enzyme-linked immunoassay (ELISA) kits, etc [14].

Recently, for the sensitive detection of infectious diseases, SERS has emerged as a suitable platform with a wide range of integrated assays. In SERS-based LFIA kits, there is an additional component to the basic colorimetric LFIA strip. The use of SERS nanotags enhances the standard detection of the target analyte with a change in color with better color contrast and sensitivity [15]. The intensity variation in Raman spectra for the reporters is used to quantitatively estimate the target molecules. The integration of SERS with LFIA is also advantageous, resulting in a miniaturized device for point-of-care (POC) testing in clinical settings. The systematic investigation of this integration technique, associated challenges, and possible commercial applications is required to fulfill the current demand and future needs to diagnose infectious diseases [16]. Recently, Yadav *et al* published an extensive review on the nanomaterial-integrated SERS-based LFIA platform for the

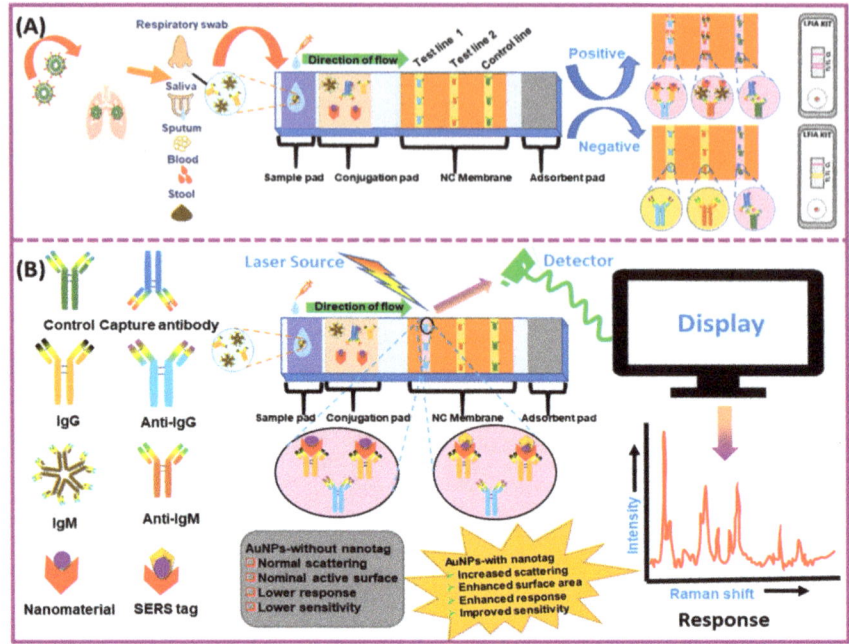

Figure 8.2. Schematic illustration of the fabrication and working principle of (A) the traditional LFIA technique and (B) the SERS-based LFIA platform for the detection of SARS-CoV-2 virus. (Reproduced with permission from [17]. Copyright 2021 American Chemical Society.)

detection of the SARS-CoV-2 virus in clinical samples. As shown in figure 8.2, the AuNP embedded SERS hotspot functionalized LFIA substrate provide rapid, more scattered Raman signals and highly sensitive results [17].

This chapter deals with the individual advantages of LFIA and SERS over traditional approaches and further discusses the advantages of integrating the LFIA technique with SERS for more efficient and sensitive detection of infectious diseases. There is a systematic and elucidative description of the advantages associated with the integration of SERS and LFIA providing quantitative as well as qualitative results. The concerning advancements in biosensing strategies enable swift and effective control over several catastrophic illnesses have been addressed. The technological challenges associated with the proposed SERS-based LFIA integrated diagnostic approach are mentioned. The information provided here will make researchers aware of the advancements in POC-based diagnostics involving combined quantitative and qualitative approaches for infectious diseases [18].

8.2 Traditional diagnostic approaches

Laboratory-based standard detection techniques for viral infections include RT-PCR [19], ELISA [20], CRISPR [21], etc, viral separations, immunofluor-escence, and others that are only suitable for a single primary analysis. The conventional approaches are complex, slow, tedious, and require expert handling and analysis, which is inadequate for clinical trials [22]. The longer completion duration and high cost of the above techniques make them unsuitable to fight the social spread of diseases. As a result, there is a pressing need for fast, accurate, and stable diagnostic approaches to combat the transmission of infectious diseases. The use of biosensors has demonstrated effective performance in biological samples. They are being pursued as an alternative method for the detection of infectious diseases for prompt assistance in managing widespread adverse events [23]. Ongoing traditional methods include gold standard RT-PCR, RT-LAMP, CRISPR, ELISA, mass spectroscopy, etc. Initially, these techniques were exclusively available for the diagnosis of viral infections. With the increase in the number of cases and the high demand for sensitive primary investigatory tests, the above-mentioned approaches lacked the high-throughput, rapidity, cost-effectiveness, simplicity, and point-of-care tests needed for clinical samples [24]. The conventional methods are predominantly used for confirmation in cases where no alternative diagnostic method can detect or confirm the illness despite prevailing symptoms. The detection of target analytes using such sophisticated instruments further restricts their use in large-scale clinical trials [25]. In cases such as the COVID-19 pandemic and other infectious diseases, traditional approaches have taken a back-foot and recent biosensing techniques support detection leading to an effective treatment strategy. A comparative overview of traditional approaches for the diagnostics of infectious diseases is shown in figure 8.3 [17].

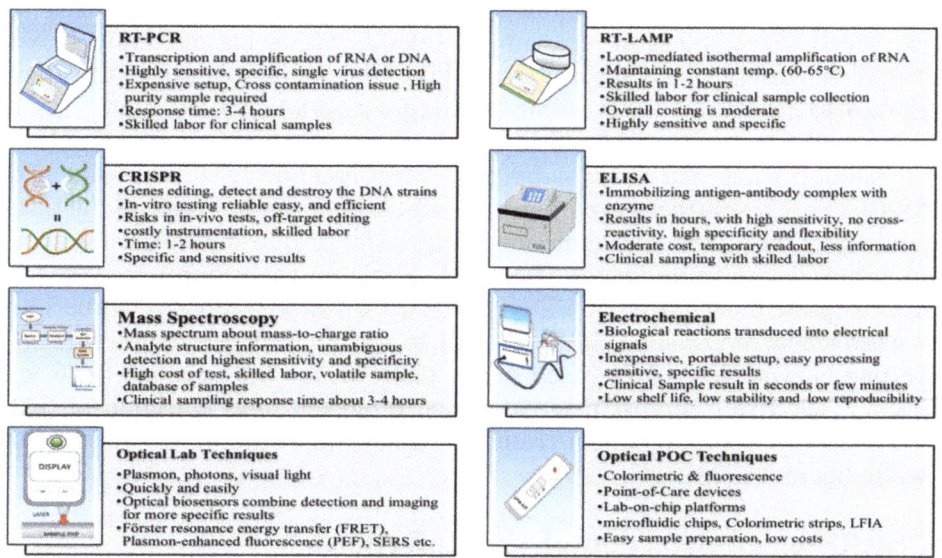

Figure 8.3. Overview of the working principles, advantages, and disadvantages of existing diagnostic techniques. (Reproduced with permission from [17]. Copyright 2021 American Chemical Society.)

8.3 LFIA-based detection of viral infections

LFIA has numerous benefits, such as being economical, quick, and easy to use, with low sample volumes and flexible multiplex detection which support POC use for effective diagnostics [26]. The basic structure of an LFIA device comprises different parts governing a flow channel that works through the capillary effect. The sections include a nitrocellulose membrane, sample pad, absorbent pad, and conjugate pad assisting in the systematic flow of the molecules [27]. A resistance-free flow of the sample with additional components is dependent on the glass or cellulose membrane of the sample pad. Further, the distribution of a biorecognition element is done on the conjugate pad. Customary LFIA utilizes gold nanoparticles (AuNPs) as labels in conjugate pads, which comes in contact with the moving sample molecules. The use of specific labels and a nitrocellulose membrane directly influences the sensitivity of the LFIA set-up. The binding of capture analytes (complementary to target analytes) is favored by the test and control lines on the membrane. The absorbent pad affects the results and plays an important role to prevent the backflow of the liquid, retain the flow rate, act as a sink, and define the absorbing capacity of the assay [28]. Further, the LFIA gives quantitative results by visualizing the color intensities. Qualitative screening of positive and negative samples can be identified by the color observed on the test and control lines [29]. Another advantage of the use of LFIA devices is the lack of complex processing, heavy instrumentation, and skilled personnel. The overall process is rapid, reliable, and simple. In addition to the advantages of LFIA in a broad variety of practical applications, its several drawbacks include low sensitivity, narrow detection range, and inadequate reproducibility [30]. The practical applicability of LFIA as a POC device was demonstrated during the high demand of the COVID-19 pandemic. To detect SARS-CoV-2 IgM and IgG antibodies in real samples (blood, serum, plasma, etc) LFIA kits provide distinguishable and specific results [31]. For example, a rapid detection kit based on LFIA delivers results within 10 min for anti-SARS-CoV-2 IgG in serum samples. Additionally, another work demonstrates that LFIA is compatible with whole blood, plasma, and serum samples to detect IgG and IgM antibodies against SARS-CoV-2 [32]. Further development in LFIA by Yen *et al* utilized the distinct size and optical behavior of silver nanoparticles to fabricate a multiplexed system for simultaneous detection of dengue virus NS1, Ebola virus glycoprotein, and yellow fever virus protein. The detection limit of these viruses was reported to be 150 ng ml^{-1} when recorded visually [33]. Recently, Lee *et al* reported a human angiotensin-converting enzyme 2 (ACE2) based LFIA platform for the sensitive (1.86×10^5 copies/ml), selective (no-cross reactivity), and rapid (20 min) detection of SARS-CoV-2 S22 antigens in real patient samples. A schematic of the ACE2-based LFIA is shown in figure 8.4 [34].

8.4 SERS-based detection of viral infections

Since the discovery of SERS in 1973 it has gained immense popularity in advanced diagnostics owing to its ability to detect single molecules with high accuracy. It has huge potential in the development of POC devices for various target analytes such as

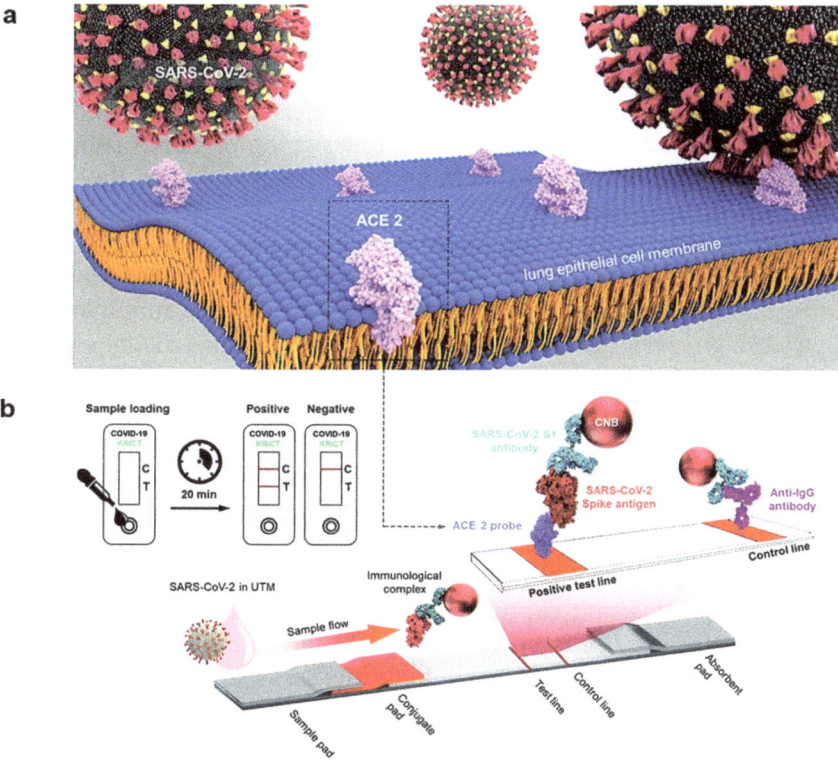

Figure 8.4. (a) The detection of SARS-CoV-2 spike 1 antigens using a cellular receptor (ACE2)-based LFIA. (b) In the design of the ACE2-based LFIA, the detection result was obtained in 20 min. (Reproduced with permission from [34]. Copyright 2020 Elsevier.)

viruses, bacteria, fungi, etc. It has a high possibility to detect trace amounts of target analytes with ultra-low sensitivity and measure the signals without complex sampling procedures [35]. Moreover, SERS is a detection tool that mainly depends upon the improvement in the Raman scattering of molecules adsorbed on the rough metal substrates. Today SERS-based detection of biomolecules has emerged as a technique with great potential due to its non-destructive nature, ultra-sensitivity, great enhancement factors up to 10^{10}–10^{11}, and high capability to detect a single molecule [36]. SERS can also offer a large number of vibrational spectra of adsorbed molecules and be applicable for the detection of multiple analytes to the lowest possible well-defined peaks. Recently, SERS has been utilized extensively in the analysis of biological analytes such as nucleic acids, viruses, biomarkers, and cells. In the past few years, SERS-based ultrasensitive biosensors have been developed for specific detection at the nanoscale due to their numerous advantages such as narrow line width, non-destructive biosensing, and selective target analysis [37]. Generally, the presence of a target analyte near the metal surface leads to the emergence of SERS signals. Different components are responsible for the optimization of SERS measurements. including adsorbed target analytes, laser sources, and plasmonic nanostructured materials [38]. Additionally, the constituents of nanostructured materials have greatly influenced the SERS signal intensities, such as the composition, size, and shape of the nanomaterials, permitting the broad optimization of SERS parameters. Currently, plasmonic nanomaterials such as AuNPs, AgNPs, magnetic NPs, etc, are utilized largely in the designing of SERS substrates which have great chemical and thermal stability and further enhance the SERS signal intensities and other optimizing parameters [39]. In this context, flexible SERS substrates have gained a lot of attention among researchers owing to their several advantages, such as high sensitivity and flexibility and their applicability in real-life conditions, e.g. the healthcare sector. Figure 8.5 shows the multiplex sensing of bioanalytes using plasmonic nanomaterials and simultaneous diagnosis of COVID-19 with enhanced SERS signals with the incorporation of flexible SERS substrates and SERS nanotags [40].

Owing to its advantages, Sun *et al* developed a highly sensitive SERS-based immunoassay to detect the avian influenza virus H3N2. They fabricated the sandwich model SERS platform by layering the SERS tags, magnetic supported substrates, and the target analyte, i.e. H3N2. Therein, SERS tags were composed of 4-mercaptobenzoic acid (MBA)-labeled AuNPs, and Fe_3O_4/AuNPs acted as highly SERS-active supporting and capturing substrates. The fabricated SERS platform exhibited low detection limits up to 10^2 $TCID_{50}$/ml for the H3N2 virus [41]. In another study Zhang *et al* reported a multivariate-statistical analysis that integrated the SERS technique to detect the SARS-CoV-2 virus. The performance of SERS has been determined through the binding of receptor binding domain (RBD) of spike glycoprotein and the ACE2 receptor of the S1 component which acts as both a

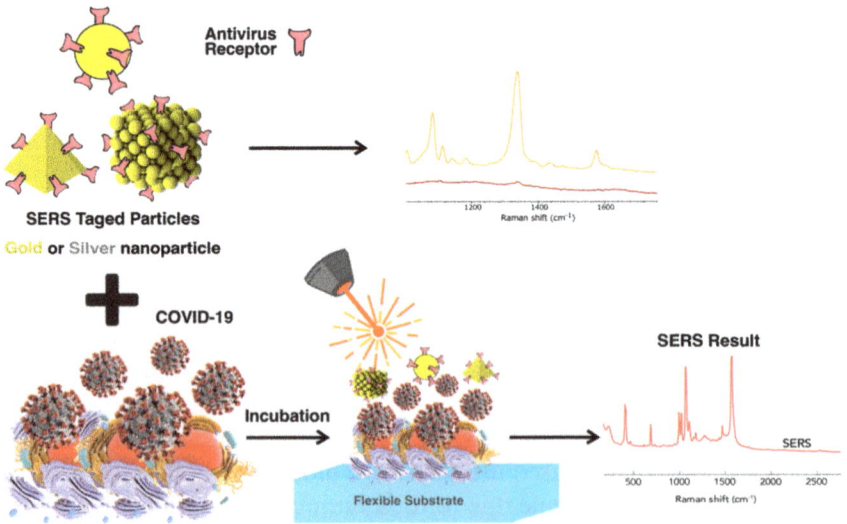

Figure 8.5. Advancement in the SERS detection technique from single biomarker detection to multiple analyte detection. The role of the flexible SERS substrate and plasmonic nanoparticles in the SERS signal enhancement for the diagnosis of COVID-19. (Reproduced with permission from [40]. CC BY 4.0.)

biorecognition molecule as well as a Raman reporter. The Raman intensities were suppressed after the successful binding of ACE2 and RBD at a 738 nm laser from which it could be concluded that the SARS-CoV-2 virus has been detected with high sensitivity [42]. In another study, Kukushkin *et al* developed an aptamer functionalized SERS platform for the investigation of the influenza (H3N2) virus. To achieve the 10^6–10^9 times SERS signal amplification, primary aptamer, influenza virus, and secondary aptamers were assembled using the sandwich approach. Primary aptamers were bonded with the SERS substrate, and influenza viruses were captured and attached with secondary aptamer functionalized Raman reporters. The SERS signal intensity was greatly influenced by the amount of both primary and secondary aptamers used. Hence the LOD observed for the platform was 10^{-4} hemagglutination units per probe as tested for the H3N2 virus [43].

8.5 SERS-based LFIA for sensitive detection of viral infections

In recent decades, the demand for developing highly specific and sensitive POC devices has increased for early diagnostics and other purposes. LFIA gained a lot of attention from researchers owing to its flexible, simple, and high-throughput screening characteristics [44]. Until now, most of the data obtained from conventional LFIA kits, i.e. colloidal AuNP-based LFIA testing kits, provided visual changes in color intensities of target analytes. However, the lower sensitivity results of the assay limited its utilization for highly sensitive detection and further diagnostic applications [45]. Meanwhile, several studies were performed for improving the sensitivity through different sensitivity enhanced platforms such as enzyme amplified signal systems, signal enhancement through fluorescence systems, magnetic particle embedded systems, and near-infrared dyes as reporters, but these systems may experience optical interference and need extra steps for the measurement of signals [46].

Despite several excellent features of the LFIA platform for the diagnosis of viral infections, they have some limitations, such as low sensitivity, poor selectivity, and the inability to perform multiple detections of analytes [47]. These disadvantages can be overcome by integrating the LFIA with a high-performance biosensing system such as SERS. SERS is a frequently used powerful sensing method that is dependent on the scattering of enhanced inelastic light by biomolecules adsorbed onto roughened metal surfaces [48]. Significantly, the SERS-based biosensing method can detect a single molecule with the incorporation of noble-metal nanoparticles. Hence, SERS has been widely utilized in different biomedical applications. SERS-based biosensors have also been explored extensively for the POC detection of various infectious diseases, primarily viruses [49]. However, SERS has several limitations, such as the large-scale synthesis of SERS nanotags, chemical and thermal stability, reusability, and reproducibility of SERS substrates. If SERS is integrated with immunoassay platforms, then the resulting technique can achieve high specificity, multiplex detection ability, and ultra-low sensitivity. In addition, SERS-based immunoassay platforms can detect multiple analytes simultaneously which certainly increases the usefulness of the technique [50].

Since 2007 the integration of SERS with LFIA has emerged as a highly sensitive detection technique for viral infections. The conjugation of Raman reporters with SERS nanotags enhanced the multiple detection ability of the LFIA system and provided enhanced Raman signals at the test line. Currently, the emergence of distinguished SERS nanotags overcame the challenges associated with AuNP-based conventional LFIA techniques and amplify the quantification of results with high sensitivity and specificity [51]. In addition, SERS-based LFA strips are simple assays projected to determine the sensitivity of target analytes. The technique has gained attention owing to its various advantages, such as rapidity, simplicity, and high stability [52]. For the integration of SERS into the LFIA platform, Raman reporter or SERS tags are labeled with detection nanoparticles and biorecognition moieties such as antibodies, proteins, nucleic acids, etc. The Raman reporter molecules should exhibit a high Raman scattering cross section and encompass thiolates or amino groups for high binding affinity to noble metals such as Au, Pt, or Ag to increase the enhancement factor of the SERS technique [53]. The electromagnetic enhancement factor mainly occurred due to the electromagnetic effect between the surface of nanoparticles and Raman reporter molecules [54]. In addition, the enhancement factor can also be induced by adjusting the excitation wavelength with absorption spectra of Raman reporters which led to surface-enhanced resonance Raman scattering (SERRS), which has high sensitivity [50]. To calculate the LOD of the LFIA, the test line should be analyzed through a Raman spectrometer with suitable laser excitation. Usually, SERS-based LFIA has been analyzed by Raman mapping of the test zone of the LFIA with a large Raman spectrometer set-up. The decrease in concentrations of target analytes leads to a lower intensity of SERS signals that can be visualized across the test zone via generating heat maps of signals [55]. For example, AuNPs labeled with Raman reporter malachite green isothiocyanate (MGITC) have been reported as SERS nanotags for the highly sensitive detection of oligonucleotides (DNA probe detection), i.e. HIV-1 DNA. Subsequently, it was observed that the reported SERS nanotags were more efficient than conventional AuNPs functionalized LF strips. MGITC exhibited a high enhancement factor that affected the SERS intensity of the fabricated MGITC–AuNPs–DNA SERS nanotags. The quantitative detection of the target HIV-1 DNA was observed by a change in the SERS intensity at the test line [56].

Traditionally, LFIA devices were thermally unstable and have not been utilized effectively in tropical regions. Therefore, silica-embedded AuNP-based SERS integrated LFIA kits have been developed for the effective diagnosis of viral diseases in tropical regions. For instance, Wang and co-workers developed SERS-based LFIA kits for the multiplex detection of two oligonucleotide DNAs from the herpes virus and bacillary angiomatosis (BA) simultaneously. The fabricated kit was composed of a 1:1 mixture of target analytes, i.e. immobilization of SERS nanotags with DNA of herpes virus and BA at the conjugate pad followed by two test lines and one control line. The SERS-based LFIA kits have high sensitivity compared to previously reported aggregation-based colorimetric techniques with an LOD of 0.043 pM and 0.074 pM for the herpes virus and BA, respectively [37]. In another study, Maneeprakorn and their group used highly roughened surface Au nanostars in a SERS-based LFIA array for the detection of the influenza A virus. Au nanostars have a multi-branched morphology and tunable surface plasmons which have good SERS performance. In addition, the Au nanostars were integrated with 4-amino thiophenol Raman reporter molecules and influenza A nucleoprotein specific antibody as the SERS detection probe. Furthermore, a SERS-based LFIA system has been developed based on the detection probe. The developed test system exhibited high sensitivity for the detection of the influenza A virus with an LOD of 6.7 ng ml^{-1} [46]. Recently Chen *et al* developed a highly sensitive SERS-based LFIA for the detection of both IgG and IgM antibodies simultaneously. They utilized gap-improved SERS nanotags with a 1 nm gap between the shell and core resulting in SERS hotspots that enhance the performance of the platform by 30-fold compared to traditional nanotags. In addition, the conjugated SARS-CoV-2 protein with gap-enhanced Raman nanotags replaced the conventional Au nanotags and provided highly sensitive Raman detection of both IgG and IgM antibodies with an LOD of 0.1 ng ml^{-1} and 1 ng ml^{-1}, respectively [52]. Recently, a portable SERS-based LFIA has been reported for the multiplexed detection of different analytes such as alpha-fetoprotein (AFP), prostate-specific antigen (PSA), and carcinoembryonic antigen (CEA) [30]. Xiao *et al* developed a rapid, portable, cost-effective, and POC SERS-based LFIA for highly sensitive determination of avian influenza virus (AIV H7N9). They fabricated the LFIA via functionalizing the AuAg^{4-}^{ATP}@AgNPs with AIV-specific antibodies and goat anti-mouse IgG antibodies on the test and control line, respectively, at the nitrocellulose membrane as shown in figure 8.6. The change in color on the test line confirmed the existence of AIV H7H9.

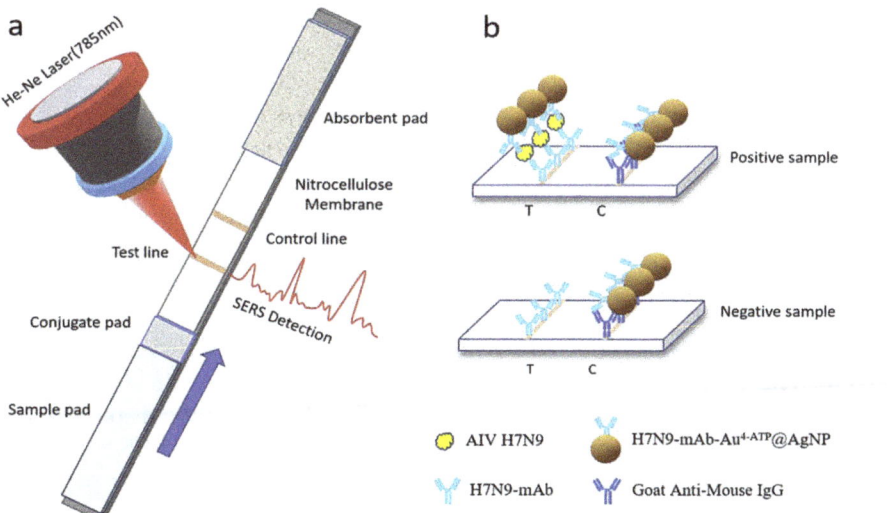

Figure 8.6. (a) Pictorial representation of SERS-based LFIA detection of AIV H7N9. (b) The depiction of two brown lines on the test line and control line indicates the detection of AIV H7N9 and only one line observed at the control line indicates the absence of AIV H7N9 in the sample analysis. (Reproduced with permission from [57]. Copyright 2019 Elsevier.)

For quantification of the target, the SERS laser would strike the test line and provide highly sensitive detection of AIV H7N9 with an LOD of 0.0018 HAU [57]. Antibacterial drugs such as neomycin and lincomycin have been used effectively in the treatment of bacterial infectious diseases. However, increasing antibiotic resistance poses a serious threat to mankind. Hence, Shi *et al* developed a fast and multiplexed SRS-based LFIA platform for ultrasensitive detection of neomycin and lincomycin in milk samples. They detected both neomycin and lincomycin within 15 min with an LOD of 0.33 pg ml^{-1} and 0.29 pg ml^{-1}, respectively, in a lower volume of 100 ml [58].

Recently, Bai *et al* synthesized three types of citrate-capped bimetallic Ag–AuNPs SERS probes, i.e. core–shell (Ag shell at Au core), rattle-like Ag–Au shell@Au core, and Ag–AuNPs, and utilized these for SERS activities. The experimental results revealed that the citrate-capped Au@Ag–AuNPs have the highest SERS enhancement factor amongst all synthesized SERS probes for various target analytes [55]. In another study, Wang and the group demonstrated SERS-based LFIA for simultaneous detection of influenza A H1N1 virus and human adenovirus (HAdV) by utilizing the Fe_3O_4@Ag nanoparticles as magnetic SERS nanotags. The developed magnetic nanotags specific recognized and magnetically enriched viral targets in the sample and detected the virus on the LFIA strip with SERS. Hence the developed platform has the lowest detection limit up to 50 and 10 pfu ml^{-1} for H1N1 and HAdV, respectively, which was 2000-fold more sensitive than conventional colloidal AuNP modified LFIA strips. The modification of the LFIA strips with magnetic SERS nanotags and the immobilization of antibodies of the target viruses with a detection route is shown in figure 8.7 [53].

In recent times, Zhang *et al* reported a rapid, sensitive, and quantitative SERS-based immunochromatic assay (ICA) for the detection of rotavirus by using dual Raman labeled Ag@AuNPs. The Raman signal was observed at a characteristic peak at 1334 cm^{-1} for ICA color change at the test line for rotavirus detection. The fabricated quantitative immunoassay had a detection limit of 80 pg ml^{-1} and 8 pg ml^{-1} for visual and SERS detection in a wide linear range of 8–40 000 pg ml^{-1} for rotavirus. In addition, the results obtained from this assay were compared with RT-PCR tested clinical samples and commercially available colloidal AuNPs-based immunoassay kits to validate the fabricated platform. The developed SERS-based ICA quantitatively demonstrated the highly specific, sensitive, accurate, and precise results for the determination of rotavirus [59]. In another study, a highly sensitive SERS-based LFIA was reported for the determination of SARS-CoV-2 spike RBD antigen. The SERS nanotag was prepared by integrating the anti-SARS-CoV-2 spike antibodies with MBA-modified AuNPs. The analytical parameters were optimized, such as the concentration of antibodies used in SERS nanotags, the loading of Raman reporters, and material for a membrane for better performance of the fabricated SERS-based LFIA platform. Moreover, the analytical outcomes were compared with traditional techniques such as ELISA and LFIA for the detection of the SARS-CoV-2 virus. The reported method has a lowest detection limit of 0.1 ng ml^{-1} with a short time within 20 min as compared to ELISA having 0.4 ng ml^{-1}

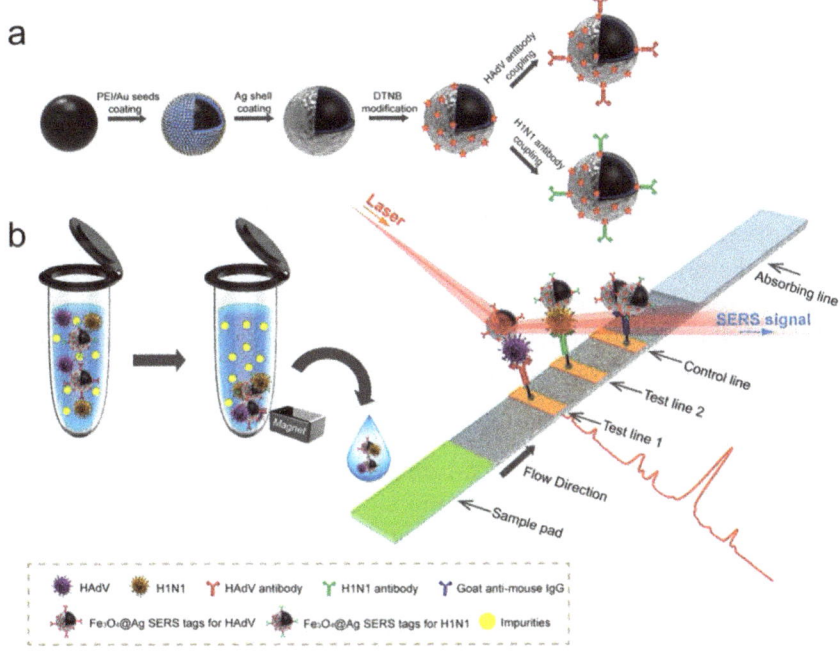

Figure 8.7. (a) Preparation strategy of antibody-modified Fe$_3$O$_4$@Ag magnetic tags and (b) schematic representation of a magnetic SERS-strip for simultaneous detection of both H1N1 and HAdV viruses. (Reproduced with permission from [53]. Copyright 2019 American Chemical Society.)

within 3.5 h and LFIA having 1 ng ml^{-1} within 15 min [60]. Recently, Liu *et al* developed a highly sensitive SERS-based LFIA method for simultaneous detection of both IgM/IgG SARS-CoV-2 antibodies. They prepared excellent Raman scattering SERS nanotags by labeling the double layer of 5,5-dithiobis-(2-nitrobenzoic acid) (DTNB) Raman dye and SiO$_2$ core coated with Ag shell (SiO$_2$@Ag). The synthesized SERS nanotags are highly stable with good mono dispersity and exceptional SERS signals. The surface of SiO2@Ag was altered with SARS-CoV-2 spike protein to bind with a specific target analyte, i.e. SARS-CoV-2 spike protein antibodies. Afterward, the two test zones of the analytical membrane were modified with anti-human IgM and IgG antibodies to bind simultaneously and detect anti-SARS-CoV-2 IgM/IgG on one test line. The developed assay provided 800 times higher sensitivity than the traditional AuNP-based LFIA method for the detection of both IgM and IgG antibodies simultaneously. Further, the fabricated method has potential applicability in clinical samples and has been validated in serum samples with highly precise and 100% accurate results [61].

Recently, a portable SERS-based LFIA tool has been developed for the automatic detection of West Nile virus (WNV) with good specificity and high sensitivity. The detection technique employed SERS nanotags prepared through labeling of Au@AgNPs on dual-layer Raman molecules that were specifically developed for detecting WNV. The reported method has 100-fold more sensitivity than naked eye signals with an LOD of 0.1 ng ml^{-1} for the WNV. The SERS-based LFIA platform exhibited comparable results to fluorescence and RT-PCR methods with high sensitivity and good specificity for WNV [62].

8.6 Challenges

The integration of cross-cutting research and development on both SERS and LFIA technologies has gained a lot of attention from the scientific community. Although the combination of SERS and LFIA provides highly sensitive and specific results for the determination of various viral infections, the integrated technology has some limitations, such as how to achieve a uniform thickness of SERS substrates and precise quantified results, and how to reduce the fabrication cost of SERS substrates. Moreover, merging SERS with LFIA is also able to detect target analytes in POC settings with varied concentrations and quantified results, but there is need for a simple and user-friendly set-up to provide interpretable and accurate results to the clinicians and patients. Moreover, SERS-based LFIA could provide a rapid and cost-effective measurement of viral biomarkers with existing set-ups in healthcare industries, e.g. ambulances, doctor's practices, and pharmaceutical sectors. There is also a need for awareness to reorganize clinical trials and personalized data collection of patients. This offers more comprehensive, inexpensive, and possibly harmless detection at an early stage of viral infections. The SERS-based LFIA platform is well-suited to POC settings where it could be utilized to detect viral biomarkers associated with the toxicity of drugs, allowing the technique to be improved for POC usage. In addition, SERS-based LFIA could be very valuable in permitting the instant making of decisions in the least developed countries as there the availability of data is very limited. However, to date the research and development has mainly focused on laboratory-based SERS-based LFIA owing to the existing benchtop set-ups to perform the Raman analysis of the LFIA strips. Hence, research should emphasize the development of portable and hand-held Raman instruments to obtain Raman signal readout across the LFIA kits and on the translation of SERS-based LFIA platforms from laboratory to POC settings.

The portability and stability of the SERS-based LFIA systems have been limited by the complex sampling procedure and if this system is to be converted into a routine screening or diagnostic method like LFIA analysis, then it is mandatory to develop the Raman system into hand-held devices which permit the LFIA and SERS measurements to occur in more confined settings. Further, this system would deliver fast responses at the patient location which leads to much quicker decision-making in time sensitive situations. Confined sampling procedures will also lessen issues regarding the safety measures against harmful laser beams which are present in the open laser microscopic systems. Another challenge faced by SERS-based LFIA settings is the usage of a calibration model before the detection of biomolecules to provide accurate results. However, the calibration of the tools is a complex data analysis that requires trained personnel or spectroscopists to interpret the results accurately. Hence SERS-based LFIA cannot be used in POC testing due to the complex calibration model. Therefore, it needs to be simplified and give simpler readable results to the patient who will not be skilled personnel. In addition, the integration of nanomaterials in LFIA strips has led to the agglomeration of biorecognition elements at the test zone which can provide exaggeratedly high SERS signal intensities which results in false-negative results. The stability and shelf-life of nanomaterial incorporated Raman reporters or hotspots are the key components that need to be considered carefully to obtain reproducible outcomes. In addition, the control zone of the LFIA strip must be calibrated before the testing to normalize the results. Even though several other challenges need to be solved to develop a highly sensitive, selective, multiplexed, miniaturized, and portable SERS-based LFIA platform, this technique may present a promising alternative for the advanced diagnostics of viral infections. If we address the current issues, the SERS-based LFIA may be used for rapid and accurate POC quantitation of viral infections in the near future.

8.7 Summary

To summarize, the search for a highly sensitive, selective, rapid, accurate, stable, and point-of-care diagnostic technique is highly motivated in times like the COVID-19 pandemic. The available approaches that detect infectious diseases face various drawbacks such as being expensive, time-consuming, complex, less sensitive, and requiring heavy instruments. Alternative methods including the development of biosensors have tried to deal with such concerns by providing simple, quick, and cost-effective solutions. However, the demands of current times require further investigation and integration of multi-skilled techniques that can overcome the bottlenecks of available biosensing methods. One such approach has been discussed in this chapter, i.e. the integration of SERS with LFIA. This combinational diagnostic approach offers dual benefits of quantitative as well as qualitative results with the advantages of high sensitivity, a high degree of quantification, accuracy via the SERS platform, and simple, cost-effective, and rapid results via LFIA integration. The use of SERS utilizes the peculiar features of plasmonic nanoparticles, and the optical properties and surface functionalities of the modified SERS substrates. The use of LFIA strips enables point-of-care, miniaturized, smooth, simple, rapid, cheap, and high-throughput outcomes of the diagnostic tests. Numerous infectious diseases impact human lives around the globe, which require advanced diagnostic techniques such as SERS-based LFIA to help fight pandemics and future health hazards. Further, the exploitation of the remarkable attributes of nanomaterials and nano-systems is needed to be utilized for ultra-low detection levels of viruses, highly selective binding of bioanalytes, and the development of accurate, prompt, affordable, and economic diagnostic platforms. The integration of SERS and LFIA technologies gives numerous advantages, such as rapid responses, good selectivity, high sensitivity, small sample volume, low cross-contamination, and simple operation. With the incorporation of emerging functional nanomaterials, SERS-based LFIA platforms will continue to be enhanced and be established rapidly toward portability, integration, miniaturization, and commercialization.

Acknowledgments

The authors thank the Director of CSIR-AMPRI Bhopal, India, for his interest in this work. SY thanks CSIR, India, for the award of a JRF. MAS thanks DST-SERB for a JRF. PR thanks CSIR, India, for an SRF. NK thanks UGC, India, for an SRF. RK acknowledges SERB and CSIR for providing funds in the form of the IPA/2020/000130 project and MLP-0049, respectively.

References

[1] Sadique Mohd A *et al* 2021 High-performance antiviral nano-systems as a shield to inhibit viral infections: SARS-CoV-2 as a model case study *J. Mater. Chem.* B **9** 4620–42

[2] Souf S 2016 Recent advances in diagnostic testing for viral infections *Biosci. Horiz.* **9** hzw010

[3] Ranjan P *et al* 2021 Rapid diagnosis of SARS-CoV-2 using potential point-of-care electro-chemical immunosensor: toward the future prospects *Int. Rev. Immunol.* **40** 126–42

[4] Choi H K, Lee M J, Lee S N, Kim T H and Oh B K 2021 Noble metal nanomaterial-based biosensors for electrochemical and optical detection of viruses causing respiratory illnesses *Front. Chem.* **9** 1–9

[5] Abubakar Sadique Mohd Y S, Ranjan P, Akram Khan Mohd, Kumar A and Khan R 2021 Rapid detection of SARS-CoV-2 using graphene-based IoT integrated advanced electro-chemical biosensor *Mater. Lett.* **305** 130824

[6] Ribeiro B V, Cordeiro T A R, Oliveira e Freitas G R, Ferreira L F and Franco D L 2020 Biosensors for the detection of respiratory viruses: a review *Talanta Open* **2** 100007

[7] Ranjan P, Singhal A, Sadique M A, Yadav S, Parihar A and Khan R 2022 Scope of biosensors, commercial aspects, and miniaturized devices for point-of-care testing from lab to clinics applications *Biosensor Based Advanced Cancer Diagnostics: From Lab to Clinics* ed R Khan, A Parihar and S K Sanghi (New York: Academic) ch 24 pp 395–410

[8] Hamm L, Gee A and Indrasekara A S D S 2019 Recent advancement in the surface-enhanced Raman spectroscopy-based biosensors for infectious disease diagnosis *Appl. Sci.* **9** 1448

[9] Saviñon-Flores F *et al* 2021 A review on SERS-based detection of human virus infections: influenza and coronavirus *Biosensors* **11** 66

[10] Dieringer J A *et al* 2006 Surface enhanced Raman spectroscopy: new materials, concepts, characterization tools, and applications *Faraday Discuss.* **132** 9–26

[11] Shanmukh S, Jones L, Driskell J, Zhao Y, Dluhy R and Tripp R A 2006 Rapid and sensitive detection of respiratory virus molecular signatures using a silver nanorod array SERS substrate *Nano Lett.* **6** 2630–6

[12] Sitjar J, Liao J, der, Lee H, Tsai H P, Wang J R and Liu P Y 2021 Challenges of SERS technology as a non-nucleic acid or -antigen detection method for SARS-CoV-2 virus and its variants *Biosens. Bioelectron.* **181** 113153

[13] Hsiao W W W *et al* 2021 Recent advances in novel lateral flow technologies for detection of COVID-19 *Biosensors* **11** 295

[14] Sloan-Dennison S, O'Connor E, Dear J W, Graham D and Faulds K 2022 Towards quantitative point of care detection using SERS lateral flow immunoassays *Anal. Bioanal. Chem.* **414** 4541–9

[15] Wang L *et al* 2021 SERS-based test strips: principles, designs and applications *Biosens. Bioelectron.* **189** 113360

[16] Wu Z 2019 Simultaneous detection of *Listeria monocytogenes* and *Salmonella typhimurium* by a SERS-based lateral flow immunochromatographic assay *Food Anal. Methods* **12** 1086–91

[17] Yadav S *et al* 2021 SERS based lateral flow immunoassay for point-of-care detection of SARS-CoV-2 in clinical samples *ACS Appl. Biomater.* **4** 2974–95

[18] Premraj A, Aleyas A G, Nautiyal B and Rasool T J 2020 Nucleic acid and immunological diagnostics for SARS-CoV-2: processes, platforms and pitfalls *Diagnostics* **10** 866

[19] Ichzan A M *et al* 2021 Solid-phase recombinase polymerase amplification using an extremely low concentration of a solution primer for sensitive electrochemical detection of hepatitis B viral DNA *Biosens. Bioelectron.* **179** 113065

[20] Fabiani L *et al* 2021 Magnetic beads combined with carbon black-based screen-printed electrodes for COVID-19: a reliable and miniaturized electrochemical immunosensor for SARS-CoV-2 detection in saliva *Biosens. Bioelectron.* **171** 112686

[21] Ranjan P, Sadique Mohd A, Yadav S, Parihar A and Khan R 2022 Miniaturized analytical system for point-of-care coronavirus infection diagnostics *Advanced Biosensors for Virus Detection: Smart Diagnostics to Combat SARS-CoV-2* ed R Khan, A Parihar, A Kaushik and A Kumar (New York: Academic) ch 17 pp 305–40

[22] Ranjan P, Sadique Mohd A, Yadav S and Khan R 2022 Approaches for fabrication of point-of-care biosensors for viral infection *Advanced Biosensors for Virus Detection: Smart Diagnostics to Combat SARS-CoV-2* ed R Khan, A Parihar, A Kaushik and A Kumar (New York: Academic) ch 19 pp 353–71

[23] Sharma A *et al* 2021 Optical biosensors for diagnostics of infectious viral disease: a recent update *Diagnostics* **11** 2083

[24] Sadique Mohd A, Ranjan P, Yadav S and Khan R 2022 Advanced high-throughput biosensor-based diagnostic approaches for detection of severe acute respiratory syndrome-coronavirus-2 *Computational Approaches for Novel Therapeutic and Diagnostic Designing to Mitigate SARS-CoV-2 Infection: Revolutionary Strategies to Combat Pandemics* ed A Parihar, R Khan, A Kumar, A K Kaushik and H Gohel (New York: Academic) ch 8 pp 147–69

[25] Singhal A, Parihar A, Kumar N and Khan R 2022 High throughput molecularly imprinted polymers based electrochemical nanosensors for point-of-care diagnostics of COVID-19 *Mater. Lett.* **306** 130898

[26] Liu X *et al* 2020 Fe_3O_4@Au SERS tags-based lateral flow assay for simultaneous detection of serum amyloid A and C-reactive protein in unprocessed blood sample *Sens. Actuators* B **320** 128350

[27] Tripathi P, Upadhyay N and Nara S 2018 Recent advancements in lateral flow immunoassays: a journey for toxin detection in food *Crit. Rev. Food Sci. Nutr.* **58** 1715–34

[28] Sajid M, Kawde A N and Daud M 2015 Designs, formats and applications of lateral flow assay: a literature review *J. Saudi Chem. Soc.* **19** 689–705

[29] Khlebtsov B and Khlebtsov N 2020 Surface-enhanced Raman scattering-based lateral-flow immunoassay *Nanomaterials* **10** 2228

[30] Xiao R *et al* 2020 Portable and multiplexed lateral flow immunoassay reader based on SERS for highly sensitive point-of-care testing *Biosens. Bioelectron.* **168** 112524

[31] Ragnesola B, Jin D, Lamb C C, Shaz B H, Hillyer C D and Luchsinger L L 2020 COVID-19 antibody detection using lateral flow assay tests in a cohort of convalescent plasma donors *BMC Res. Notes* **13** 372

[32] Kim K *et al* 2021 Recent advances in sensitive surface-enhanced Raman scattering-based lateral flow assay platforms for point-of-care diagnostics of infectious diseases *Sens. Actuators* B **329** 129214

[33] Yen C W *et al* 2015 Multicolored silver nanoparticles for multiplexed disease diagnostics: distinguishing dengue, yellow fever, and Ebola viruses *Lab Chip* **15** 1638–41

[34] Lee J H *et al* 2021 A novel rapid detection for SARS-CoV-2 spike 1 antigens using human angiotensin converting enzyme 2 (ACE2) *Biosens. Bioelectron.* **171** 112715

[35] Ambartsumyan O, Gribanyov D, Kukushkin V, Kopylov A and Zavyalova E 2020 SERS-based biosensors for virus determination with oligonucleotides as recognition elements *Int. J. Mol. Sci.* **21** 1–15

[36] Hassanain W A, Spoors J, Johnson C L, Faulds K, Keegan N and Graham D 2021 Rapid ultra-sensitive diagnosis of: clostridium difficile infection using a SERS-based lateral flow assay *Analyst* **146** 4495–505

[37] Chen H *et al* 2020 Recent advances in surface-enhanced Raman scattering-based micro-devices for point-of-care diagnosis of viruses and bacteria *Nanoscale* **12** 21560–70

[38] Zhang D, Huang L, Liu B, Ge Q, Dong J and Zhao X 2019 Rapid and ultrasensitive quantification of multiplex respiratory tract infection pathogen via lateral flow microarray based on SERS nanotags *Theranostics* **9** 4849–59

[39] Mosier-Boss P A 2017 Review of SERS substrates for chemical sensing *Nanomaterials* **7** 142

[40] Mousavi S M *et al* 2022 Highly sensitive flexible SERS-based sensing platform for detection of COVID-19 *Biosensors* **12** 466

[41] Sun Y *et al* 2017 A promising magnetic SERS immunosensor for sensitive detection of avian influenza virus *Biosens. Bioelectron.* **89** 906–12

[42] Li Y, Lin C, Peng Y, He J and Yang Y 2022 High-sensitivity and point-of-care detection of SARS-CoV-2 from nasal and throat swabs by magnetic SERS biosensor *Sens. Actuators* B **365** 131974

[43] Kukushkin V I *et al* 2019 Highly sensitive detection of influenza virus with SERS aptasensor *PLoS One* **14** e0216247

[44] Kim H, Chung D R and Kang M 2019 A new point-of-care test for the diagnosis of infectious diseases based on multiplex lateral flow immunoassays *Analyst* **144** 2460–6

[45] Quesada-González D and Merkoçi A 2015 Nanoparticle-based lateral flow biosensors *Biosens. Bioelectron.* **73** 47–63

[46] Maneeprakorn W, Bamrungsap S, Apiwat C and Wiriyachaiporn N 2016 Surface-enhanced Raman scattering based lateral flow immunochromatographic assay for sensitive influenza detection *RSC Adv.* **6** 112079–85

[47] Li F *et al* 2020 Paper-based point-of-care immunoassays: recent advances and emerging trends *Biotechnol. Adv.* **39** 107442

[48] Liang X *et al* 2021 Carbon-based SERS biosensor: from substrate design to sensing and bioapplication *NPG Asia Mater.* **13** 8

[49] Wang C, Liu M, Wang Z, Li S, Deng Y and He N 2021 Point-of-care diagnostics for infectious diseases: from methods to devices *Nano Today* **37** 101092

[50] Achadu O J *et al* 2021 Molybdenum trioxide quantum dot-encapsulated nanogels for virus detection by surface-enhanced Raman scattering on a 2D substrate *ACS Appl. Mater. Interfaces* **13** 27836–44

[51] Ye H, Liu Y, Zhan L, Liu Y and Qin Z 2020 Signal amplification and quantification on lateral flow assays by laser excitation of plasmonic nanomaterials *Theranostics* **10** 4359–73

[52] Chen S *et al* 2021 SERS-based lateral flow immunoassay for sensitive and simultaneous detection of anti-SARS-CoV-2 IgM and IgG antibodies by using gap-enhanced Raman nanotags *Sens. Actuators* B **348** 130706

[53] Wang C *et al* 2019 Magnetic SERS strip for sensitive and simultaneous detection of respiratory viruses *ACS Appl. Mater. Interfaces* **11** 19495–505

[54] Qian X M and Nie S M 2008 Single-molecule and single-nanoparticle SERS: from fundamental mechanisms to biomedical applications *Chem. Soc. Rev.* **37** 912–20

[55] Bai T *et al* 2018 Functionalized Au@Ag–Au nanoparticles as an optical and SERS dual probe for lateral flow sensing *Anal. Bioanal. Chem.* **410** 2291–303

[56] Fu X, Cheng Z, Yu J, Choo P, Chen L and Choo J 2016 A SERS-based lateral flow assay biosensor for highly sensitive detection of HIV-1 DNA *Biosens. Bioelectron.* **78** 530–7

[57] Xiao M *et al* 2019 Ultrasensitive detection of avian influenza A (H7N9) virus using surface-enhanced Raman scattering-based lateral flow immunoassay strips *Anal. Chim. Acta.* **1053** 139–47

[58] Shi Q, Tao C and Kong D 2022 Multiplex SERS-based lateral flow assay for one-step simultaneous detection of neomycin and lincomycin in milk *Eur. Food Res. Technol.* **248** 2157–65

[59] Zhang Y *et al* 2021 Rapid and sensitive detection of rotavirus by surface-enhanced Raman scattering immunochromatography *Microchim. Acta.* **188** 3

[60] Serebrennikova K V *et al* 2021 Lateral flow immunoassay of SARS-CoV-2 antigen with SERS-based registration: development and comparison with traditional immunoassays *Biosensors* **11** 510

[61] Liu H *et al* 2021 Development of a SERS-based lateral flow immunoassay for rapid and ultra-sensitive detection of anti-SARS-CoV-2 IgM/IgG in clinical samples *Sens. Actuators* B **329** 129196

[62] Jia X, Liu Z, Peng Y, Hou G, Chen W and Xiao R 2021 Automatic and sensitive detection of West Nile virus non-structural protein 1 with a portable SERS-LFIA detector *Microchim. Acta.* **188** 206

Chapter 9

SERS-based microfluidics for real sample detection

Jijo Lukose, Santhosh Chidangil and Sajan D George

The quest to develop easy-to-operate systems that require minimal sample volume for accurate and specific detection of analytes or biomolecules has paved the way for synergic integration of microfluidics and surface-enhanced Raman spectroscopy. The advances in nanotechnology facilitate the reproducible fabrication of plasmonic platforms that allow fingerprinting of the molecule of interest, while progress in microfluidic fabrication technologies allows the separation of the target molecule in ultra-small volumes in an automated way. Here, we present the fundamentals of the surface-enhanced Raman spectroscopic technique followed by an account of continuous and droplet-based microfluidic platforms and their integration with the surface-enhanced Raman spectroscopic technique. Further, the progress in sensing real samples using the synergically integrated microfluidics–surface-enhanced Raman spectroscopy devices is discussed with a special emphasis on biosensing, pathogen detection, heavy metal detection, etc.

9.1 Introduction

The increasing demand for the miniaturization and integration of specific and accurate detection moieties to probe the target molecules of interest in an analytical assay platform has paved the wave for the emergence of microfluidics-assisted lab-on-a-chip (LOC) technologies. The utilization of the samples in micron-scale confined channels or open microfluidic platforms not only results in a decrease in analysis time, sample volume, and reagent consumption, but also improves the sensitivity and allows parallel measurements without increasing the complexity or system footprint [1]. With the proper design of the microfluidic platforms, currently, measurements using picoliter sample volumes and less are possible. Apart from being an efficient analytical assay platform, the potential of these techniques is demonstrated in diverse areas including virology, biotechnology, micro-propulsion, environmental sensing, energy applications, lab-on-a-chip (LOC) devices, etc [2–5]. The microfluidic-assisted platforms are now emerging as an efficient alternative to the conventional bio-fluid analysis platforms (e.g. 96 well plates assisted probing of biological interactions in conventional ELISA tests) as they do not require the tedious manual dilution process [6]. In addition, the microfluidics platforms facilitate desired concentration gradients. The technique can be used for real-life applications via the development of point-of-care (POC) sensors for the chemical as well as biological detection of the target molecules. Despite the great promise that microfluidics technology offers, most LOC devices still rely on external and complex instrumentation for accurate and specific detection of the target analyte. Therefore, these devices are still largely considered to be lab-based systems wherein stand-ardized laboratory protocols are in order and they often fail outside the controlled laboratory environment. However, the integration of transducers such as electro-chemical, magnetic, or optics/photonics enables the sensitive and selective probing of the biological/chemical interaction in real-life samples [7–12]. Amongst these different transducers, the optical transducers offer the unique advantage of having a non-contact nature and consequent maintenance of sample sterility. Researchers have integrated various modalities such as laser-induced fluorescence (LIF) and Raman spectroscopy with microfluidic systems for carrying out investigations on real samples [13–17]. The potential of microfluidics-assisted techniques in point-of-care sensing applications is well reviewed in the recent literature [18, 19].

In this chapter, we focus mainly on surface-enhanced Raman spectroscopy (SERS) and its integration with microfluidics for diverse applications with an emphasis on biological applications. The chapter provides a brief introduction to the progress in the field of surface-enhanced Raman spectroscopy and the strategies used for the improvement of the Raman signal. Further, an account of the continuous flow and droplet-based platforms used in conjunction with Raman spectroscopy is given. In addition, an overview of the progress happening in the field of colloidal and solid-substrate fabrication for microfluidics-integrated SERS plat-forms is given. Additionally, the various applications of the microfluidics-integrated SERS technique, particularly in the field of biosensing, pathogen detection, and detection of pollutants, pesticides, drugs, and heavy metal ions, are discussed in detail. Finally, the conclusion and the future perspectives in microfluidics integrated with the SERS technique are also discussed.

9.2 Surface-enhanced Raman spectroscopy

Spectroscopic modalities, in particular Raman spectroscopy, have been of great interest due to their highly sensitive and non-destructive sample analysis capability. This technique relies on the collection of scattered light from a sample in response to the incidence of a monochromatic light source on it. Following the elimination of the elastically scattered light with the usage of an appropriate optical filter, the analysis of collected inelastic scattered light can provide information that allows molecular fingerprinting of the sample of interest. The Raman spectroscopy technique is highly sensitive to the environmental perturbations occurring inside and outside the sample. The application of the vibrational spectroscopic technique in solving real-world problems has turned into reality only in recent years, even though the Raman effect was discovered as far back as the late 1920s. It can be attributed to the low-Raman scattering cross-section of most of the molecules as only 1 out of 10^8 incident photons are scattered inelastically. Nevertheless, the utility of Raman spectroscopy and its different variants can increase exponentially as the technology proves its efficacy in diverse areas including environmental monitoring, biosensing, chemical sensing, forensics, disease detection, etc [21–24]. The advances in nano-science and nanotechnology caused a major renaissance in the field of Raman spectroscopy by exploiting the plasmonic field around metallic nanoparticles upon excitation with an appropriate resonance wavelength optical radiation [20]. The integration of nanoscience along with Raman spectroscopy mitigates the issue of a low-Raman scattering cross-section to a large extent and currently enables the measurement of analyte molecules of concentrations as low as femto- to attomoles. The approach wherein the Raman spectroscopy is integrated with nanoparticles or nanostructures is popularly known as the surface-enhanced Raman spectroscopic technique (SERS). The enhancement in the SERS signal is generally attributed to chemical enhancement or electromagnetic enhancement or a combination of the two, as demonstrated in figure 9.1 [20]. The electromagnetic enhancement (EM) originates from the field enhancement of incident as well as scattered fields as a result of localized surface plasmon resonance (LSPR) excitation of metallic nanoparticles or nanostructures [25, 26]. On the other hand, the chemical transfer mechanism (CT) stems from the molecular structure of the sample and the specific interaction

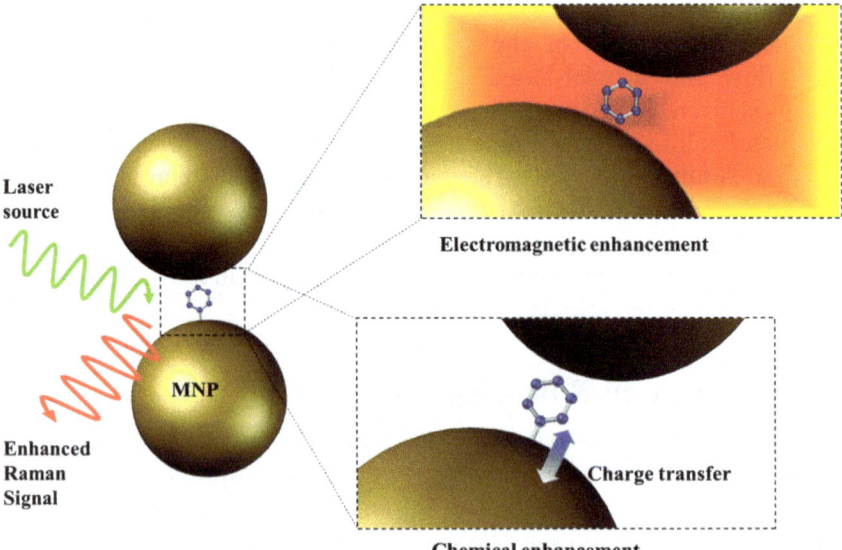

Figure 9.1. Schematic of the electromagnetic and chemical enhancement mechanism of Raman scattering. (Reproduced with permission from [20]. Copyright 2019 Springer.)

between the sample and the nanostructures [27]. The enhancement in the Raman signal occurs when the analyte molecule is placed in the proximity of nanoparticles called 'hotspots'. Recent studies report an average enhancement factor of 11–12 orders and an order of 14 for single-molecule detection [28, 29]. With the integration with optical microscopes, Raman spectroscopy can be used for imaging biochemical changes with a higher spatial resolution that cannot be normally achieved via conventional infrared spectroscopy. Detection via the SERS technique can be performed via direct or indirect strategies, as demonstrated in figure 9.2. In the direct approach, the Raman spectra are acquired directly from the target analyte, which is kept close to the nanoparticle surface. Indirect strategies for SERS detection can be performed using host–guest interaction wherein spectra will be acquired from the host molecule placed in close contact with the nanomaterial surface. The presence of the target analyte can induce variations in the Raman spectra of the host material, which normally manifest as a change in the Raman spectrum. In another indirect approach, specific Raman probes which can selectively bind the target analyte will be attached to nanomaterials. Direct detection strategies are employed in cases where the nanoparticle has a higher affinity toward the target of interest. Conversely, analytes with a lower affinity toward metallic nanostructures can be detected using an indirect SERS approach [30–32].

SERS substrates can be fabricated via various routes which include the replication of the substrates from pulsed laser patterned surfaces using soft lithography in combination with the reduction of plasmonic nanoparticles as mentioned in our earlier work [33]. Researchers have also employed the potential of superhydrophobic gold-loaded nanoporous anodic alumina as efficient substrates which can provide an enhancement factor of ~6.9×10^5 [31]. Another alternative is to create a wettability contrast surface in a superhydrophobic material to generate a plasmonic droplet assay for sensing applications [32]. Despite the great promise of the SERS technique, the real-life application of the technique is largely limited by the lack of substrate reproducibility and the high cost of analysis. To mitigate these issues, the scientific

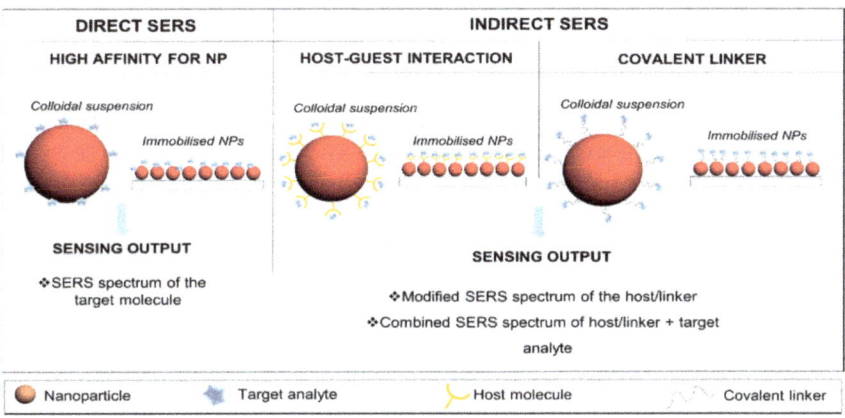

Figure 9.2. Surface-enhanced Raman scattering (SERS) detection strategies. (Reproduced with permission from [30]. CC BY 4.0.)

community is currently exploring the advantages of microfluidics and to integrate with them the sensitive SERS technique (MF-SERS). However, the integration of SERS substrates into a microfluidic chip requires complicated fabrication techniques, and the substrate is often exposed to additional stress such as fluid flow which can adversely affect the physicochemical stability. Nevertheless, several strategies have been employed to create the SERS effect in a microfluidic channel. The commonly adopted techniques involve SERS substrates dispersed in a flowing medium, and integration or immobilization of the SERS substrates via a top-down or bottom-up approach.

The first strategy requires pre-synthesis of nanomolar assemblies of differently shaped plasmonic nanoparticles and their dispersion in the microfluidic channel and concentration enrichment of the particles and analytes at desired locations. The advantage of this approach is the ease of operation and the possibility of recovering back the plasmonic nanoparticles. The second strategy exploits the advances in microfabrication technologies to create nanostructures such as nanopillars inside the microfluidic channels to which plasmonic nanomaterials can be sputtered. Such substrate fabrication provides better reproducibility in the Raman signal due to more homogeneous absorption of the analyte molecules. Direct laser writing, nanoprinting, etc, are popularly employed to create plasmonic SERS substrates inside a microfluidic channel [34, 35]. The last bottom-up strategy employs spatial deposition of single metal nanoparticles or nanostructured materials inside the microfluidic channel. This approach includes the utilization of surface functionalization chemistry or polymer/glass writing via various lithographic techniques. Depending upon the purpose, homogeneous or heterogeneous patterns can be created easily on these kinds of substrates.

9.3 Continuous flow and droplet-based platforms

Integration of SERS with microfluidic technologies can be realized via continuous flow platforms or droplet-based digital platforms (figure 9.3). The continuous flow microfluidic platform can be coupled with active SERS (*in situ* aggregation of plasmonic particles to create hotspots and SERS platforms) as well as passive platforms (SERS platforms are already integrated with microfluidic channels). As the continuous flow system can mitigate the issue of localized temperature rise due to various factors including exciting Raman laser-induced heating, these systems are particularly beneficial for highly temperature-sensitive measurements of samples such as biological samples. However, the memory effect due to the enrichment of the analyte molecules onto the walls of the channel is a major limitation in continuous flow microfluidic platforms. In addition, most of the continuous flow microfluidic channel-assisted SERS approaches rely on diffusion-driven flow and consequent mixing. This makes the measurements much slower compared to the conventional approaches. Droplet-based microfluidics, also called segmented flow platforms, can be a reliable alternative in this scenario, which involves the separation of nanoparticle suspension and sample droplets of an immiscible fluid phase (water/oil two phases segmented continuous flow). As the droplets do not permit significant liquid exchange between

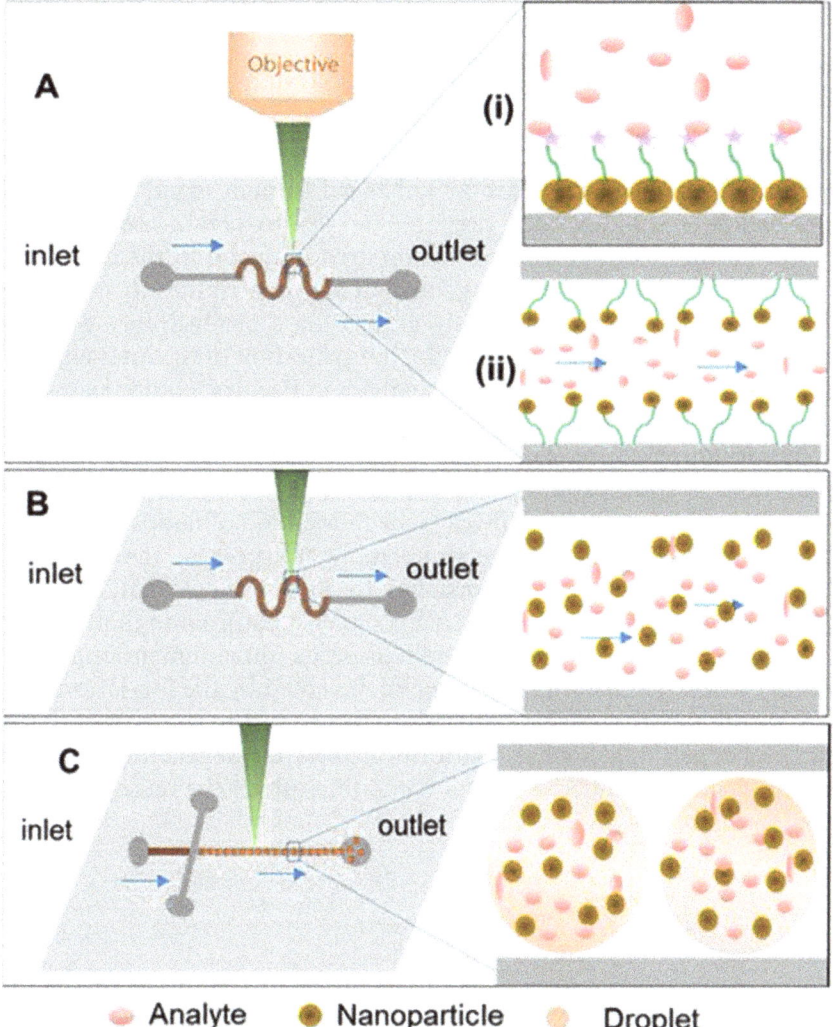

Figure 9.3. Different strategies employed in lab-on-a-chip (LOC)-SERS devices. (A) Nanoparticle function-alization in channels in (i) static or (ii) continuous flow approach, (B) colloidal dispersions and continuous flow approach, and (C) in segmented flow. (Reproduced from [30]. CC BY 4.0.)

both segments, the memory effect is not considered a significant problem here. The convective flow profile inside the microfluidic platform ensures the proper mixing of the nanostructure and the sample of interest. The challenge of colloidal adhesion is averted here via chaotic advection due to repeated stretching as well as folding of the two fluids in the oil and water phase, respectively [25]. The mixing between colloidal nanoparticles and analytes can be done easily using droplet-based SERS-microfluidic platforms, as the convective flow of analytes happens within the droplets. The limitation in integrating with solid SERS substrates is considered to be a major drawback in droplet-based microfluidic platforms.

9.4 Colloidal and solid substrates for MF-SERS studies

As mentioned, depending upon the nature of the plasmonic substrate, the MF-SERS can be classified into colloidal MF-SERS and solid-substrate MF-SERS [36]. In the case of colloidal MF-SERS, the plasmonic nanoparticles are prepared externally and administrated through fluidic pathways in the microfluidic channel wherein they mix it with analyte molecules to give an enhanced Raman signal. Alternatively, the plasmonic colloidal solutions are prepared *in situ* to create the required SERS hotspots for sensing. However, the diffusion-driven mixing in the case of colloidal MF-SERS not only makes the process slow but also contributes toward large signal fluctuations and consequently adversely affects the reproducibility of the Raman spectroscopic studies [37]. Additionally, the long duration of the interaction between the plasmonic nanoparticles and the analyte molecules could lead to sample contamination. As particles are dispersed in colloidal MF-SERS, the memory effect plays an important role here, and impacts the efficacy of the technique negatively. These limitations to some extent can be tackled by replacing the colloidal substrates with solid SERS substrates, which involve the fabrication of nanostructures onto the microfluidic channel surface. To generate more hotspots in the probing region, researchers are exploring zero-dimensional to three-dimensional complex nano-architectures, which include nanodots (zero-dimensional), nanopillars (one-dimensional), nanodisks (two-dimensional), and nanoseeds (three-dimensional) [38–41]. In an interesting work, the memory effect is circumvented by the ink-jet printing of Ag nanoparticles onto an indium tin oxide electrode placed in the bottom layer of the microfluidic channel [42]. Such a platform enables the regeneration of the target analytes with electrically aided desorption and thus allows the reuse of the substrate, as depicted in figure 9.4.

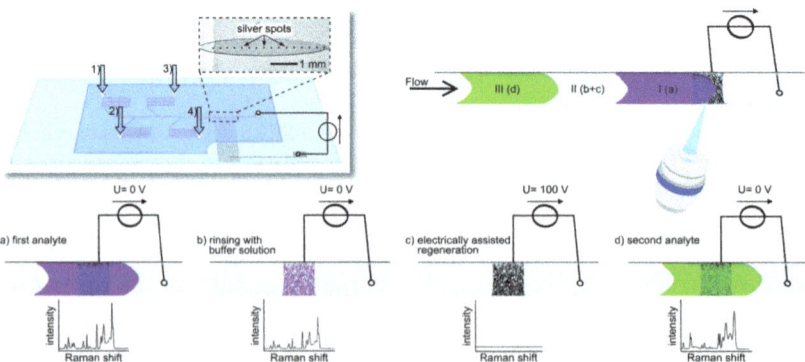

Figure 9.4. Electrochemical-assisted regeneration of integrated SERS substrates in a microfluidic chip (a), the SERS spectrum is achieved once the sample crosses the detection region (b). The residues of samples persist at the detection surface, even after the passage which results in withstanding the Raman signal (c). Rapid sample removal is realized by inducing a high electrical potential (d) allowing for detection of the following compound zone. (Reproduced with permission from [42]. CC BY-NC.)

9.5 MF-SERS for sensing applications

The integration of sensitive SERS spectroscopic techniques with microfluidic technologies resulted in the development of miniaturized analytical sensing platforms wherein the analyte fluids are controlled and analysed within the microchannels. The efficacy of these sensing methods relies on the interaction of analyte molecules with the externally added or built-in micro–nanoscale structures. It means that the specific topographical morphologies play a critical role in specific functionalities such as mixing, cell studies, separation columns, and catalysis. With the combination of advanced subjects and techniques such as SERS, the research field of MF-SERS is now extending the possible applications in the field of sensing. For instance, with progress in *in situ* preparation and pre-treatment strategies, the MF-SERS sensors are finding a plethora of applications in the field of biological sciences where the sample volume is a critical parameter. Since the SERS signal suffers a sharp decrease when increasing the distance between the substrate and sample molecules, much of the effort in recent years has been put toward to developing approaches that drive the analyte molecules closer to the hotspots via techniques such as dielectrophoresis. A few important and emerging applications of the MF-SERS are discussed here.

9.5.1 Biosensing

The emergence of biotechnology and its integration with nanotechnology made it possible to have specific targeting of MF-SERS systems. Herein, the sensitivity and specificity can be increased by decorating plasmonic structures with antibodies that can detect corresponding antigens or bacteria [43–45]. In another interesting application, the labeled DNA oligonucleotides were specifically identified in regions wherein the SERS microchannels were decorated with complementary nucleotides [47]. The aggregation of amyloid beta-peptide and the structural evolution of the aggregate were investigated using a label-free-SERS active nanofluidic device wherein micro- as well as nanofluidic junctions and Au-NP-based SERS active surfaces were employed for the studies [48]. In an interesting work, Kaminska *et al* demonstrated multiplexed detection of interleukins from blood plasma using a SERS-based microfluidic assay. They were able to detect IL-6, IL-8, and IL-18 in blood plasma by incorporating bimetallic SERS substrate inside the microfluidic channel, as demonstrated in figure 9.5. In the initial phase, the bimetallic Ag–Au substrate functionalized with an alkane thiol monolayer can bind antibodies via amine coupling. These antibodies can facilitate the selective binding of corresponding interleukins [49].

Cui *et al* have designed and fabricated a droplet SERS-microfluidic device for conducting thiocyanate detection from blood serum and saliva samples. The whole detection procedure can be performed within a few minutes with only a minimal sample volume ($\sim\mu$l) requirement. The band at 2100 cm^{-1}, contributed by –C$\equiv$N stretch in thiocyanate, has been explored for quantitative detection [50]. In another interesting work, Meinhart *et al* demonstrated a microfluidic-SERS substrate that can detect trace concentrations of the drug methamphetamine in human saliva [51].

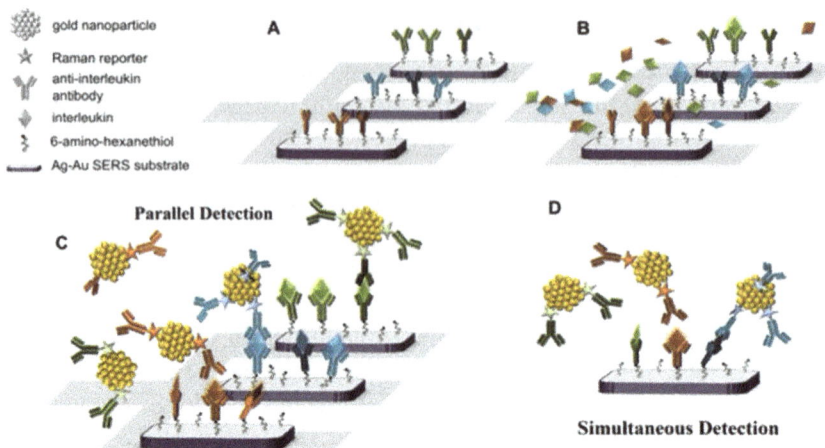

Figure 9.5. Steps involved in a SERS-based immunoassay for multiplex detection of interleukins (IL-6, IL-8, IL-18) in human blood plasma. (Reproduced with permission from [49]. Copyright 2017 Springer.)

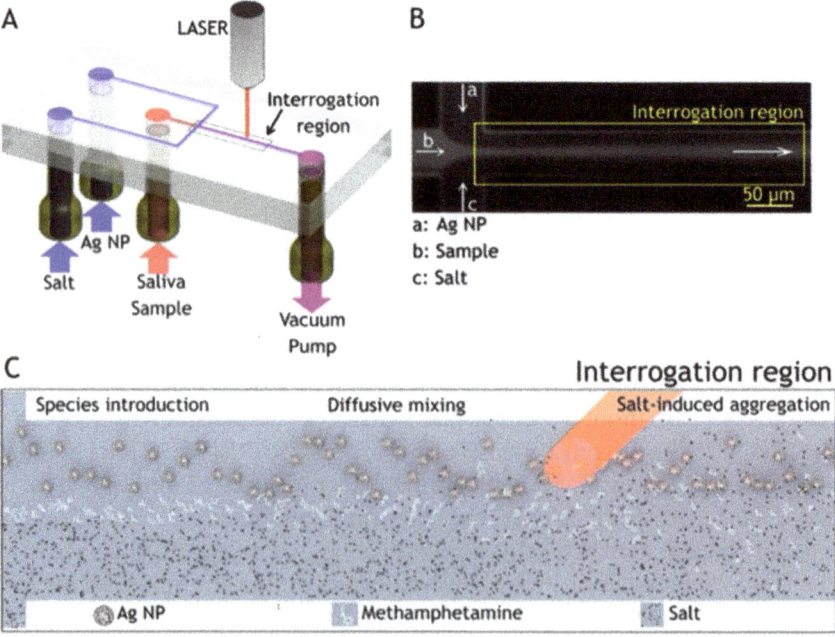

Figure 9.6. The flow-focusing microfluidic device is employed for controlled AgNP aggregation. (Reproduced with permission from [51]. Copyright 2013 American Chemical Society.)

This approach permits the target molecule to diffuse into the nanoparticle-containing sidestream, adsorbed on it, followed by salt ions, causing nanoparticle aggregation to obtain enhanced Raman signals. The schematic of the employed approach is given in figure 9.6. In this approach, partial separation of these target molecules from complex samples was possible to achieve due to the slow diffusion of larger-sized molecules. The aggregating agents in this approach, salt ions needed to travel more distance to reach the nanoparticle-containing sidestream. Even though salt ions diffuse faster, this distance ensured that the salt ion-induced aggregation occurs only after the analyte adsorption happened onto the nanoparticle surface.

Cui *et al* demonstrated a microfluidic biosensor capable of detecting breast cancer biomarkers from serum samples [52]. Silver nanoparticles were injected onto the PDMS-based microfluidic substrate to generate SERS active parallel channels, which were further immobilized by peculiar antibodies that can target reliable cancer biomarkers simultaneously. This platform was capable of detecting a list of biomarkers comprising CA153, CA125, and CEA with a detection limit of 0.01 U ml^{-1}, 0.01 U ml^{-1}, and 1 pg ml^{-1} in serum. The detection limit was sufficient for its utility in clinical diagnostics when compared with ELISA kits, which was demonstrated by testing the real samples from patients. Li *et al* developed a microfluidic platform that can provide more bioanalyte adsorption sites for sensing via increasing the whole surface area of nanostructures, by integrating a nanoporous gold disk (NPGD) array onto the surface [40]. The advantage of having nanoscale pores and ligaments three-dimensionally distributed in the gold disk array demonstrated huge potential for the detection of biomolecules such as dopamine and urea. The application of the SERS-microfluidic platform for single-cell analysis was demonstrated first in 2018 by Willner *et al* [53]. Wheat germ agglutinin (WGA)-functionalized nanoprobes have been used for the analysis of prostate cancer cells in this study. The aim to employ WGA in the study was to target the glycan features on the surface of cancer cells. Both the nanoprobes and cancerous cells were encapsulated in a microfluidic chip for these investigations.

9.5.2 Pathogen detection

The commonly adopted methods for pathogen detection are based on immobilization using specific antigens, antibodies, labeling molecules, etc, and to obtain significant biomass for accurate detection several approaches of capturing/concentration/filtration are employed. However, the integration of SERS tags with microfluidics allows not only advantages such as miniaturization and automation, but also reduces the time for labor-intensive pathogen detection in the conventional approaches. Li *et al* have performed waterborne pathogen detection using a nanodielectrophoretic (nano-DEP) SERS-microfluidic platform. The integration of the nano-DEP mechanism inside the platform facilitated the pathogen concentration enrichment before mixing with nanoprobes so that a detection limit down to 10^0 CFU ml^{-1} for an *Escherichia coli* strain was achieved [52]. Cheng *et al* have also employed AC electric field-induced dielectrophoresis (DEP) and an electrohydrodynamics mechanism simultaneously to achieve bacterial enrichment from blood samples over a rough electrode surface to carry out SERS measurements [55]. The whole process of selective isolation and concentration enrichment was completed in a few minutes (3 min), and researchers were able to identify *E. coli*, *Staphylococcus aureus*, and *Pseudomonas aeruginosa* with LODs of 1×10^4, 3×10^3, and 5×10^3 CFU ml^{-1}, respectively.

Belder *et al* designed a nanoporous membrane connected two stacked perpendicular microfluidic channel based SERS LOC platform for pathogen sensing in drinking water [56]. In this sensing device, the sample and the silver nanoparticles were supplied through the first channel (sample channel). The second channel (extraction channel) was kept grounded as compared to the first channel which was kept under a positive voltage (300 V). This resulted in a high electro-osmotic flow of the sample solution towards the second channel. This miniaturized sensing platform with dimensions 2.5 × 2.5 cm had been effective in sensing *Pseudomonas taiwanensis* VLB120 and *E. coli* DH5α in tap water. Sakalys *et al* introduced a novel, cost-effective approach that employed a combination of 3D printing and soft lithography for fabricating cavity array-based reproducible SERS substrates and later integrated these with a microfluidic chip for sensing applications [57]. This approach involved the creation of a master template using two-photon 3D printing, which can further facilitate the replication of reproducible arrays and cavity structures with sub-micron resolution via the soft-lithography technique. The integration of these plasmonic hotspot arrays resulted in obtaining an enhancement factor of ~6.7×10^7. The proposed approach using two-photon 3D printing demonstrated a four-fold enhancement in Raman intensity in comparison with sphere lithography. Walter *et al* were the first one to carry out SERS-based bacterial detection using a lab-on-a-chip device in flow-through conditions [58]. The researchers verified the potential of this platform by conducting 5600 measurements altogether from nine different *E. coli* strains. The SVM algorithm model generated from these measurements demonstrated a classification accuracy of ~93%. The SERS spectral measurement duration was rapid and the measurement took a time of ~1 s only, which was highly beneficial for rapid bacterial strain identification. In another work, Neethirajan *et al* developed a SERS-based microfluidic sensor for the detection of foodborne pathogens [59]. The use of chemometric (PCA-LDA) analysis over the recorded spectral data elucidated the potential to detect and discriminate eight common foodborne pathogens (*E. coli*, *S. typhimirium*, *S. enteritis*, *Pseudomonas aeruginosa*, *Listeria monocytogenes*, *L. innocua*, *MRSA 35,* and MRSA 86) from the complex polymicrobial mixture. *E. coli* detection from drinking water was reported using a microarray flow-through system integrated with the SERS imaging technique [60]. Recently, Konkel *et al* designed an automatic optofluidic SERS device for the detection and discrimination of methicillin-resistant *Staphylococcus aureus* (MRSA) using human clinical isolates from the United States of America and China [61]. MRSA detection was also reported using a cost-effective, disposable microfluidic sensor, which relies on evaporation-induced meniscus dragging to concentrate bacterial samples within a nanoliter volume to generate enhanced Raman signals [62]. In a recent literature review, Khan *et al* have detailed the possibilities, highlights, and challenges of employing the combination of SERS with lateral flow immunoassay (LFIA) for the sensitive detection of SARS-CoV-2 from clinical samples [63].

9.5.3 Pollutants, pesticides, and drugs

Research findings elucidate that pollutants in the aquatic environment and food products are complex chemical mixtures of various groups (biocides, pharmaceuticals, industrial chemicals, pesticides, etc). The determination of the pollutants is normally conducted via sampling, extraction, and separation of chemicals from the medium using high-performance liquid-phase chromatography followed by detection using advanced techniques such as mass spectroscopy. Although this approach provides high sensitivity, good specificity, and outstanding precision, the technique is complex in nature and laborious in operation. The aqueous sample of interest could undergo a physical and chemical transformation during the operation that can lead to inaccurate results. Therefore, researchers are now exploring a sensitive technique such as MF-SERS as a simpler and portable on-site analytical platform. Huang *et al* have introduced an interesting plasmonic substrate (AgNPs@basil-seeds), in which silver nanoparticles have been loaded on a 3D porous framework of natural basil seeds, and these plasmonic seeds were loaded into a microfluidic chip for the real-time measurement of melamine from milk samples [41]. The porosity of the natural seeds facilitated the adsorption of melamine and the placement of the analyte molecules in the vicinity of the plasmonic hotspot. This sensor obtained a detection limit of ~0.68 μM for melamine in milk samples. This 3D SERS substrate was also effective in the detection of methyl parathion in juice with an LOD of 10^{-7} M. Meinhart *et al* developed a SERS-microfluidic device for the rapid detection of trace concentrations of ampicillin in raw milk samples from a minimal sample volume of around 20 μl [64]. Ampicillin at a concentration up to 10 ppb was detected by monitoring the phenyl ring associated Raman bands present at 1007 and 1035 cm^{-1}. Parisi *et al* have proposed galvanic replacement reactions as a cheap, reproducible pathway for the *in situ* fabrication of silver nanoparticles inside a microfluidic channel for SERS applications [65]. The efficacy of the fabricated SERS substrate was verified using crystal violet as the reference sample and obtained an enhancement factor of ~2.2 $\times$ 10^7. This substrate was then tested against pesticides such as Carbofuran and Alachlor and found a detection limit down to 5 ppb using the MF-SERS set-up. Direct laser writing using a femtosecond laser was proposed as an efficient alternative way for controlled and precise *in situ* fabrication of nanostructures in a microfluidic device. Xu *et al* have integrated such a SERS substrate inside the fluidic channel using the laser-generated photoreduction of silver ions [34]. An enhancement factor of 10^8 was achieved while p-aminothiophenol (p-ATP) and flavin adenine dinucleotide (FAD) were taken as analyte samples. In general, the poor concentration of nanoparticles in an open microfluidic channel is a limitation as shown in figure 9.7(a). Because of this, researchers have improved SERS performance by incorporating a nanoporous silica matrix inside the optofluidic channel for concentrating nanoparticles and analytes before the measurement (figures 9.7(b) and (c)). Moreover, by adopting this approach the researchers were able to achieve a stable fluidic transport without clogging [66]. The need for tedious optical alignment and focusing was also eliminated in the device by using fiber optic cables for excitation and collection and making the system suitable for field

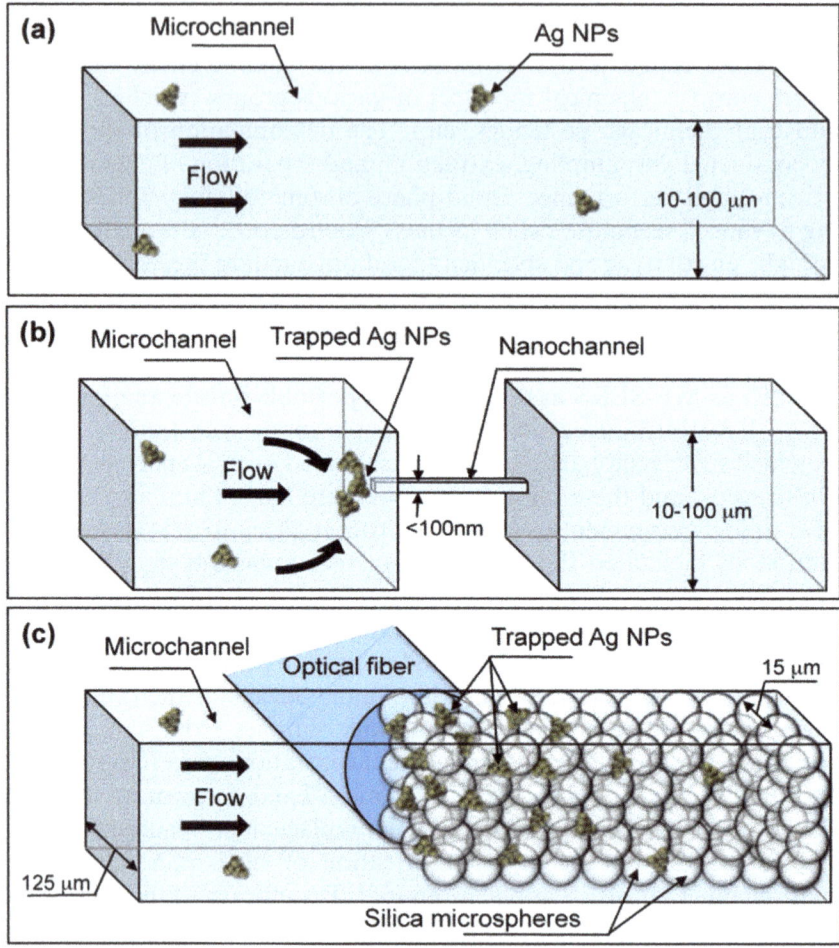

Figure 9.7. Nanofluidic trapping versus open-channel microfluidics. (Reproduced with permission from [66]. Copyright 2012 AIP Publishing.)

applications. Incorporating a passive mixture into the optofluidic channel eradicated the requirement of manual sample mixing procedures and made possible the detection of melamine and fungicide thiram with an LOD of 63 ppb and 50 ppt, respectively, in an automatic manner [67]. Researchers have also improved the portability of the system by replacing the syringe pump with a pipette for sample loading [68]. This easy-to-use system was able to perform multiplexed detection of three aquaculture fungicides (methyl parathion, thiram, and malachite green) with an LOD of 5 ppm, 5 ppb, and 0.1 ppb, respectively. Xu *et al* have also performed multiplexed detection of thiram and adenine using a microfluidic chip patterned with well-ordered silver nanodot arrays [38]. Contrary to the usual approach of focusing the laser line through the channel side, this device has explored an inverted Raman configuration to eliminate the background signals originating from PDMS material while focusing on the analyte. A detection limit of $\sim 5 \times 10^{-7}$ was obtained for thiram and adenine using this sensing platform.

9.5.4 Heavy metal ions

The hazardous nature of heavy metals in our environment is posing serious health concerns from mental health issues to malnutrition. Plants absorb the heavy metals from soil pores in the form of ions. The prime dietary origin of mercury (Hg) ions is aquatic products whereas Pb toxicity stems from meats, beverages, cereals, etc. With the integration of microfluidic technologies, SERS has proven to be of enormous potential for detecting ultra-low concentrations of toxic metals in food owing to its high sensitivity, rapid response, and clear fingerprinting capability. The well-known interaction between gold nanoparticles and mercury ions has been exploited to develop a digital microfluidic-SERS sensor for Hg ion detection [69]. The interaction resulted in changes in the SERS signals of the dye molecule (rhodamine B), which acts as a reporter molecule, in response to varying mercury concentration. The samples in the form of nanoliter droplets passing through microchannels ensured effective mixing of components and, in addition, the use of a continuous oil phase that isolates the droplets avoided memory effects. In another work on mercury ion detection from drinking water using a microdroplet sensing platform, Chung *et al* used oligo nucleic acid (aptamer) functionalized Au/Ag core–shell nanoparticles [70]. The approach depended on the reaction between mercury ions and an aptamer and it can be a potential candidate for field applications due to its portability and low detection limit (10 pM). Chen *et al* developed a PDMS-based microfluidic-SERS sensor for the detection of arsenic ions in water [71]. In this work, silver nanoparticles were functionalized with glutathione (GSH) with 4-mercaptopyridine (4-MPY), which has a strong affinity toward arsenic ions. The applicability of this platform for real sample cases has been verified using drinking water spiked with heavy metal ions with a concentration of 30–100 ppb and the obtained results were very well correlated with the ICP-MS technique. Wang *et al* have demonstrated the application of semi-conductor–noble-metal nanocomposites inside a SERS-microfluidic platform for exploring Raman enhancement of semiconductor material due to both electro-magnetic and chemical effects [72]. Aptamer functionalized on sea urchin ZnO–Ag arrays fabricated using monolayer colloidal crystal template technique (figure 9.8) has demonstrated high specificity and sensitivity for UO_2^{2+} ion detection in tap water and river water. The proposed cost-effective platform can be reused after cleaning the microfluidic surface with phosphate buffer saline and supplementation of aptamer substrate strands.

9.6 Conclusions

The MF-SERS technique demonstrated great potential in developing miniaturized devices that can be explored for sensitive and selective measurements of an analyte from different kinds of samples, ranging from biological cells to environmental samples. The performance of the label-free approach of the MF-SERS technique relied much on the size, shape, composition, and architecture of the SERS substrate

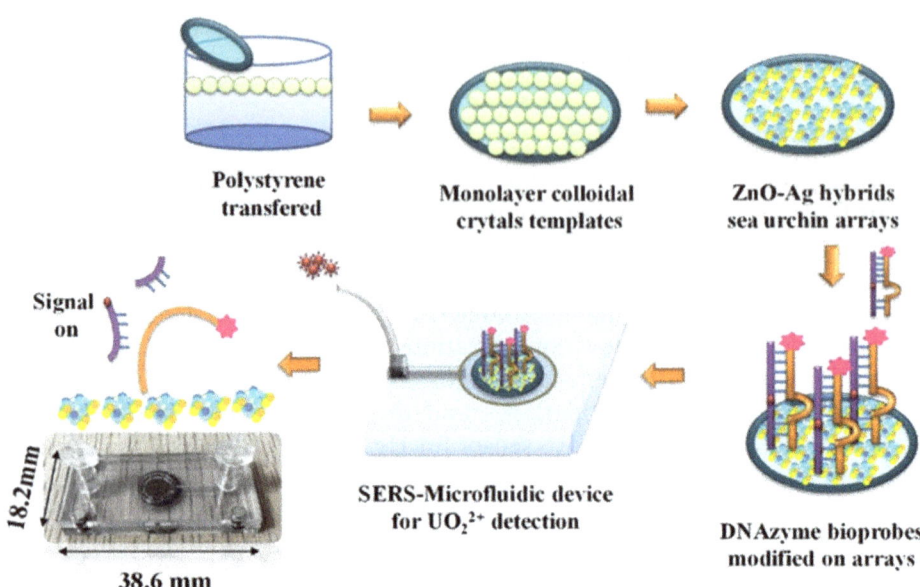

Figure 9.8. A SERS-based microfluidic device employed for UO_2^{2+} ion sensing. (Reproduced with permission from [72]. Copyright 2020 Elsevier.)

and its efficient integration with the microfluidic channel. Different plasmonic particles such as Ag, Au, Au/AgNPs, etc were used in fabricating the SERS platforms in the microfluidic channel. The possibility of automation in the MF-SERS technique allowed higher reproducibility of the Raman signal which was considered to be a major challenge in conventional Raman studies. The research work done so far unambiguously shows that the MF-SERS technique provides a novel way to analyse samples with great control of the small volume of that sample. Such integration of MF with the SERS technique provides a wide range of possibilities that can result in new knowledge in the field of chemistry, biology, and medicine. With the impetus obtained from the advances in miniaturization technology and machine learning, we believe that MF-SERS technologies will soon become a cost-effective analytic tool for real-life sensing applications.

9.7 Challenges and future outlook

The research work done so far on MF-SERS is mainly focused on improving the reliability and feasibility of the approach or the device. For example, the studies using MF-SERS are focused on having an on-demand and reversible assembly of plasmonic nanoparticles, efficient adsorption of analyte molecules onto the plasmonic substrate, and the development of facile strategies for *in situ* synthesis of SERS substrates, the creation of well-defined solid-state SERS substrates, etc. In addition, the potential of the technique in diverse areas, particularly where the sample volume is a critical parameter, is demonstrated by exploring the potential of the small volume requirement of microfluidics and the sensitive fingerprinting capability of the Raman spectroscopic technique. Despite the great promise that the approach of MF-SERS holds, implementation of a new technique where numerous well-established devices already exist is a challenging task. Thus, the existing MF-SERS technique should be developed with field-ready hardware and test kits that allow multiplexed testing capability with great accuracy and sensitivity. The multiplexed MF-SERS detection can find application in medical diagnosis wherein multiple biomarker detection can be used to confirm a particular disease. The multiplexed analysis often requires the SERS tags and thus analyses non-label-free SERS. Apart from the mentioned requirements, the efficient utilization of MF-SERS also requires advances in chemometric tools for deconvoluting and classifying the obtained Raman signatures for developing it as a routine sensor. With the advances in photonics and fiber technologies, it is expected that the footprint and cost of the MF-SERS technique can be reduced considerably. Thanks to advances in the lithographic technique and soft lithography to replicate the master structures, the scaling up of the SERS substrates in microfluidic channel fabricating material, polydimethylsiloxane, is now possible and thus provides a pathway for the scaling up of MF-SERS devices. The current trend is to exploit the capillary force-driven microfluidic flow instead of the syringe pump-created fluid flow thereby reducing the cost of MF-SERS devices. However, the real-life application of MF-SERS still has to meet challenges such as the quality of SERS active substrates, the high chemical variability of clinical and environmental samples, the surface nature dependence of the SERS technique, etc.

Acknowledgments

SDG acknowledges the financial support through (i) CRG/2020/002096 funded by SERB, DST, Government of India, (ii) IDP/BDTD/ 20/2019, and SR/FST/PSI-174/ 2012 from DST, Government of India.

References

[1] Lin C-C, Wang J-H, Wu H-W and Lee G-B 2010 Microfluidic immunoassays *J. Assoc. Lab. Autom.* **15** 253–74
[2] Liu W, He H and Zheng S-Y 2020 Microfluidics in single-cell virology: technologies and applications *Trends Biotechnol.* **38** 1360–72
[3] Luka G, Ahmadi A, Najjaran H, Alocilja E, DeRosa M, Wolthers K, Malki A, Aziz H, Althani A and Hoorfar M 2015 Microfluidics integrated biosensors: a leading technology towards lab-on-a-chip and sensing applications *Sensors* **15** 30011–31
[4] Ortseifen V, Viefhues M, Wobbe L and Grünberger A 2020 Microfluidics for biotechnology: bridging gaps to foster microfluidic applications *Front. Bioeng. Biotechnol.* **8** 589074
[5] Aryasomayajula A, Bayat P, Rezai P and Selvaganapathy P R 2017 Microfluidic devices and their applications *Springer Handbook of Nanotechnology* ed B Bhushan 4th edn (Berlin: Springer) pp 487–536
[6] Wang G, Das C, Ledden B, Sun Q, Nguyen C and Kumar S 2017 Evaluation of disposable microfluidic chip design for automated and fast Immunoassays *Biomicrofluidics* **11** 014115

[7] Zhu L, Liu X, Yang J, He Y and Li Y 2020 Application of multiplex microfluidic electrochemical sensors in monitoring hematological tumor biomarkers *Anal. Chem.* **92** 11981–6

[8] Huang Y and Mason A J 2013 Lab-on-CMOS integration of microfluidics and electrochemical sensors *Lab Chip* **13** 3929–34

[9] Bechstein D J B, Ng E, Lee J-R, Cone G S, Gaster R S, Osterfeld S J, Hall D A, Weaver J A, Wilson R J and Wang S X 2015 Microfluidic multiplexed partitioning enables flexible and effective utilization of magnetic sensor arrays *Lab Chip* **15** 4273–6

[10] Cardoso S, Leitao D, Dias T, Valadeiro J, Silva M, Chicharo A, Silveiro V, Gasper J and Freitas P P 2017 Challenges and trends in magnetic sensor integration with microfluidics for biomedical applications *J. Phys. D: Appl. Phys.* **50** 213001

[11] Chen Y, Yu F, Yang C, Song J, Tang L, Li M and Hi J J 2015 Label-free biosensing using cascaded double-microring resonators integrated with microfluidic channels *Opt. Commun.* **344** 129–33

[12] Wang Y, Yuan W, Kimber M, Lu M and Dong L 2018 Rapid differentiation of host and parasitic exosome vesicles using microfluidic photonic crystal biosensor *ACS Sens.* **3** 1616–21

[13] Parker H E, Sengupta S, Harish A V, Soares R G, Joensson H N, Margulis W, Russom A and Laurell F 2022 A lab-in-a-fiber optofluidic device using droplet microfluidics and laser-induced fluorescence for virus detection *Sci. Rep.* **12** 3539

[14] Shrinivasan S, Norris P M, Landers J P and Ferrance J P 2007 A low-cost, low-power consumption, miniature laser-induced fluorescence system for DNA detection on a microfluidic device *Clin. Lab. Med.* **27** 173–81

[15] Dochow S, Beleites C, Henkel T, Mayer G, Albert J and Clement J 2013 Quartz microfluidic chip for tumour cell identification by Raman spectroscopy in combination with optical traps *Anal. Bioanal. Chem.* **405** 2743–6

[16] Dochow S, Krafft C, Neugebauer U, Bocklitz T, Henkel T, Mayer G, Albert J and Popp J 2011 Tumour cell identification by means of Raman spectroscopy in combination with optical traps and microfluidic environments *Lab Chip* **11** 1484–90

[17] Jadhav S A, Biji P, Panthalingal M K, Krishna C M, Rajkumar S, Joshi D S and Sundaram N 2021 Development of integrated microfluidic platform coupled with surface-enhanced Raman spectroscopy for diagnosis of COVID-19 *Med. Hypotheses* **146** 110356

[18] Ranjan P, Sadique M A, Parihar A, Dhand C, Mishra A and Khan R 2022 Commercialization of microfluidic point-of-care diagnostic devices *Advanced Microfluidics-Based Point-of-Care Diagnostics* ed R Khan, C Dhand, S K Sanghi, D S T Salammal and A P Mishra (Boca Raton, FL: Taylor and Francis/CRC Press) pp 383–98

[19] Parihar A, Parihar D S, Ranjan P and Khan R 2022 Role of microfluidics-based point-of-care testing (POCT) for clinical applications *Advanced Microfluidics-Based Point-of-Care Diagnostics* ed R Khan, C Dhand, S K Sanghi, D S T Salammal and A P Mishra (Boca Raton, FL: Taylor and Francis/CRC Press) pp 39–60

[20] George S D 2019 Surface-enhanced Raman scattering substrates: fabrication, properties, and applications *Self-Standing Substrates: Materials and Applications. Engineering Materials Series* ed R Inamuddin, Boddula and A Asiri (Cham: Springer) pp 83–118

[21] Notingher I 2007 Raman spectroscopy cell-based biosensors *Sensors* **7** 1343–58

[22] Wang N, Ren F, Li L, Wang H, Wang L, Zeng Q, Song Y, Zeng T, Zhu S and Chen X 2022 Quantitative chemical sensing of drugs in scattering media with Bessel beam Raman spectroscopy *Biomed. Opt. Express* **13** 2488–502

[23] Braz A, López-López M and García-Ruiz C 2013 Raman spectroscopy for forensic analysis of inks in questioned documents *Forensic Sci. Int.* **232** 206–12

[24] Virkler K and Lednev I K 2010 Forensic body fluid identification: the Raman spectroscopic signature of saliva *Analyst* **135** 512–7

[25] Schlücker S 2014 Surface-enhanced Raman spectroscopy: concepts and chemical applications *Angew. Chem.* **53** 4756–95

[26] Le R E and Etchegoin P 2008 *Principles of Surface-Enhanced Raman Spectroscopy: And Related Plasmonic Effects* (Amsterdam: Elsevier) pp 1–14

[27] Stiles P L, Dieringer J A, Shah N C and Van Duyne R P 2008 Surface-enhanced Raman spectroscopy *Annu. Rev. Anal. Chem.* **1** 601–26

[28] Kneipp K 2007 Surface-enhanced Raman scattering *Phys. Today* **60** 40–6

[29] Pérez-Jiménez A I, Lyu D, Lu Z, Liu G and Ren B 2020 Surface-enhanced Raman spectroscopy: benefits, trade-offs and future developments *Chem. Sci.* **11** 4563–77

[30] Kant K and Abalde-Cela S 2018 Surface-enhanced Raman scattering spectroscopy and microfluidics: towards ultrasensitive label-free sensing *Biosensors* **8** 62

[31] Choudhari K, Sinha R K, Kulkarni S D, Santhosh C and George S D 2022 Facile fabrication of superhydrophobic gold loaded nanoporous anodic alumina as surface-enhanced Raman spectroscopy substrates *J. Opt.* **24** 044002

[32] Peethan A, Aravind M, Unnikrishnan V, Chidangil S and George S D 2022 Facile fabrication of plasmonic wettability contrast paper surface for droplet array-based SERS sensing *Appl. Surf. Sci.* **571** 151188

[33] George J E, Unnikrishnan V, Mathur D, Chidangil S and George S D 2018 Flexible superhydrophobic SERS substrates fabricated by *in situ* reduction of Ag on femtosecond laser-written hierarchical surfaces *Sensors Actuators* B **272** 485–93

[34] Xu B-B *et al* 2011 Localized flexible integration of high-efficiency surface enhanced Raman scattering (SERS) monitors into microfluidic channels *Lab Chip* **11** 3347–51

[35] Liu G L and Lee L P 2005 Nanowell surface enhanced Raman scattering arrays fabricated by soft-lithography for label-free biomolecular detections in integrated microfluidics *Appl. Phys. Lett.* **87** 074101

[36] Guo J, Zeng F, Guo J and Ma X J 2020 Preparation and application of microfluidic SERS substrate: challenges and future perspectives *J. Mater. Sci. Technol.* **37** 96–103

[37] Jahn I, Žukovskaja O, Zheng X-S, Weber K, Bocklitz T, Cialla-May D and Popp J 2017 Surface-enhanced Raman spectroscopy and microfluidic platforms: challenges, solutions and potential applications *Analyst* **142** 1022–47

[38] Chen G, Wang Y, Wang H, Cong M, Chen L, Yang Y, Geng Y, Li H, Xu S and Xu W 2014 A highly sensitive microfluidics system for multiplexed surface-enhanced Raman scattering (SERS) detection based on Ag nanodot arrays *RSC Adv.* **4** 54434–40

[39] Zhao Y, Zhang Y-L, Huang J-A, Zhang Z, Chen X and Zhang W 2015 Plasmonic nanopillar array embedded microfluidic chips: an *in situ* SERS monitoring platform *J. Mater. Chem.* A **3** 6408–13

[40] Li M, Zhao F, Zeng J, Qi J, Lu J and Shih W-C 2014 Microfluidic surface-enhanced Raman scattering sensor with monolithically integrated nanoporous gold disk arrays for rapid and label-free biomolecular detection *J. Biomed. Opt.* **19** 111611

[41] Zhou Q, Meng G, Wu N, Zhou N, Chen B, Li F and Huang Q 2016 Dipping into a drink: basil-seed supported silver nanoparticles as surface-enhanced Raman scattering substrates for toxic molecule detection *Sensors Actuators* B **223** 447–52

[42] Meier T-A, Poehler E, Kemper F, Pabst O, Jahnke H-G, Beckert E, Robitzki A and Belder D 2015 Fast electrically assisted regeneration of on-chip SERS substrates *Lab Chip* **15** 2923–7

[43] Wang Y, Rauf S, Grewal Y S, Spadafora L J, Shiddiky M J, Cangelosi G A, Schlücker S and Trau M 2014 Duplex microfluidic SERS detection of pathogen antigens with nanoyeast single-chain variable fragments *Anal. Chem.* **86** 9930–8

[44] Lee M, Lee K, Kim K H, Oh K W and Choo J 2012 SERS-based immunoassay using a gold array-embedded gradient microfluidic chip *Lab Chip* **12** 3720–7

[45] Choi N, Lee K, Lim D W, Lee E K, Chang S-I and Oh K W 2012 Simultaneous detection of duplex DNA oligonucleotides using a SERS-based micro-network gradient chip *Lab Chip* **12** 5160–7

[46] Yazdi S H, Giles K L and White I M 2013 Multiplexed detection of DNA sequences using a competitive displacement assay in a microfluidic SERRS-based device *Anal. Chem.* **85** 10605–11

[47] Strelau K K, Kretschmer R, Möller R, Fritzsche W and Popp J 2010 SERS as tool for the analysis of DNA-chips in a microfluidic platform *Anal. Bioanal. Chem.* **396** 1381–4

[48] Choi I, Huh Y S and Erickson D J M 2012 Ultra-sensitive, label-free probing of the conformational characteristics of amyloid beta aggregates with a SERS active nanofluidic device *Microfluid. Nanofluid.* **12** 663–9

[49] Kamińska A, Winkler K, Kowalska A, Witkowska E, Szymborski T, Janeczek A and Waluk J 2017 SERS-based immunoassay in a microfluidic system for the multiplexed recognition of interleukins from blood plasma: towards picogram detection *Sci. Rep.* **7** 10656

[50] Wu L, Wang Z, Zong S and Cui Y 2014 Rapid and reproducible analysis of thiocyanate in real human serum and saliva using a droplet SERS-microfluidic chip *Biosens. Bioelectron.* **62** 13–8

[51] Andreou C, Hoonejani M R, Barmi M R, Moskovits M and Meinhart C D 2013 Rapid detection of drugs of abuse in saliva using surface enhanced Raman spectroscopy and microfluidics *ACS Nano* **7** 7157–64

[52] Zheng Z, Wu L, Li L, Zong S, Wang Z and Cui Y 2018 Simultaneous and highly sensitive detection of multiple breast cancer biomarkers in real samples using a SERS microfluidic chip *Talanta* **188** 507–15

[53] Willner M R, McMillan K S, Graham D, Vikesland P J and Zagnoni M 2018 Surface-enhanced Raman scattering based microfluidics for single-cell analysis *Anal. Chem.* **90** 12004–10

[54] Wang C, Madiyar F, Yu C and Li J 2017 Detection of extremely low concentration waterborne pathogen using a multiplexing self-referencing SERS microfluidic biosensor *J. Biol. Eng.* **11** 9

[55] Cheng I-F, Chang H-C, Chen T-Y, Hu C and Yang F-L 2013 Rapid (<5 min) identification of pathogen in human blood by electrokinetic concentration and surface-enhanced Raman spectroscopy *Sci. Rep.* **3** 2365

[56] Krafft B, Tycova A, Urban R D, Dusny C and Belder D 2021 Microfluidic device for concentration and SERS-based detection of bacteria in drinking water *Electrophoresis* **42** 86–94

[57] Šakalys R, Kho K W and Keyes T E 2021 A reproducible, low cost microfluidic microcavity array SERS platform prepared by soft lithography from a 2 photon 3D printed template *Sensors Actuators B* **340** 129970

[58] Walter A, März A, Schumacher W, Rösch P and Popp J 2011 Towards a fast, high specific and reliable discrimination of bacteria on strain level by means of SERS in a microfluidic device *Lab Chip* **11** 1013–21

[59] Mungroo N A, Oliveira G and Neethirajan S 2016 SERS based point-of-care detection of food-borne pathogens *Microchim. Acta.* **183** 697–707

[60] Knauer M, Ivleva N P, Niessner R and Haisch C 2012 A flow-through microarray cell for the online SERS detection of antibody-captured *E. coli* bacteria *Anal. Bioanal. Chem.* **402** 2663–7

[61] Lu X, Samuelson D R, Xu Y, Zhang H, Wang S, Rasco B A, Xu J and Konkel M E 2013 Detecting and tracking nosocomial methicillin-resistant *Staphylococcus aureus* using a microfluidic SERS biosensor *Anal. Chem.* **85** 2320–7

[62] Zhang J Y, Do J, Premasiri W R, Ziegler L D and Klapperich C M 2010 Rapid point-of-care concentration of bacteria in a disposable microfluidic device using meniscus dragging effect *Lab Chip* **10** 3265–70

[63] Yadav S, Sadique M A, Ranjan P, Kumar N, Singhal A, Srivastava A K and Khan R 2021 SERS based lateral flow immunoassay for point-of-care detection of SARS-CoV-2 in clinical samples *ACS Appl. Bio Mater.* **4** 2974–95

[64] Andreou C, Mirsafavi R, Moskovits M and Meinhart C D 2015 Detection of low concentrations of ampicillin in milk *Analyst* **140** 5003–5

[65] Parisi J, Dong Q and Lei Y 2015 *In situ* microfluidic fabrication of SERS nanostructures for highly sensitive fingerprint microfluidic-SERS sensing *RSC Adv.* **5** 14081–9

[66] Yazdi S H and White I M 2012 A nanoporous optofluidic microsystem for highly sensitive and repeatable surface enhanced Raman spectroscopy detection *Biomicrofluidics* **6** 014105

[67] Yazdi S H and White I M 2012 Optofluidic surface enhanced Raman spectroscopy microsystem for sensitive and repeatable on-site detection of chemical contaminants *Anal. Chem.* **84** 7992–8

[68] Yazdi S H and White I M 2013 Multiplexed detection of aquaculture fungicides using a pump-free optofluidic SERS microsystem *Analyst* **138** 100–3

[69] Wang G, Lim C, Chen L, Chon H, Choo J, Hong J and Demello J A 2009 Surface-enhanced Raman scattering in nanoliter droplets: towards high-sensitivity detection of mercury (II) ions *Anal. Bioanal. Chem.* **394** 1827–32

[70] Chung E, Gao R, Ko J, Choi N, Lim D W and Lee E K 2013 Trace analysis of mercury (II) ions using aptamer-modified Au/Ag core–shell nanoparticles and SERS spectroscopy in a microdroplet channel *Lab Chip* **13** 260–6

[71] Qi N, Li B, You H, Zhang W, Fu L, Wang Y and Chen L 2014 Surface-enhanced Raman scattering on a zigzag microfluidic chip: towards high-sensitivity detection of As (III) ions *Anal. Methods* **6** 4077–82

[72] He X, Zhou X, Liu Y and Wang X 2020 Ultrasensitive, recyclable and portable microfluidic surface-enhanced Raman scattering (SERS) biosensor for uranyl ions detection *Sensors Actuators* B **311** 127676

Chapter 10

IoMT-based SERS detection as advanced diagnostics

N E Dina, A M R Gherman and I Brezeştean

This chapter reviews the development in the field of surface-enhanced Raman scattering (SERS)-based approaches, including point-of-care (POC) strategies for viruses, namely SARS-CoV-2, and bacteria-caused infections as well as other life-threatening pathologies. We intend to cover the progress in developing SERS-based biosensors with their great potential for multiplexing, rapid testing, and biomolecular screening at a clinical level. We are currently facing an avalanche of existing or under-development computational techniques, digital tools, and devices as fit-to-purpose solutions meant to manage the current challenges in healthcare systems. From AI-based monitoring of health indicators to wearable biosensors that register medical parameters and treat certain pathologies through the smart release of drugs, our body fluids, temperature, and O_2 saturation have become omnipresent values in our modern lives. Like every up-to-date analytical technique with high potential for advanced diagnostics and treatment, SERS has evolved into a futuristic asset in POC analysis. We will provide the latest input resulting from synergistic approaches such as SERS and machine learning, SERS-based spectral pathology enhanced by chemometrics, or SERS-based set-ups that integrate digital technology. The role of handling big spectral data by considering the clinically relevant variables for medical decisions and obtaining high accuracy diagnoses will be emphasized.

10.1 Introduction

The Internet of Medical Things (IoMT) is the medical version of the Internet of Things (IoT) with applications in healthcare systems. The IoT is to be implemented in healthcare systems to provide smart healthcare services by connecting and exchanging data over different network communications, including the Internet, between available medical devices, hardware infrastructure, and software resources. It aims to lower patient care costs and also targets a better healthcare level in terms of more accurate diagnosis and a reduced number of errors in medical acts. The IoMT can manipulate healthcare-related information, making it a useful tool for treating and monitoring chronic patients in unusual circumstances such as a pandemic, when the healthcare system is overburdened, or its focus is switched to pandemic-related pathologies while the rest of the patients are placed second.

POC device development revolves around remote and low-resource areas, in particular off-site laboratories meant for testing patients in underserved regions. There is also a special focus on creating rapid and reliable diagnostic tests (within minutes), equivalent to the sensitivity of laboratory-based ones. Low-cost paper diagnostics as an extensive, off-site, robust alternative could improve healthcare access and address most of the POC challenges. A user-friendly interface, no complex analysis, multiplex capacity for detecting several biomarkers from a single test, portable or easy-to-use handheld devices, and cell phone-based design are key aspects in meeting the current clinical standards. The criteria of POC technology are defined under the ASSURED acronym (affordable, sensitive, specific, user-friendly, rapid, equipment-free, and deliverable).

10.2 Spectral pathology for advanced diagnostics

Raman spectroscopy (RS) is a promising methodology for microbial fingerprinting with many advantages, including multi-resistant clinical species identification at strain level [1], rapid and label-free differentiation of clinical pathogens [2], and a portable strategy for *in vitro* species identification of biofilm-related infections [3], etc. RS provides a wealth of structural information and is successfully used in biomolecule detection and molecular dynamic studies due to its molecular specificity. In this context, attempts to gather microbial biosignature databases are envisioned; for instance, by using unsupervised K-means clustering as a statistical approach based on the spectral patterns specific to biomolecules found in bacteria [4].

Currently, it is practical to use Raman for diagnosis, monitoring, prevention, and treatment of infections and inflammatory diseases as described comprehensively in the most recent studies assessed by the J Popp group [5–8]. RS, using a fiber-optic probe, combines contact- and label-free molecular fingerprinting with high applicability for biomedical [9] and clinical applications [10]. The acquisition of images is used to determine the molecular distribution and provide real-time imaging of the sample. In combination with simultaneous data processing and analysis, it is possible to achieve a real-time augmented chemical reality image built from the molecular distribution of the sample surface [7]. Yang *et al* [7] demonstrated experimentally that by using the Raman ChemLighter approach it is possible to determine and distinguish the borders of different bimolecular compounds in a short time. Thus, implementing Raman imaging using handheld fiber-optic probes, built around computer-vision-based interpretation of simultaneous acquisition of spectroscopic information, is already critically impacting clinical applications.

Recently, a handheld fiber-optic Raman probe coupled with a 785 nm excitation source with a bandpass filter was designed for biomolecular imaging [6]. The approach is well suited for clinical tissue boundary demarcation within minutes. The multistep procedure of deciphering the acquired Raman signal involves brightfield imaging with no molecular boundaries visible, then reconstruction by Raman imaging, computer-vision-based positional tracking of the laser, and evaluating the performance of the mixed Raman reality and the spatial resolution by the beam spot. Raman signals can now be used in a variety of applications on *ex vivo* and *in vivo* biological samples in combination with optical coherence tomography (OCT) modules [11], or for a rapid and intuitive assessment of molecular boundaries by using optical fibers [6] (figure 10.1).

However, Raman scattering is an inherently weak effect *per se*, with technical limitations for routine microbiological use [12]. The Raman signal is effectively exploited in the particular case of surface-enhanced Raman scattering (SERS). In SERS, Raman intensities are dramatically amplified when a molecule is adsorbed onto nano-roughened noble metal surfaces such as silver, gold, or platinum. The degree of enhancement enables single-molecule detection [13], which offers the potential for the unambiguous identification of pathogens at the single-cell level [14], on-site trace analysis by SERS [15], the study of cellular uptake in complex environments [16], and real-time monitoring of bacteria for testing their antimicrobial resistance [17]. SERS is also used in the absence of labels, tags, or reporter molecules [18, 19], enabling a wide variety of investigations: sensing and imaging in live cells [20], POC diagnosis, and tissue imaging [21].

Most recently, Wang *et al* [22] fabricated a simple, flexible microsphere-coupled SERS (MCSERS) substrate designed with a dielectric microsphere cavity array (MCA) and random gold nanoparticle (AuNP) capping on a PDMS film, obtaining a giant Raman enhancement on flexible substrates for practical use. The role of the

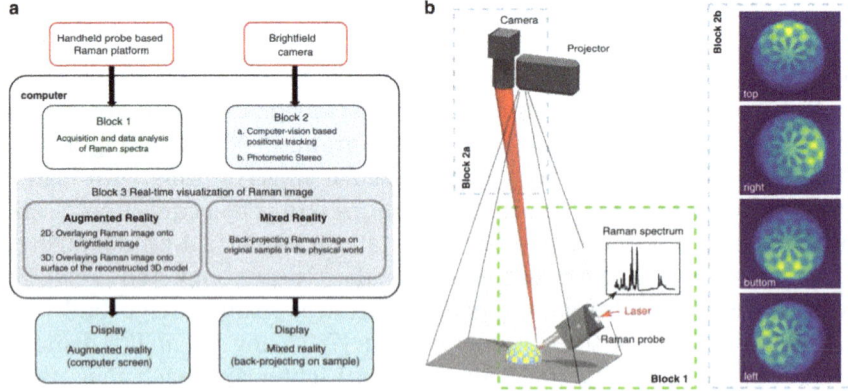

Figure 10.1. Raman spectra acquisition (Block 1) and computer-vision-based positional information for the spectra acquired (Block 2a). The spectral data are processed in real-time and along with the positional tracking provide the Raman image reconstruction for molecular distribution mapping. Furthermore, by using photometric stereo, a 3D map of the sample surface (Block 2b), is obtained and overlaid with the Raman-based visualization of the molecular composition. (Reproduced with permission from [6]. Copyright 2022 Springer Nature.)

MCA capped on the AuNPs is to boost the Raman signal via the multiple optical manipulation processes to an enhancement factor (EF) of up to 10^7. Moreover, the flexible MCSERS substrate exhibits outstanding durability and compatibility as an ultrasensitive Raman test strip and represents a facile strategy to fabricate SERS substrates with high flexibility for optical trace detection in real-world applications [22].

The SERS performance of a substrate is the key aspect of high-sensitivity detection and diagnosis. The SERS performance of noble metal nanomaterials highly depends on their size, morphology, composition, and nanopatterning [23], or other design effects that are known to deliver a huge electric field enhancement. The same noble metal (Au- or Ag-based) nanomaterial can render an EF of various magnitudes when designed with different morphology: multibranched [24], nanostars [25–27], nanodendrites [28], bipyramid nanostructures [29], flower-like nanostructures [30, 31], berry-like nanostructures [32], urchin-shaped nanostructures [33], nanopancakes [34], etc. Two-layer based nanoparticles (NPs) such as core–shell structures [35] or solid substrates (sandwich structures [36], laminated films [23]) are the most exploited due to their unique optical properties and high chemical stability. Spherical gold and silver nanoparticles, easy to prepare with tuneable size, are used extensively as SERS substrates, capped or uncapped, due to the favorable local scattering field enhancement, potential surface chemical modification, biocompatibility, and bioavailability. In other circumstances, the covering layer has a completely different scope, as Zhou *et al* demonstrated in their latest work [34]. The multiple functions of PBS-stimulated Au–Ag stuffed nanopancakes (AAS-NPs) were bacterial sensing, by employing the widely used 4-MPBA as both an internal standard and SERS tag, inactivation of pathogens in human blood samples, and successful bacterial biofilm disruption. Figure 10.2 shows schematically the triple function features of the newly designed Au–Ag stuffed nanostructures.

With the recent advancement in developing reliable, wearable, ready-to-use, and integrated SERS-active substrates, bacterial metabolomics and SERS-based *resistograms* [37] are envisioned with every new study in this field as alternatives for current clinical routine testing. This convenient method should prove useful for high-throughput surveillance of multidrug-resistant species, the 'superbugs' found on hospital premises.

The single-cell and label-free nature of the detection methods imply wide applicability for rapid POC bacterial and viral diagnosis. Sometimes a few pathogens are sufficient to induce chronic conditions. The SERS-based approaches have the potential to identify uncultivable bacteria and avoid inter-species competition while culturing heterogeneous populations. The advantages of SERS reside primarily in its low cost, ultra-sensitivity, reliability, and performance, even outdoors, and multiplex capacity. Reagentless and straightforward approaches usually involve the synthesis of colloidal suspensions, with high stability in human fluids [38–42] for the early diagnosis of chronic pathologies.

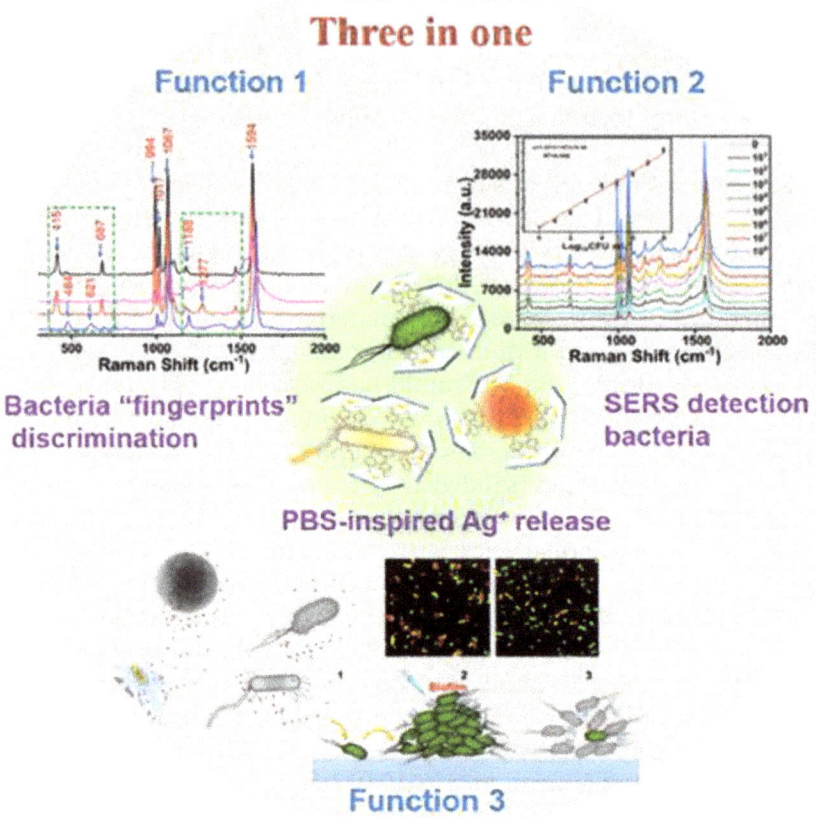

Figure 10.2. Scheme showing the three-in-one design for Au–Ag-Stuffed nanopancakes: discrimination of pathogens by using SERS fingerprinting (Function 1), SERS-based detection of bacteria (Function 2), and inactivation of multiple bacteria by silver ions released in their biofilm (Function 3). (Reproduced with permission [34]. Copyright 2022 American Chemical Society.)

10.3 PoC SERS-based strategies for advanced diagnostics

10.3.1 Microfluidic SERS-based diagnosis of infections

Microfluidics is usually integrated with portable vibrational spectroscopy systems in POC devices meant to monitor and analyse the biochemicals found in the surroundings of microorganisms or released by those. SERS-based biosensing allows for real-time and non-destructive analysis with almost no sample preparation and high sensitivity. The spectral output obtained is usually complex and Raman identifier band (RIB) strategies are employed to decipher the spectral area of interest and to avoid overlapping of structurally similar analytes.

A microfluidic device contains interconnected microscale channels designed into or on top of a solid (glass slide, silicon) or flexible (PC, PDMS, PMMA) substrate. The analytes can flow through the microchannels due to the hydrostatic pressure or can be injected by using a peristaltic pump or syringe. Currently, these microdevices are used in POC to examine chemical and biological processes with a high level of precision and in a carefully controlled microenvironment [43, 44]. The key advantages of such portable systems are minimal sample volume, design flexibility, increased throughput, low-cost fabrication, and short analysis time.

In the case of SERS combined with microfluidics, the samples are controlled and analysed inside the microchannels, where the analyte interacts with the previously prepared SERS substrate or the built-in micro- or nanostructured noble metal. This leads to a dramatic increase in the microfluidic device's performance [45]. The IoMT SERS measurements are envisioned as semi- or fully automatic, exploiting the reproducibility of the technique and benefiting microfluidic platforms able to sense small volumes [46].

The majority of the approaches combining SERS and microfluidics are either based on costly patterning techniques or on nanostructured wafers, which are not usually lucrative for scaling up. In fabricating PoC devices that can be connected easily to digital platforms, it is feasible to consider smart, multiplex, polymer-based, or paper-based low-cost SERS substrates for analysing human fluids by spectral and biological recognition. IoMT-based advanced diagnostics are being developed to enable ultrasensitive detection and replace culture-based testing.

Usually, the pathogen's detection is based on immobilization using specific antigens, antibodies, labels, etc. Moreover, several approaches to capturing, concentration, or filtration are used to obtain significant biomass for accurate detection. For instance, the online SERS detection of prostate-specific antigen (PSA) from blood samples at a trace level has been realized by a microfluidic chip integrated with the dielectrophoresis (DEP) biosensing strategy [44].

Muhlig et al [47] successfully differentiated six types of mycobacteria using silver nanoparticles (AgNPs) as a SERS substrate in a glass microfluidic system. Other authors [48] reported the use of a microfluidic chip capable of continuously sorting and concentrating bacteria via 3D DEP and in situ SERS. The microchannels were made as a sandwich structure between two glass slides and the microelectrodes used in DEP. In this way, Staphylococcus aureus and Pseudomonas aeruginosa bacteria were effectively discriminated against, while S. aureus was continuously separated and concentrated via DEP out of a sample of blood cells.

Bloodstream infections (BSIs) are among the most costly and high mortality public health issues to tackle, as they are the primary cause of sepsis. Modern methods are proposed for rapid turn-around time (TAT) in cases of infection using biomarkers of bacterial metabolic responses to antibiotics. SERS-based consistent antibiotic susceptibility test (AST) results from clinical blood-culture samples are assessed within hours [49, 50]. The rapid SERS-based resistogram is the clinical outcome targeted since at least 12 h (overnight, medical shift long cultures) are needed to reach a highly concentrated living bacteria source for strain identification. A novel biochip integrated with microelectrodes was fabricated for filtration and enrichment of airborne microbes and further in situ detection and identification based on electrical impedance spectroscopy (EIS) in combination with SERS (figure 10.3). The PDA-co-CS composite gel provides good permeability for the

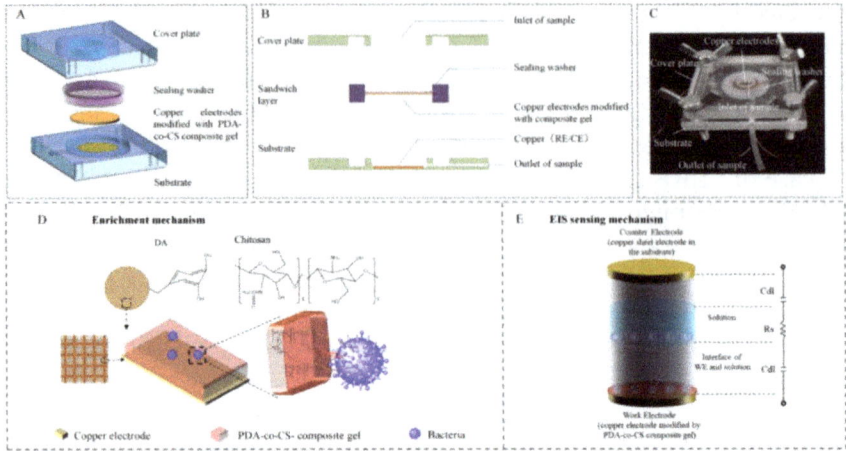

Figure 10.3. Scheme of a biochip integrated with microelectrodes modified by PDA-co-CS composite gel (A), sectional view (B), and photograph (C) of the biochip. Diagram of enrichment mechanism (D) and EIS test unit (E) of the biochip. (Reproduced with permission from [51]. Copyright 2021 Elsevier.)

air and is also used for capturing the target microbe [51]. In this set-up, the changes in the numbers of the captured microbes on the copper electrode surface would be reflected by changes in the value of the electrical impedance of the system. Thus, the quantitative assessment of microbial concentration found in aerosol by using EIS as possible down to the single-microbe level. The electrical impedance signal of the biochip was found to be inversely dependent on the pathogens' concentration.

In situ enrichment followed by detection of airborne pathogens is required due to their very low concentrations in practical applications. Simple sedimentation or filtration may not be sufficient. It is surprising, however, that in this case, as in many others, the *in situ* SERS-based sensing approach relies on a common silver solution, while the highest effort and the most elaborate parts of the device are meant to pre-concentrate and capture the microbial sample. This aspect underlies the great potential of colloidal suspensions in practice, mostly outdoors, due to their SERS performance, high stability in time, online use inside microfluidic channels, and cost-efficiency as compared to solid SERS-active substrates fabricated using sophisticated, expensive equipment. While notable progress has been made in the field in the last decade, challenges or drawbacks in their applications such as pathogen detection and biomolecular screening remain to be overcome [52].

Another recent approach for rapid AST of bacteria from patients' blood samples using SERS was demonstrated by testing 75 clinical strains of *S. aureus* and *E. coli*. The authors developed a SERS-AST clinical protocol including pre-concentration of the samples, inoculation and antibiotic testing for 2 h, sample centrifugation to separate cells from drugs, and SERS measurements for determining bacterial metabolic response with and without treatment [37]. The spectral peaks found at 730 cm^{-1} and 724 cm^{-1} were defined as biomarkers for *S. aureus* and *E. coli* species, respectively, and their intensity signal ratios for antibiotic-treated and untreated samples were further analysed. A cut-off signal ratio was defined so that each SERS biomarker signal ratio would be carefully compared to it and specific MICs and susceptibilities would result from this assessment. A receiver operating characteristic (ROC) analysis was adopted, and the area under the curve (AUC) was considered for determining the SERS-AST method's accuracy.

The rationale for the rapid response offered by the spectral profiling of the bacteria's metabolism is supported by studies indicating that independent of the class of antibiotic (β-lactams, aminoglycosides, quinolones, etc), the treatment will induce similar metabolic modifications after 30 min [53]. Practically, the concentration of the purine-like molecules defined as the biomarkers' SERS bands in the method's working principle is greatly reduced due to antibiotic exposure. The drawback is that the time required for a blood culture to become statistically relevant in terms of antimicrobial activity biomarker concentration is still around half a shift.

A noteworthy aspect of this proof-of-principle AST assay is that the SERS signals for both Gram-positive and Gram-negative species are obtained with high reproducibility, so those SERS marker peaks are consistent in their position. The schematic flow of experimental work and data analysis was clearly described by the authors even in their first AST study based on SERS biomarker monitoring [54]. In the following study [37], the most recent one, the group managed to describe mathematically the extraction protocol for the biomarker SERS signals and their clinically relevant interpretation with high accuracy. Such assays relying on the bacterial metabolic response with SERS from blood samples represents a major step in the implementation of the SERS-AST method in clinical routine analysis, as an alternative to conventional methods.

For instance, a deep-learning-based spectroscopic analysis for determining the *resistogram* of UTI pathogens was implemented by Fu *et al* [55]. An intelligent identification model and a multidrug resistance algorithm based on convolutional neural networks (CNN) were constructed, achieving 96% accuracy in classification. The authors used the SERS profiles of six UTI pathogens as the input layers. The construction of the CNN model was assessed by using 70% of the SERS spectra for training the model, then 20% was employed for training the model, and 10% for testing the model. The CNN model uses the convolutional layer to take out features from the input dataset, and the mapping of these features is then transmitted to the next layer until the fully connected layer. Each step is an improvement of the non-linear classification deviations made by using corrections based on an activation function. In comparison with PCA or PCA combined with KNN algorithms, the CNN model showed higher accuracy in classification and bacteria recognition. The drug sensitivity of pathogenic species can also be assessed with an accuracy above 95%, as shown by the authors. This approach has great potential to be applied to clinical isolates for unknown species recognition, drug susceptibility testing, and multidrug resistance.

Regarding the applications of SERS-based microfluidic devices for detecting COVID-19, Zhao and co-workers developed the eSIREN platform, consisting of an integrated system combining reconfigurable enzyme–DNA nanostructures and

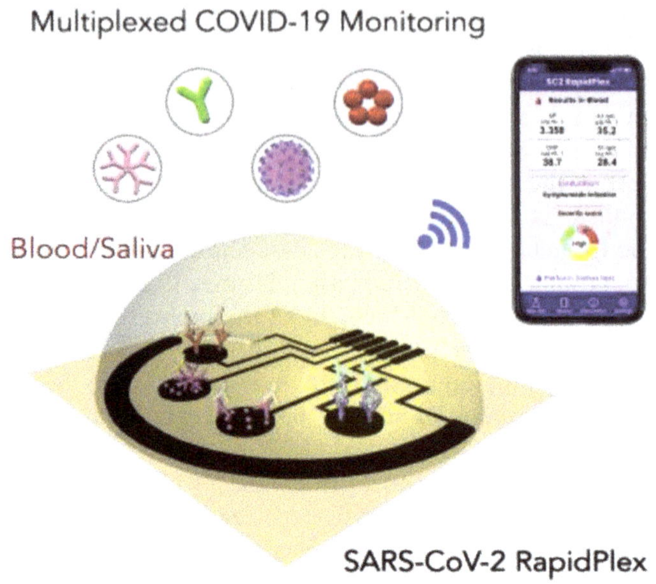

Figure 10.4. The SARS-CoV-2 RapidPlex is a graphene-based multiplexed platform for rapid and low-cost COVID-19 diagnosis and monitoring. (Reproduced with permission from [61]. Copyright 2020 Elsevier.)

automated microfluidics. The system can provide a rapid and accurate diagnosis [56]. The results were obtained in less than 20 min, and the microfluidic system was tested both on extracted RNA samples and swab lysates, overcoming the need for any purification or extraction.

Most of the available kits for COVID testing that are biosensors-based are reviewed by Parihar *et al* [57], including their practical limitations and strong points in practice. The platforms for electrochemical, colorimetric, and plasmonic biosensing are designed to test biological samples and to provide a fast, reliable diagnosis. Biomarkers, such as biomolecules associated with COVID-19, are either viral proteins, specific antibodies, or viral nucleotide sequences. These can be detected by immuno-assay tests, portable electrochemical biosensors, or more recently by SERS coupled with LFIA [58], in low sample volumes with 100% accuracy [59]. Future advancements in SERS-based testing, as one of the most efficient and fast spectroscopies, is towards integration with IoT for accessible, on-site use for local communities. The rapid detection of SARS-CoV-2 is already IoT integrated for electrochemical graphene-based immunoassays [60, 61] (see figure 10.4).

10.3.2 Raman imaging for advanced diagnostics

Advanced digital pathology is now possible as presented by the CytoViva hyper-spectral microscopy imaging (HSI)-based latest studies. Their hyperspectral micro-scope systems include custom microscopy configurations, such as patented enhanced darkfield and traditional brightfield imaging for tissue specimens. Stained cells or stained negative control tissues as well as spectral mapping of specific cancerous elements in tissues can be monitored by HSI [62–64]. Even human coronaviruses (HCoVs) in infected cells were detected by this non-invasive, label-free diagnostic tool, providing rapid and accurate identification of two strains of HCoVs [65].

Raman imaging is a quantitative and qualitative analysis used for in-line measurements by employing fiber-optics or probes. In contrast to hyperspectral imaging, the experimental progress in Raman imaging needs further validation to be approved for commercial use [66].

The automatic scanning mode of recent Raman systems can map significant areas in a short time, providing an inherently chemical distribution of the most relevant components in biological samples. These unique characteristics of Raman imaging offer great benefits in applications such as pathogen detection and biomolecular screening.

Ongoing troubleshooting in Raman imaging is focused on finding ways to reconstruct images when the spectra acquisition is achieved using optical fibers instead of benchtop systems, for medical applications. Real-time molecular imaging based on a computer-vision-based positional tracking system is proposed by the Popp group as part of the Raman4Clinics strategy. Employing augmented reality molecular imaging and direct visualization of the molecular boundaries of 3D surfaces, such as tissues, is possible. The implementation of fiber-optic probe-based RS in medical premises is constantly present at the leading edge of hot research topics [67].

A very useful solution was recently proposed for Raman data handling, including the big datasets resulting from mapping heterogeneous samples [68]. The Raman Light is a single app designed to handle complex spectral datasets and analyse them, also considering the Raman images resulting from scanning the surface of the sample as a mixture of different pure compounds with modified contributions within the thousands of spectra. The Raman identifying bands strategy is once again considered a relevant, reliable interpretation of the Raman images and their associated spectral data as end-members of the analysis model. The capabilities of the app to assess hyperspectral images and to visualize the spatial abundances of known compounds were demonstrated for RS, as an established analysis method. Thus, a free, widely available MATLAB app is already produced for the use of experts in the research area. The product was successfully tested for processing Raman hyperspectral images of pharmaceutical mixtures, biomedical tissue, and mixed polymer coating materials. The accuracy of the product is guaranteed by including the most common pre-processing protocols for spectral data when using eight independent unsupervised algorithms, adapted for these types of data.

10.4 The role of data analysis in advanced diagnostics

The data analysis is crucial regardless of whether we are analysing SERS spectra of living microorganisms or just the specific spectral response to their presence. Data analysis can help improve the TAT for medical decisions but can also make the adopted methodologies more effective, accurate, and automated. Skvortsova *et al* [50] recently proposed an advanced diagnostic approach for bacterial AST.

The method can detect a specific oligonucleotide sequence encoding the β-lactam antibiotic resistance in picomolar concentrations by using SERS combined with a specially designed decision system (DS). The DS consists of a Siamese neural network coupled with robust statistics and the Bayes decision rule and provides a 99% level of confidence. The high accuracy was reached by employing a feedback function within the DS, relying on spectral *regions of interest (ROI)*. As intuitive as it may sound, while we are as experts used to exploiting the same spectral features, the process of decision is, in this case, fully automatic, so time and human resources are required at a minimum.

10.4.1 AI and smartphone-based readout of the spectral signal

SERS is omnipresent in biomedical applications as a reliable candidate for both quantitative and multiplex sensing of known or unknown analytes. The full automatization of a SERS experiment has not yet been realized, but an attempt at liquid sample handling by a robot followed by a SERS assay was proposed by Grys *et al* [69]. The so-called SERSbot is an optical system integrating the robot sampling component. The robot is also assigned with the *in situ* synthesis of AuNPs during sampling, which gives it a high reproducibility and short analysis time. The key advantages of this approach are that the optimized parameter aggregation and incubation times are controlled. Nowadays, the standardization of SERS experiments is of great research interest [70, 71] and this could become a good way to reduce human-associated errors in sampling and also pave the pathway to SERS as a standardized clinical methodology.

PoC devices should be designed as equivalent to laboratory-based approaches: rapid, low-cost, user-friendly, and not lacking in specificity or sensitivity. A smartphone-based microplate reader was designed and fabricated as a portable device enabling colorimetric, fluorescence, luminescence, and turbidity analyses [72]. The Bluetooth module and optical system consisting of one UV SMD LED and four white LEDs provide useful information for detecting a variety of relevant molecular analytes (antibodies, toxins, drugs, and classic fluorophore dyes). Moreover, its analytical performance is comparable to that of a commercial microplate reader. The greatest advantage remains to incorporate a cheap, low-consumption, and tuneable light source such as an LED into a microplate reader that can be easily miniaturized and integrated into a portable device. As a solution to a current issue, the device was successfully tested for bacterial cultures and their specific bactericidal drug screening. The device's automatic operation and interface design are assured by a microcontroller adapted for smartphone-based reading through a dedicated app (figure 10.5(a)). As a gold standard analytical assay, the device was tested as an ELISA for the detection of a SARS-CoV-2 N-protein, a stringent need within POC rapid testing. Another POC test device comprising a giant magnetoresistance (GMR) was used to detect the magnetic intensity of anti-SARS-CoV-2 IgG and IgM antibodies previously labeled with superparamagnetic nanoparticles (SMNP) in a lateral flow immunoassay (LFIA) strip. The obtained data can be transmitted to a smartphone through Bluetooth technology, providing a

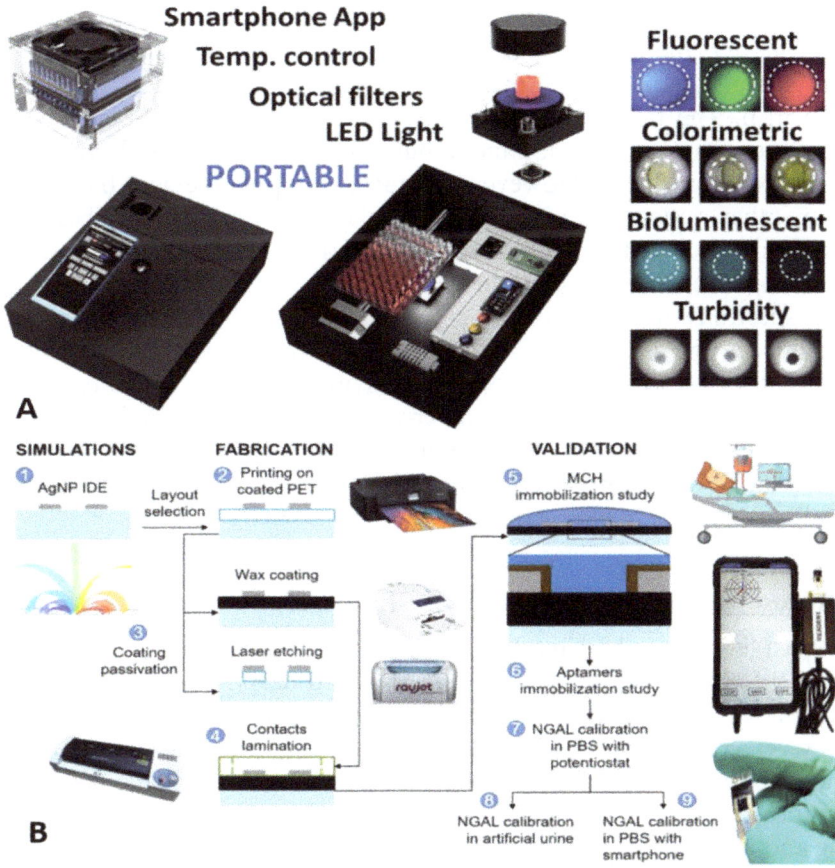

Figure 10.5. (A) Smartphone-based microplate reader designed and fabricated as a portable device for colorimetric, fluorescence, luminescence, and turbidity analyses. (Reproduced with permission from [72]. Copyright 2022 American Chemical Society.) (B) Smartphone-based quantification and impedance readout for acute kidney injury biomarker from urine. (Reproduced with permission from [75]. Copyright 2022 Elsevier.)

diagnosis within 10 min, and a concentration of IgG and IgM of 5 ng mL^{-1} and 10 ng ml^{-1} [73]. Bokemann and co-workers [74] developed the Cap-iLAMP—capture and improved looped-mediated isothermal amplification, the improved version of iLAMP, a POC device for the detection of positive SARS-CoV-2 samples. The initial version, iLAMP, was susceptible to false-positive results. The technology behind the device is based on a combination of RNA extraction from the gargle lavage samples based on hybridization capture. The LAMP components are further mixed with SYBR Green, allowing the visual detection of the virus from a change in color ranging from red to yellow. By using the Palette Cam app on a smartphone, the obtained color was further transformed into a numerical hue value, which, in the end, was attributed to a COVID-19 'positive' or 'negative' result.

The facile and rapid smartphone-based readout was also used for clinical diagnosis of acute kidney injury via biosensing an important marker in urine [75].

After the sensitivity of the impedance measurements to the coverage of the electrodes was achieved, the surface was validated, the device was adapted for specific aptamer sensing, and the smartphone-based quantification was assessed (figure 10.5(b)). The fabrication steps are transferable for SERS-active substrates designed for sensing, such as aptamers, but a similar SERS-based portable device has not yet been produced. However, wearable electronic devices based on SERS readout or other optical techniques with similar performance have been designed and thoroughly discussed for glucose sensing [76]. Moreover, super-resolution SERS imaging was performed on metallic and silica particles embedded in fixed cells for obtaining spectrally resolved SERS images of biological samples. The homebuilt experimental set-up designed by Schultz *et al* [77] is one step forward towards non-invasive SERS microscopy for monitoring living subjects and *in operando* conditions. The complex technique of super-resolution SERS imaging is exploiting localization algorithms such as those used in stochastic optical reconstruction microscopy (STORM) for deciphering the intense SERS signals obtained from biological samples.

10.4.2 Robust models for data analysis of SERS spectra

Over the past few years, there has been an increase in using artificial intelligence (AI) and, more specifically, machine learning (ML) and deep learning (DL) to perform classification tasks of Raman spectral data on clinical samples. Spectral insight is complex when considering that of the abundant data, not all are clinically relevant to the classification model and, thus, it should be trained to consider only the diagnosis/prognosis or monitoring parameters of interest. ML is very good at adapting and identifying patterns in large amounts of complex data and has already been implemented for broad real-world applications. This has been done mostly because of the availability of data and the need for medical experts to obtain the most rapid, accurate, and personalized response for a fair clinical decision.

With almost 520 million positive cases and over 6 million deaths registered up to May 2022 (coronavirus.jhu.edu/map), disregarding all the negative aspects of the COVID-19 pandemic, one of its positive contributions to IoMTs was to generate a enormous amount of data at the global level in a short period, providing valuable raw material for specialists in data analytics. Several such databases combining data analytics and SERS/Raman fingerprints of various media contaminated with SARS-CoV-2 were used to create statistical models used as pillars of COVID-19 diagnosis.

By using a database provided by Yin *et al* [78], comprising 250 Raman spectra recorded on human serum, Chen [79] aimed to develop a classification model of healthy and COVID-19-positive patients. Out of nine ML and artificial neural network (ANN) models tested in the study, the stacked subassembly model proved to have the best performance (98% accuracy).

Huang *et al* [80] combined Raman spectra of SARS-CoV-2's spike protein and the deep-learning RNN model performed on a database of SERS spectra recorded on throat swabs from both healthy and COVID-19 confirmed patients. Moitra *et al* [81] developed a set of antisense oligonucleotides designed to efficiently bind to a segment of the nucleocapsid phosphoprotein gene of SARS-CoV-2. Since the genetic segment used as a target is common to all SARS-CoV-2 variants, a database containing SERS fingerprints of the resulting systems was further used to create a classification model able to discriminate between a positive and negative COVID-19 test, by employing both classical multivariate methods and algorithms based on support vector machine (SVM) analysis coupled with standard normal variate (SNV) pre-processing. The rapid (within 30 min) detection protocol comprises a mixture of the sample collected from nasopharyngeal aspiration with antibody-conjugated magnetic beads and hollow gold nanoparticles (AuNPs) with malachite green isothiocyanate (MGITC) tested by using a portable Raman spectrometer to collect the data, and then identification of COVID-19-positive patients is made in the clinical setting [82].

A combination of SERS spectra of wild-type, alpha, and beta variants of SARS-CoV-2 with ML tools managed to identify the presence of the virus with more than 95% sensitivity and specificity. Samples' fingerprints were collected from the original biosensor previously developed by Torun and co-workers, which is an oligonucleotide presenting high affinity to the receptor-binding domain of spike protein in SARS-CoV-2. To identify the virus, the original aptamer was modified by adding a Cy5.5 fluorescent marker as a second aptamer. The database comprises PCR clinical samples of both saliva and nasopharyngeal exudate and the analysis model distinguishes between the three variants of the virus [83].

In vivo collected spectra tend to be noisier, and far more difficult to discriminate. For this, we can use one of the many digital filters available, the most popular for spectra pre-processing being the Savitzky–Golay filter already implemented in Python libraries such as Scypy [84].

One last key aspect which should be addressed when analysing SERS spectral datasets is that the number of features (wavenumbers) is higher for small and medium-sized data than the number of spectra (hundreds to thousands of registered spectra). In most tabular data used for ML classification, feature selection is employed to increase the scores, because some characteristics are in strong relation with one another. A similar approach was proposed by Kemmler *et al* [85], as they selected discriminative characteristics or more explicitly biomarkers to see the variability of the accuracy for different bacterial datasets. This approach could solve the approach shortcomings of spectra in ML and increase the relevant classification metrics.

10.5 Conclusions

SERS is a competitive, ultrasensitive technique, very suitable for viral and bacterial fingerprinting, pathogenicity barcoding, and monitoring, mostly in sub-lethal antibiotic concentrations. Scenarios of susceptibility, resistance, pseudo-resistance, and tolerance can be reflected by analysing SERS spectral data with robust chemometrics.

The development of SERS-based biosensors and rapid testing platforms for clinical use requires standardization of the methodology and versatility toward multidrug-resistant pathogens or the ever-growing variety of viral mutations of the SARS-CoV. The high-throughput features of biosensors (speed, portability, trace level sensitivity, multiplex capacity, low cost, reusability, digitization) enable rapid POC testing of infections in clinical applications.

Constant effort is invested in biosensing technological progress and availability for on-site monitoring of biomarkers indicating chronic diseases from a direct sampling of biofluids. Moreover, the interpretation of the SERS spectral output and diagnosis potential is significantly helped by the latest AI-based and ML models adapted for big dataset analysis with clinical relevance.

The high demand for rapid testing caused mainly by the recent viral outbreaks is reflected by the hundreds of scientific solutions developed as paper-based, single-use, strip-like antigenic tests translated from the lab premises directly to the clinical setting. SERS in combination with microfluidics, DEP, or magnetic separation in miniaturized devices can detect cellular components as well as immunogenic material in label-based approaches (LFIA, enzymatic assays).

Hence, further experimental validation of simple, ready-to-use SERS-based approaches is needed but the critical mass involved in this research direction is building step-by-step the pathway towards IoMT-based SERS detection as advanced diagnostics.

Acknowledgments

This work was funded by the Ministry of Research, Innovation, and Digitization through Programme 1—Development of the National Research and Development System, Subprogramme 1.2—Institutional Performance—Funding Projects for Excellence in RDI, Contract No. 37PFE/30.12.2021. and Subprogramme 1.1—Human resources—Research projects to stimulate young independent teams—project number PN-III-P1-1.1-TE-2019-0910.

References

[1] Nakar A, Pistiki A, Ryabchykov O, Bocklitz T, Rösch P and Popp J 2022 Detection of multi-resistant clinical strains of *E. coli* with Raman spectroscopy *Anal. Bioanal. Chem.* **414** 1481–92

[2] Nakar A, Pistiki A, Ryabchykov O, Bocklitz T, Rösch P and Popp J 2022 Label-free differentiation of clinical *E. coli* and Klebsiella isolates with Raman spectroscopy *J. Biophoton.* **15** e202200005

[3] Shen H, Rösch P, Pletz M W and Popp J 2022 *In vitro* fiber-probe-based identification of pathogens in biofilms by Raman spectroscopy *Anal. Chem.* **94** 5375–81

[4] Messmer M W, Dieser M S, Parker H J, Foreman A E and Christine M 2022 Investigation of Raman spectroscopic signatures with multivariate statistics: an approach for cataloguing microbial biosignatures *Astrobiology* **22** 14–24

[5] Pahlow S *et al* 2018 Application of vibrational spectroscopy and imaging to point-of-care medicine: a review *Appl. Spectrosc.* **72** 52–84

[6] Yang W, Knorr F, Latka I, Vogt M, Hofmann G O, Popp J and Schie I W 2022 Real-time molecular imaging of near-surface tissue using Raman spectroscopy *Light Sci. Appl.* **11** 90

[7] Yang W, Mondol A S, Stiebing C, Marcu L, Popp J and Schie I W 2019 Raman ChemLighter: fiber optic Raman probe imaging in combination with augmented chemical reality *J. Biophoton.* **12** e201800447

[8] Lorenz B, Guo S, Raab C, Leisching P, Bocklitz T, Rösch P and Popp J 2022 Comparison of conventional and shifted excitation Raman difference spectroscopy for bacterial identification *J. Raman Spectrosc.* **53** 1285–92

[9] Shaik T A *et al* 2022 Structural and biochemical changes in pericardium upon genipin cross-linking investigated using nondestructive and label-free imaging techniques *Anal. Chem.* **94** 1575–84

[10] Shen H, Rösch P and Popp J 2022 Fiber probe-based Raman spectroscopic identification of pathogenic infection microorganisms on agar plates *Anal. Chem.* **94** 4635–42

[11] Ren X, Lin K, Hsieh C-M, Liu L, Ge X and Liu Q 2022 Optical coherence tomography-guided confocal Raman microspectroscopy for rapid measurements in tissues *Biomed. Opt. Express* **13** 344–57

[12] Lee K *et al* 2021 Raman microspectroscopy for microbiology *Nat. Rev. Methods Primers* **1** 80

[13] Kneipp J, Kneipp H and Kneipp K 2008 SERS—a single-molecule and nanoscale tool for bioanalytics *Chem. Soc. Rev.* **37** 1052–60

[14] Liu S *et al* 2021 Wide-range, rapid, and specific identification of pathogenic bacteria by surface-enhanced Raman spectroscopy *ACS Sens.* **6** 2911–9

[15] Guo J, Liu Y, Ju H and Lu G 2022 From lab to field: surface-enhanced Raman scattering-based sensing strategies for on-site analysis *TrAC Trends Anal. Chem.* **146** 116488

[16] Kapara A, Brunton V, Graham D and Faulds K 2020 Investigation of cellular uptake mechanism of functionalised gold nanoparticles into breast cancer using SERS *Chem. Sci.* **11** 5819–29

[17] Lin S-J, Chao P-H, Cheng H-W, Wang J-K, Wang Y-L, Han Y-Y and Huang N-T 2022 An antibiotic concentration gradient microfluidic device integrating surface-enhanced Raman spectroscopy for multiplex antimicrobial susceptibility testing *Lab Chip* **22** 1805–14

[18] Bonifacio A 2022 *Principles and Clinical Diagnostic Applications of Surface-Enhanced Raman Spectroscopy* ed Y Wang (Amsterdam: Elsevier) pp 125–70

[19] Liu C, Popp J and Cialla-May D *World Scientific Reference on Plasmonic Nanomaterials* (Singapore: World Scientific) pp 125–61

[20] Kneipp J 2022 *Principles and Clinical Diagnostic Applications of Surface-Enhanced Raman Spectroscopy* ed Y Wang (Amsterdam: Elsevier) pp 303–25

[21] Zhang Y, Tran V, Adanalic M and Schlücker S 2022 *Principles and Clinical Diagnostic Applications of Surface-Enhanced Raman Spectroscopy* ed Y Wang (Amsterdam: Elsevier) pp 327–72

[22] Wang M, Yan Y, Mi Y and Jiang Y 2022 Flexible microsphere-coupled surface-enhanced Raman spectroscopy (McSERS) by dielectric microsphere cavity array with random plasmonic nanoparticles *J. Raman Spectrosc.* **53** 1238–48

[23] Colniţă A, Marconi D, Dina N E, Brezeştean I, Bogdan D and Turcu I 2022 3D silver metallized nanotrenches fabricated by nanoimprint lithography as flexible SERS detection platform *Spectrochim. Acta* A **276** 121232

[24] Verma A K and Soni R K 2022 Ultrasensitive surface-enhanced Raman spectroscopy detection of explosive molecules with multibranched silver nanostructures *J. Raman Spectrosc.* **53** 694–708

[25] Qian J, Xing C, Ge Y, Li R, Li A and Yan W 2020 Gold nanostars-enhanced Raman fingerprint strip for rapid detection of trace tetracycline in water samples *Spectrochim. Acta A* **232** 118146

[26] Thu V T, Cuong N M, Cao D T, Hung L T and Ngan L T-Q 2022 Trace detection of ciprofloxacin antibiotic using surface-enhanced Raman scattering coupled with silver nanostars *Optik* **260** 169043

[27] Becerril-Castro I B, Calderon I, Pazos-Perez N, Guerrini L, Schulz F, Feliu N, Chakraborty I, Giannini V, Parak W J and Alvarez-Puebla R A 2022 Gold nanostars: synthesis, optical and SERS analytical properties *Anal. Sens.* **2** e202200005

[28] Tang M, Zheng P, Wu Y, Zhu P, Qin Y, Jiang Y, Sun R, Wong C P and Li Z 2020 Silver dendrites based electrically conductive composites, towards the application of stretchable conductors *Compos. Commun.* **19** 121–6

[29] Wu H, Luo Y, Hou C, Huo D, Zhou Y, Zou S, Zhao J and Lei Y 2019 Flexible bipyramid-AuNPs based SERS tape sensing strategy for detecting methyl parathion on vegetable and fruit surface *Sens. Actuators* B **285** 123–8

[30] Ma M, Sun J, Chen Y, Wen K, Wang Z, Shen J, Zhang S, Ke Y and Wang Z 2018 Highly sensitive SERS immunosensor for the detection of amantadine in chicken based on flower-like gold nanoparticles and magnetic bead separation *Food Chem. Toxicol.* **118** 589–94

[31] Nguyen M C, Ngan Luong T Q, Vu T T, Anh C T and Dao T C 2022 Synthesis of wool roll-like silver nanoflowers in an ethanol/water mixture and their application to detect traces of the fungicide carbendazim by SERS technique *RSC Adv.* **12** 11583–90

[32] Chang C-C, Imae T, Chen L-Y and Ujihara M 2015 Efficient surface enhanced Raman scattering on confeito-like gold nanoparticle-adsorbed self-assembled monolayers *Phys. Chem. Chem. Phys.* **17** 32328–34

[33] Duan N, Yao T, Li C, Wang Z and Wu S 2022 Surface-enhanced Raman spectroscopy relying on bimetallic Au–Ag nanourchins for the detection of the food allergen β-lactoglobulin *Talanta* **245** 123445

[34] Zhou S, Guo X, Huang H, Huang X, Zhou X, Zhang Z, Sun G, Cai H, Zhou H and Sun P 2022 Triple-function Au–Ag-stuffed nanopancakes for SERS detection, discrimination, and inactivation of multiple bacteria *Anal. Chem.* **94** 5785–96

[35] Höller R P M, Jahn I J, Cialla-May D, Chanana M, Popp J, Fery A and Kuttner C 2020 Biomacromolecular-assembled nanoclusters: key aspects for robust colloidal SERS sensing *ACS Appl. Mater. Interfaces* **12** 57302–13

[36] Qu L-L, Ying Y-L, Yu R-J and Long Y-T 2021 *In situ* food-borne pathogen sensors in a nanoconfined space by surface enhanced Raman scattering *Microchim. Acta* **188** 201

[37] Han Y Y, Lin Y C, Cheng W C, Lin Y T, Teng L J, Wang J K and Wang Y L 2020 Rapid antibiotic susceptibility testing of bacteria from patients' blood via assaying bacterial metabolic response with surface-enhanced Raman spectroscopy *Sci. Rep.* **10** 12538

[38] Moisoiu V *et al* 2019 Breast cancer diagnosis by surface-enhanced Raman scattering (SERS) of urine *Appl. Sci.* **9** 806

[39] Stefancu A, Moisoiu V, Couti R, Andras I, Rahota R, Crisan D, Pavel I E, Socaciu C, Leopold N and Crisan N 2018 Combining SERS analysis of serum with PSA levels for improving the detection of prostate cancer *Nanomedicine* **13** 2455–67

[40] Moisoiu V, Badarinza M, Stefancu A, Iancu S D, Serban O, Leopold N and Fodor D 2020 Combining surface-enhanced Raman scattering (SERS) of saliva and two-dimensional shear

wave elastography (2D-SWE) of the parotid glands in the diagnosis of Sjögren's syndrome *Spectrochim. Acta* A **235** 118267

[41] Moisoiu V *et al* 2019 SERS-based differential diagnosis between multiple solid malignancies: breast, colorectal, lung, ovarian and oral cancer *Int. J. Nanomed.* **14** 6165–78

[42] Stefancu A, Badarinza M, Moisoiu V, Iancu S D, Serban O, Leopold N and Fodor D 2019 SERS-based liquid biopsy of saliva and serum from patients with Sjögren's syndrome *Anal. Bioanal. Chem.* **411** 5877–83

[43] Amin R, Knowlton S, Hart A, Yenilmez B, Ghaderinezhad F, Katebifar S, Messina M, Khademhosseini A and Tasoglu S 2016 3D-printed microfluidic devices *Biofabrication* **8** 022001

[44] Wang X, He X, He Z, Hou L, Ge C, Wang L, Li S and Xu Y 2022 Detection of prostate specific antigen in whole blood by microfluidic chip integrated with dielectrophoretic separation and electrochemical sensing *Biosens. Bioelectron.* **204** 114057

[45] Zhou Q and Kim T 2016 Review of microfluidic approaches for surface-enhanced Raman scattering *Sens. Actuators* B **227** 504–14

[46] Jahn I J, Zukovskaja O, Zheng X S, Weber K, Bocklitz T W, Cialla-May D and Popp J 2017 Surface-enhanced Raman spectroscopy and microfluidic platforms: challenges, solutions and potential applications *Analyst* **142** 1022–47

[47] Mühlig A *et al* 2016 LOC-SERS: a promising closed system for the identification of mycobacteria *Anal. Chem.* **88** 7998–8004

[48] Cheng I F, Lin C C, Lin D Y and Chang H C 2010 A dielectrophoretic chip with a roughened metal surface for on-chip surface-enhanced Raman scattering analysis of bacteria *Biomicrofluidics* **4** 034104

[49] Zhang P *et al* 2022 Dynamic insights into increasing antibiotic resistance in *Staphylococcus aureus* by label-free SERS using a portable Raman spectrometer *Spectrochim. Acta* A **273** 121070

[50] Skvortsova A, Trelin A, Kriz P, Elashnikov R, Vokata B, Ulbrich P, Pershina A, Svorcik V, Guselnikova O and Lyutakov O 2022 SERS and advanced chemometrics—utilization of Siamese neural network for picomolar identification of beta-lactam antibiotics resistance gene fragment *Anal. Chim. Acta* **1192** 339373

[51] Su X, Ren R, Wu Y, Li S, Ge C, Liu L and Xu Y 2021 Study of biochip integrated with microelectrodes modified by poly-dopamine-co-chitosan composite gel for separation, enrichment and detection of microbes in the aerosol *Biosens. Bioelectron.* **176** 112931

[52] Teng J, Yuan F, Ye Y, Zheng L, Yao L, Xue F, Chen W and Li B 2016 Aptamer-based technologies in foodborne pathogen detection *Front. Microbiol* **7** 1426

[53] Belenky P *et al* 2015 Bactericidal antibiotics induce toxic metabolic perturbations that lead to cellular damage *Cell Rep.* **13** 968–80

[54] Liu C-Y, Han Y-Y, Shih P-H, Lian W-N, Wang H-H, Lin C-H, Hsueh P-R, Wang J-K and Wang Y-L 2016 Rapid bacterial antibiotic susceptibility test based on simple surface-enhanced Raman spectroscopic biomarkers *Sci. Rep.* **6** 23375

[55] Fu Q, Zhang Y, Wang P, Pi J, Qiu X, Guo Z, Huang Y, Zhao Y, Li S and Xu J 2021 Rapid identification of the resistance of urinary tract pathogenic bacteria using deep learning-based spectroscopic analysis *Anal. Bioanal. Chem.* **413** 7401–10

[56] Zhao H *et al* 2021 Accessible detection of SARS-CoV-2 through molecular nanostructures and automated microfluidics *Biosens. Bioelectron.* **194** 113629

[57] Parihar A, Ranjan P, Sanghi S K, Srivastava A K and Khan R 2020 Point-of-care biosensor-based diagnosis of COVID-19 holds promise to combat current and future pandemics *ACS Appl. Bio Mater.* **3** 7326–43

[58] Yadav S, Sadique M A, Ranjan P, Kumar N, Singhal A, Srivastava A K and Khan R 2021 SERS based lateral flow immunoassay for point-of-care detection of SARS-CoV-2 in clinical samples *ACS Appl. Bio Mater.* **4** 2974–95

[59] Liu H *et al* 2021 Development of a SERS-based lateral flow immunoassay for rapid and ultra-sensitive detection of anti-SARS-CoV-2 IgM/IgG in clinical samples *Sens. Actuators* B **329** 129196

[60] Abubakar Sadique M, Yadav S, Ranjan P, Akram Khan M, Kumar A and Khan R 2021 Rapid detection of SARS-CoV-2 using graphene-based IoT integrated advanced electrochemical biosensor *Mater. Lett.* **305** 130824

[61] Torrente-Rodríguez R M, Lukas H, Tu J, Min J, Yang Y, Xu C, Rossiter H B and Gao W 2020 SARS-CoV-2 RapidPlex: a graphene-based multiplexed telemedicine platform for rapid and low-cost COVID-19 diagnosis and monitoring *Matter* **3** 1981–98

[62] Mehta N, Sahu S, Shaik S, Devireddy R and Gartia M R 2021 *Nanophotonics in Biomedical Engineering* ed X Zhao and M Lu (Singapore: Springer) pp 231–62

[63] Tan A, Liu Q, Septiadi D, Chu S, Liu T, Richards S-J, Rothen-Rutishauser B, Petri-Fink A, Gibson M I and Boyd B J 2021 Understanding selectivity of metabolic labelling and click-targeting in multicellular environments as a route to tissue selective drug delivery *J. Mater. Chem.* B **9** 5365–73

[64] Lawrence S 2021 Enhanced darkfield optical microscopy opens new nano-scale imaging possibilities *Microsc. Today* **29** 50–5

[65] Gosavi D, Cheatham B and Sztuba-Solinska J 2022 Label-free detection of human coronaviruses in infected cells using enhanced darkfield hyperspectral microscopy (EDHM) *J. Imaging* **8** 24

[66] Troy D J, Ojha K S, Kerry J P and Tiwari B K 2016 Sustainable and consumer-friendly emerging technologies for application within the meat industry: an overview *Meat Sci.* **120** 2–9

[67] Hilzenrat G, Gill E T and McArthur S L 2022 Imaging approaches for monitoring three-dimensional cell and tissue culture systems *J. Biophoton.* **15** e202100380

[68] Schmidt R W, Woutersen S and Ariese F 2022 RamanLIGHT—a graphical user-friendly tool for pre-processing and unmixing hyperspectral Raman spectroscopy images *J. Opt.* **24** 064011

[69] Grys D-B, de Nijs B, Huang J, Scherman O A and Baumberg J J 2021 SERSbot: revealing the details of SERS multianalyte sensing using full automation *ACS Sens.* **6** 4507–14

[70] Bell S E J, Charron G, Cortés E, Kneipp J, de la Chapelle M L, Langer J, Procházka M, Tran V and Schlücker S 2020 Towards reliable and quantitative surface-enhanced Raman scattering (SERS): from key parameters to good analytical practice *Angew. Chem. Int. Ed.* **59** 5454–62

[71] Guo S *et al* 2020 Comparability of Raman spectroscopic configurations: a large scale cross-laboratory study *Anal. Chem.* **92** 15745–56

[72] Bergua J F, Álvarez-Diduk R, Idili A, Parolo C, Maymó M, Hu L and Merkoçi A 2022 Low-cost, user-friendly, all-integrated smartphone-based microplate reader for optical-based biological and chemical analyses *Anal. Chem.* **94** 1271–85

[73] Bayin Q, Huang L, Ren C, Fu Y, Ma X and Guo J 2021 Anti-SARS-CoV-2 IgG and IgM detection with a GMR based LFIA system *Talanta* **227** 122207

[74] Bokelmann L, Nickel O, Maricic T, Pääbo S, Meyer M, Borte S and Riesenberg S 2021 Point-of-care bulk testing for SARS-CoV-2 by combining hybridization capture with improved colorimetric LAMP *Nat. Commun.* **12** 1467

[75] Rosati G *et al* 2022 A plug, print & play inkjet printing and impedance-based biosensing technology operating through a smartphone for clinical diagnostics *Biosens. Bioelectron.* **196** 113737

[76] Reda A, El-Safty S A, Selim M M and Shenashen M A 2021 Optical glucose biosensor built-in disposable strips and wearable electronic devices *Biosens. Bioelectron.* **185** 113237

[77] Shoup D N, Scarpitti B T and Schultz Z D 2022 A wide-field imaging approach for simultaneous super-resolution surface-enhanced Raman scattering bioimaging and spectroscopy *ACS Meas. Sci. Au.* **2** 332–41

[78] Yin G *et al* 2021 Data and code on serum Raman spectroscopy as an efficient primary screening of coronavirus disease in 2019 (COVID-19) (Fightshare Dataset) *J. Raman Spectrosc.* **52** 949–58

[79] Chen D 2021 Analysis of machine learning methods for COVID-19 detection using serum Raman spectroscopy *Appl. Artif. Intell.* **35** 1147–68

[80] Huang J *et al* 2021 On-site detection of SARS-CoV-2 antigen by deep learning-based surface-enhanced Raman spectroscopy and its biochemical foundations *Anal. Chem.* **93** 9174–82

[81] Moitra P, Chaichi A, Hasan S M A, Dighe K, Alafeef M, Prasad A, Gartia M R and Pan D 2022 Probing the mutation independent interaction of DNA probes with SARS-CoV-2 variants through a combination of surface-enhanced Raman scattering and machine learning *Biosens. Bioelectron.* **208** 114200

[82] Cha H *et al* 2022 Surface-enhanced Raman scattering-based immunoassay for severe acute respiratory syndrome coronavirus 2 *Biosens. Bioelectron.* **202** 114008

[83] Torun H *et al* 2021 Machine learning detects SARS-CoV-2 and variants rapidly on DNA aptamer metasurfaces medRxiv htttp://doi.org/10.1101/2021.08.07.21261749

[84] Virtanen P *et al* 2020 SciPy 1.0: fundamental algorithms for scientific computing in Python *Nat. Methods* **17** 261–72

[85] Kemmler M and Denzler J 2012 Finding discriminative features for Raman spectroscopy *Proc. 21st Int. Conf. on Pattern Recognition (ICPR2012)* pp 1823–6

Chapter 11

Optimization of SERS set-ups for high-efficiency and rapid detection of infectious diseases

Judy Z Wu and Samar Ali Ghopry

SERS has recently emerged as a promising approach for the high-efficiency detection of infections and diseases due to the recent advances in the development of SERS substrates based on two-dimensional (2D) atomic materials such as graphene, transition metal dichalcogenides, etc. van der Waals (vdW) heterostructures of the 2D materials and their hybrids with conventional metal nanostructures have provided a platform to design new SERS substrates for enhanced electromagnetic mechanism (EM) and chemical mechanism (CM). This allows high SERS sensitivity to be achieved on these SERS substrates using various probe molecules. This chapter will provide a review of the recent progress made in the development of SERS substrates based on 2D materials and remaining issues and future perspectives towards developing them for the high-efficiency, rapid detection of infectious diseases.

11.1 Introduction

Infectious diseases are illnesses caused by various harmful, outside pathogens entering into human bodies. While some infectious diseases are minor, others can be serious. In particular, an infection can spread from person to person, causing small- to large-scale damage to public health. COVID-19 is an excellent example among many other well-known infectious diseases, such as flu, measles, HIV, strep throat, and salmonella, to name only a few. Infectious diseases are highly common worldwide. For instance, each year in the United States, one out of every five people is infected with the influenza virus. For COVID-19, about 88 million infected cases have been confirmed in the US according to the Center for Disease Control. The pathogens causing infectious diseases include bacteria, viruses, fungi, parasites, etc. This means that infectious diseases can be viral, bacterial, parasitic, or fungal infections. Since the pathogens can be present in a vast variety of living environments including water, food, air, soil, the surface of infrastructures, and infected human bodies, high-efficiency and rapid detection of harmful pathogens becomes extremely critical for the treatment of infected patients and the prevention of the spread of infectious diseases.

Many techniques have been developed for pathogen or in general molecule detection. Among them, Raman spectroscopy, in particular surface-enhanced Raman spectroscopy (SERS) may provide a uniquely fast, efficient, and sensitive analytical technique for practical on-site analysis using portable Raman spectroscopy systems. A key to achieving such a goal is the development of SERS substrates that can provide significant enhancement to Raman sensitivity approaching the single molecular limit that are low-cost, portable, and disposable with a minimal environmental impact.

SERS was first observed by Martin Fleischmann, Patrick J Hendra, and A James McQuillan on a substrate of roughened silver in 1973 [1]. Since then, many studies have been carried out to probe SERS mechanisms and to improve SERS [2, 3]. In 1977 David L Jeanmaire *et al* verified the extraordinary sensitivity of Raman spectroscopy for adsorbed pyridine, nitrogen heterocycles, and amines on a rough silver surface and proposed an electromagnetic effect to explain the observed SERS sensitivity [3]. These pioneering works triggered intensive research on SERS, which has led to a demonstration of the power of SERS as an analytical tool for highly sensitive and selective detection of molecules adsorbed on nanostructures of noble metals such as gold and silver. More than 5000 research articles, 100 review articles, and numerous books on SERS have been published covering the fundamentals and applications of SERS in physics, chemistry, materials science, nanoscience, biosensor, clinical applications, and the life sciences [4–10].

Despite the progress made on the R&D of SERS, which has provided SERS with orders of magnitude enhanced sensitivity compared regular Raman spectroscopy, the full potential of SERS was not realized until the past decade or so. In the early stages of SERS, the majority of substrates were created utilizing electrochemically roughened electrodes [11] or randomly deposited metal films. For instance, vapor deposition of a thin layer of silver or gold, typically between 5 and 10 nm, onto slide-produced films offer a collection of a thin island that could provide surface plasmons. Because electrochemical roughening produced poorly defined substrates, the early SERS systems suffered greatly from irreproducibility. While a modest degree of tunability was achievable through changing the metal film thickness and solvent annealing, the difficulties in controlling the SERS substrate specifications and a lack of knowledge about the SERS active sites prohibited the quantitative use of SERS [12].

The discovery of single-molecule SERS in 1997 [13, 14] and the recent developments in nanofabrication sparked an explosion of new research on SERS, transforming SERS from a fascinating physical phenomenon into a reliable analytical approach for practical applications [15, 16]. Many of the intricate factors relating to SERS have been simplified by the ability to alter the form and orientation of metallic nanostructures on a surface using both top-down and bottom-up approaches. In addition, the discovery of graphene in 2004 by Andre Geim and Konstantin

Novoselov, who won a Nobel Prize in Physics in 2010, and the many other two-dimensional atomic materials (2D materials) discovered since have provided a unique pathway in the design of SERS with extraordinary sensitivity at a low cost. Applications of SERS have been reported in many analytical systems including pathogens associated with infectious diseases of SARS and COVID [17–19]. Therefore, significant progress has been made in advancing both SERS knowledge and applications over the last decade [20–24]. In this chapter, we highlight some of the recent progress made in the research and development of such SERS substrates, prompted in particular by the discovery of various novel 2D atomic materials.

11.2 Fundamentals in the design of SERS substrates

11.2.1 Raman spectroscopy

Raman spectroscopy is a spectroscopic tool used to identify the vibrational modes of the molecules based on the transferred energy when a molecule scatters an incident photon. Raman scattering can be interpreted physically in one of two ways: the quantum interaction and the classical interaction. In the former (figure 11.1(a)), when a molecule is hit by a photon, the electrons of the molecule will be excited to a higher energy state and relax to its initial state when the molecule re-emits the photon with no net energy transfer. This elastic scattering is known as Rayleigh scattering. However, a small fraction (one out of 10^7) of the excited molecules may land on a different energy level from their original state, resulting in a scattered photon with less (Stokes shifted) or more (anti-Stokes shifted) energy as compared to that of the excitation. This inelastic scattering was discovered in 1928 by an Indian physicist Raman and was named Raman scattering. Figure 11.1(b) shows this classical interaction, where molecular vibrations are represented by a simple

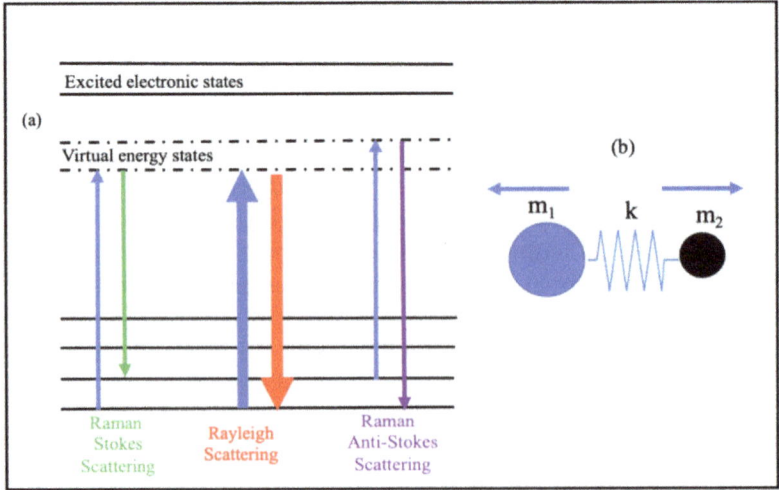

Figure 11.1. (a) Energy-level diagram representation of the energy shifts in Rayleigh and Raman scattering and (b) the harmonic oscillator representing the diatomic molecule in vibrational energy states.

diatomic molecule. Hooke's law can be utilized to express the displacement of the molecule as in

$$\frac{m_1 m_2}{m_1 + m_2}\left(\frac{d^2 x_1}{dt^2} + \frac{d^2 x_2}{dt^2}\right) = -k(x_1 + x_2), \tag{11.1}$$

where the vibration frequency depends on the spring constant (k), and the atomic mass m_1 and m_2. x and k represent the displacement and bond strength, respectively. Using $\mu = \frac{m_1 m_2}{m_1 + m_2}$, equation (11.1) could be simplified as

$$\mu\left(\frac{d^2 q}{dt^2}\right) = -k(q) \quad . \tag{11.2}$$

The solution to equation (11.2) could be given by

$$q = q_0 \cos(2\pi v_m t), \tag{11.3}$$

where $v_m = \frac{1}{2\pi}\sqrt{\frac{K}{\mu}}$.

Raman spectroscopy provides a promising tool for rapid, high-efficiency detection of molecules with the desired selectivity as needed in chemistry, biology, and medicine. This is important for the fast detection of pathogens associated with infectious diseases for the confinement of the diseases to prevent their spread on a large scale. However, Raman spectroscopy has its fundamental limit in sensitivity since the probability for the occurrence of a Raman scattering is very low due to the low cross-section of a Raman scattering event, typically more than five orders of magnitude weaker compared to the Raleigh scattering. The cross-section of Raman scattering is around 10^{-29} cm^2 which is very small compared to the cross-section of fluorescence which is on the order of 10^{-19} cm^2 [25]. This means that Raman spectroscopy would be limited only to the characterization of bulk substances unless an effective approach could be developed to enhance its sensitivity by orders of magnitude.

11.2.2 Surface-enhanced Raman spectroscopy (SERS)

To address the sensitivity issue, surface-enhanced Raman spectroscopy (SERS) has emerged recently as a scheme to obtain an enhanced cross-section of Raman scattering around 10^{-16} cm^2 orders of magnitude higher [25–29]. In particular, the enhanced sensitivity of Raman spectroscopy has been shown to have the ability to detect of a single molecule on SERS substrates [26, 30, 31]. SERS substrates differ from the regular substrates used for Raman spectroscopy by implementing two major enhancement mechanisms: the electromagnetic mechanism (EM) and chemical mechanism (CM).

The EM involves the generation of an enhanced local electromagnetic field in the proximity of probe molecules via the introduction of plasmonic nanostructures on SERS substrates. On these nanostructures, a so-called localized surface plasmonic resonance (LSPR) may be induced. As shown schematically in figure 11.2(a) using

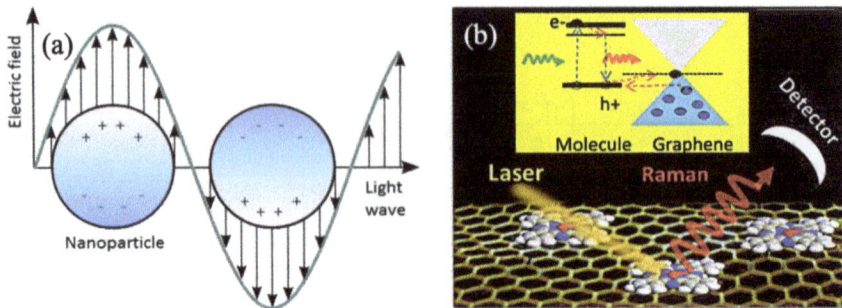

Figure 11.2. (a) Schematic description of LSPR in metallic NPs when they couple with an electric field from an incident light during SERS. Coherent oscillations of free electrons are excited, generating an evanescent electromagnetic field at the metal/dielectric interface [48]. (b) Schematic description of the SERS process with graphene-enhanced CM effect. (Reproduced with permission [45]. Copyright 2012 American Chemistry Society.)

metallic nanoparticles (NPs) as an example [32–34], the LSPR involves coherent oscillations of free charge carriers that are stimulated by the exciting illumination at the surface of the metallic NP. Molecules or chemical species located near the plasmonic nanostructures are exposed to a much-enhanced electromagnetic field (so-called near field or evanescent field) emitted by the oscillating electrons at the nanostructure surface within a distance of a few to hundreds of nanometers. The evanescent electromagnetic field could be much stronger than the incident electro-magnetic excitation. Quantitatively, the EM enhancement factor can be affected by the materials, morphology, dimension, and carrier density of the plasmonic nano-structures. In addition, the surrounding medium's dielectric properties also play a critical role in the optimization of the plasmonic nanostructures [35]. An EM enhancement factor in the range of 10^3–10^8 has been reported. This means SERS detection with high sensitivity approaching the single-molecule level could be achieved [36–38]. Metal NPs, specifically Ag and AuNPs, due to their low ohmic loss and ease in decoration, have been adopted widely on SERS substrates to achieve the SERS EM enhancement [39, 40].

The CM relies on charge transfer across the interface between the probe molecules and the attached SERS substrate. The CM enhancement factor is generally smaller than that of the EM one, in the range of 10^1–10^3 [41–43]. Quantitatively, the CM enhancement factor is dictated by the interface electronic band-edge alignment that drives the charge transfer between probe molecules and the SERS substrate. To achieve a high CM enhancement factor, the molecule/SERS substrate interface must be designed by carefully selecting a SERS substrate that would enable favorable band-edge alignment based on the probe molecule's electronic structure with consideration of the positions of the highest-occupied molecular orbital (HOMO) and the lowest-unoccupied molecular orbital (LUMO) at the molecule–SERS substrate interface. This means it is important that the SERS substrate electronic structure is tunable to allow a significant CM enhancement [44]. It should be noted that the CM effect for most molecules is negligible on a regular glass or silicon substrate. Two-dimensional (2D) atomic materials [45] provide a promising resolution to this need since they could be either transferred or grown on regular SERS substrates. This has motivated intensive research in the past decade or so on SERS substrates based on 2D materials. For example, graphene has been applied for SERS taking advantage of its unique atomically flat surface, chemical inertness, biological compatibility, and superior electronic and photonic properties. Specifically for SERS, the Fermi energy of intrinsic (or undoped) graphene at ~4.5 eV is compatible with the HOMO or/and LUMO of a large number of molecules as illustrated schematically in figure 11.2(b) [41, 43, 46, 47]. In addition, the Fermi energy of graphene could be tuned further via either p-doping or n-doping for better alignment of the electronic band edges at the molecule–graphene interface to enhance the CM for targeted molecules. Therefore, graphene, or 2D atomic materials in general, makes an excellent SERS substrate and the enhancement factor may be quantitatively tuned through tuning of the band-edge alignment at the probe molecule/2D material interface [31, 41].

11.3 Recent progress in the development of high-efficiency SERS based on 2D materials

11.3.1 Fascinating 2D atomic materials

Two-dimensional atomic materials represent a new class of materials consisting of single- or few-layer atomic sheets of crystalline materials that could be metallic, insulating, and semiconducting. Intensive research has been carried out on 2D materials for their synthesis, characterization, and applications since shortly after the discovery of graphene, one of the most popular members of the family of 2D materials, by Geim and Novoseov in 2004 [49]. Since the discovery of graphene, many other 2D materials have been discovered including transition metal dichalcogenides (TMC or TMDC), hexagonal boron nitride (h-BN), black phosphorous (BP), etc [41, 50–53]. In 2D materials, the atoms are held together by strong in-plane bonds. In contrast, their bulk layered counterparts consist of the same sheets stacked together via weak van der Waals (vdW) forces along the out-of-plane direction. This means that the layers can be separated fairly easily even using sticky tape. This so-called mechanical exfoliation method has been applied widely to generate monolayer and few-layer flakes of 2D materials with flake dimensions typically in the range of sub- to tens of micrometers. The much-enhanced quantum confinement of charge carriers towards the 2D limit in the monolayer 2D materials leads to distinctively different electronic structures from that in their bulk counterparts [54]. This leads to unique physical properties including strong interactions with light, high carrier mobility, and tunable electronic and optical properties, making 2D materials promising candidates for applications in electronic, optoelectronic, and other devices [55]. It should be noted that the bandgaps of 2D materials cover a very broad spectrum ranging from metal (zero bandgaps) to semiconductor (moderate bandgap) to insulator (large bandgap) as shown in figures 11.3(a)–(c) [56]. In addition to the single-layered form, different 2D atomic sheets can be stacked together to form vdW heterostructures as shown schematically in figure 11.3(d) in a

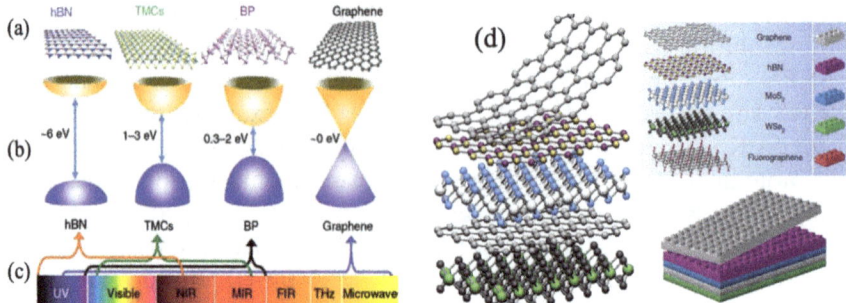

Figure 11.3. (a) Atomic crystal structures of four different 2D materials of h-BN, TMCs, BP, and graphene; (b) the corresponding electronic structures and bandgaps of the four 2D materials; and (c) accessible wavelength spectrum for each of the four 2D materials. (Reproduced with permission from [56]. Copyright 2014 Springer.) (d) Concept of assembling 2D vdW heterostructures, similar to a Lego Block for new materials with electronic structures that may not be achievable in conventional materials. (Reproduced with permission from [57]. Copyright 2013 Springer.)

similar way to assembling Lego pieces [57], permitting a theoretically infinite number of combinations of different 2D atomic materials to create a new class of materials with unprecedented properties not available in conventional materials. For SERS applications, the vdW heterostructures would provide a unique platform allowing the design of the SERS substrates for optimal enhancement based on EM as well as CM effects.

11.3.2 2D Atomic materials for SERS

11.3.2.1 Graphene-based SERS substrates

Graphene-based SERS substrates have been explored intensively in the past decade or so. Graphene can be obtained by mechanical exfoliation from graphite in the form of small flakes or by chemical vapor deposition (CVD) in large wafer-thick sheets [58]. Graphene is a gapless semiconductor or semimetal. Since graphene can absorb ~2.3% of incident light in a broad spectrum ranging from near-ultraviolet to middle-infrared (or THz) and the intrinsic plasmons in graphene are observed in the THz frequency range, the SERS EM enhancement in the visible spectrum on a SERS substrate based on graphene is negligible. This means that graphene-based SERS substrates would primarily provide the CM enhancement taking advantage of the graphene's atomically flat surface, chemical inertness, and biological compatibility. For pristine graphene without doping, the Fermi energy is located at ~4.5 eV or the so-called Dirac point that is suitable for CM enhancement of many molecules [41, 43, 46, 47]. Therefore, graphene-based SERS substrates can provide a large surface for probe molecules to attach and Fermi level tunability for a high CM enhancement factor through the alignment of the probe molecule's HOMO and/or LUMO with graphene's Fermi level. Graphene-based SERS substrates were first explored in 2010 and a SERS CM enhancement factor of 2–17 on graphene substrate has been reported by testing multiple probe molecules including R6G, pentose phosphate pathway (PPP), phthalocyanine (Pc), and crystal violet (CV) [41].

Similarly, CM enhancement factors of 13, 16, and 63 have been reported CuPc probe molecules on h-BN, MoS$_2$, and graphene, respectively [50].

11.3.2.2 SERS substrates based on other 2D atomic materials

TMD-based SERS substrates have received extensive attention recently when the mechanisms responsible for the SERS enhancement were reported. For instance, several members of the TMD family, in particular MoS$_2$ with a bandgap (E_g) in the visible spectrum ($E_g \sim 1.9$ eV for the monolayer and E_g is in the range of 1.2–1.4 eV for multilayer MoS$_2$), were reported to provide SERS enhancement [50, 59–61]. Qiu *et al* reported the synthesis of MoS$_2$ on Si-pyramid arrays by thermally decomposing the precursor (NH$_4$)$_2$MoS$_4$ [59]. On this substrate, SERS sensitivity up to 10^{-6} M was obtained on adenosine and cytidine probe molecules. The authors claimed that the higher sensitivity by a factor of ten obtained on the MoS$_2$/Si-pyramids SERS substrates may be attributed to their more favorable morphology because of enhanced excitation associated with the laser oscillation at the valleys of the pyramids as compared to that of the reference MoS$_2$ on a flat Si substrate [59]. Yin *et al* synthesized MoX$_2$ (X = S, Se) 2D materials using a chemical exfoliation method and obtained two different structures: an octahedral structure of metallic 1T-MoX$_2$ phase and a trigonal-prismatic structure for the semiconducting 2HMoX$_2$ phase. SERS enhancement on these MoX$_2$ substrates was evaluated using copper phthalocyanine, R6G, and crystal violet as probe molecules [61]. Based on the evaluation, they concluded that the metallic 1T-MoX$_2$ has a more favorable band-edge alignment to facilitate charge transfer than the semiconducting 2HMoX$_2$ as illustrated in significantly higher SERS sensitivity up to 10^{-8} M in the former on R6G molecules. It should be noted that a 532 nm excitation laser was employed in this work for the so-called resonant SERS due to the compatibility of the excitation wavelength with that of the absorption one for R6G. Similarly, Anbazhagan *et al* obtained two metallic MoS$_2$ SERS substrates: lithium-exfoliated MoS$_2$ or Li-MoS$_2$ and thioglycolic acid-exfoliated MoS$_2$ or th-MoS$_2$ [62]. Using R6G probe molecules on the former, the average CM enhancement factor is up to 3.34×10^3 on the metallic Li-MoS$_2$ based on the two Raman signature peaks at 611 cm^{-1} and 1647 cm^{-1}, respectively. On the th-MoS$_2$, similar CM enhancement factors of 1.7×10^3 and 5.6×10^2 for the R6G Raman bands of 611 cm^{-1} and 1647 cm^{-1} were also observed. The highest resonant SERS sensitivity of R6G probe molecules with 532 nm excitation are 1×10^{-8} M and 1×10^{-7} M, respectively, on the Li-MoS$_2$ and th-MoS$_2$ substrates. Basically, these results indicate that metallic or semimetallic TMD atomic materials can provide effective CM enhancement, which seems consistent with the semimetallic graphene case.

It should be noted that the 2D atomic materials represent a large family with numerous material choices. However, the bottleneck in the synthesis of the 2D materials on large scale must be removed to realize commercial applications. For example, 2D NbS$_2$ flakes (metallic) were grown on SiO$_2$/Si using CVD under ambient pressure and SERS was studied on NbS$_2$ flake decorated SiO$_2$/Si using methylene blue (MeB) probe molecules [63]. When the NbS$_2$ flakes' thicknesses changed in the range of 2.2, 3.4, 5.5, 8.2, and 11.5 nm, the SERS enhancement factor was thickness-dependent. Interestingly, the thinnest NbS_2 of ~2.2 nm exhibited the highest enhancement factor of 1.07×10^3 and a detection sensitivity up to 10^{-14} M using the soaking method into the MeB solution for 30 min. Again, CM was argued to be responsible for the observed SERS enhancement while the EM enhancement mechanism is unlikely considering the intrinsic plasmon resonance of the NbS_2 occurs in mid-infrared to terahertz spectra. Furthermore, the charge transfer across the MeB/NbS_2 interface was studied using density functional theory which has revealed a strong electronic coupling between MeB and NbS_2 at the interface in support of the CM effect. Furthermore, Nilanjan *et al* studied the SERS on h-BN films of a few layers grown on copper foil using atmospheric-pressure CVD and found the enhancement using a 532 nm excitation laser. The enhancement factors of ~10^3 and ~10^4, respectively, were reported for malachite green and methylene blue (and also R6G) [51]. Therefore, the 2D atomic materials provide outstanding platforms for molecular SERS via the enhanced CM effect. In addition, non-metallic 2D materials could allow efficient EM enhancement with reduced Ohmic loss [64, 65].

11.3.2.3 SERS substrates based on 2D vdW heterostructures

As illustrated schematically in figure 11.3(d), different 2D atomic sheets may be stacked layer by layer to form vdW heterostructures [57]. These 2D vdW heterostructures can be regarded as artificial materials with novel electronic structures that may not be realized in bulk materials. Specifically for SERS, these 2D vdW heterostructures can provide a unique platform to design SERS substrates with optimized SERS CM enhancement [66–68]. Considering that the CM effect relies on the probe molecule/SERS substrate interface electronic structures, the additional tuning of the electronic structure of the substrate in the form of vdW heterostructures is key to achieving a further enhanced CM effect [66–68].

Tan *et al* investigated the SERS CM enhancement factors of CuPc probe molecules on WSe_2 (W)/graphene (G) vdW heterostructures synthesized using CVD. A considerably higher enhancement factor of 28.6 was observed on the W/G vdW heterostructure substrates than that of 4.7 on graphene only, and 9.9 on WSe_2 only (figures 11.4(a) and (b)) [44]. They attributed the enhanced Raman scattering to the enhanced density of states through interface coupling in the W/G vdW heterostructures favorable for CM (figure 11.4(e)). In addition, the enhancement effect of the vdW heterostructures showed dependence on the sequence of the artificial stacks. For example, the SERS enhancement is greater on G/W than on W/G vdW heterostructures (figures 11.4(c) and (d)). The enhancement on four-layer vdW heterostructures of G/W/G/W (graphene on top) is comparable to the one on G/W. The enhancement on different stack sequences such as the W/G/G/W showed lower enhancement compared to that on G/W and G/W/G/W but still higher than the enhancement on the individual W and G cases. Based on these results, the authors have concluded that the different interlayer couplings in the vdW heterostructures may lead to different electron transition probability rates. Seo *et al* reported another example of the vdW heterostructure of graphene/ReO_xS_y as an ultrasensitive SERS substrate because of CT affect and exciton resonances [69].

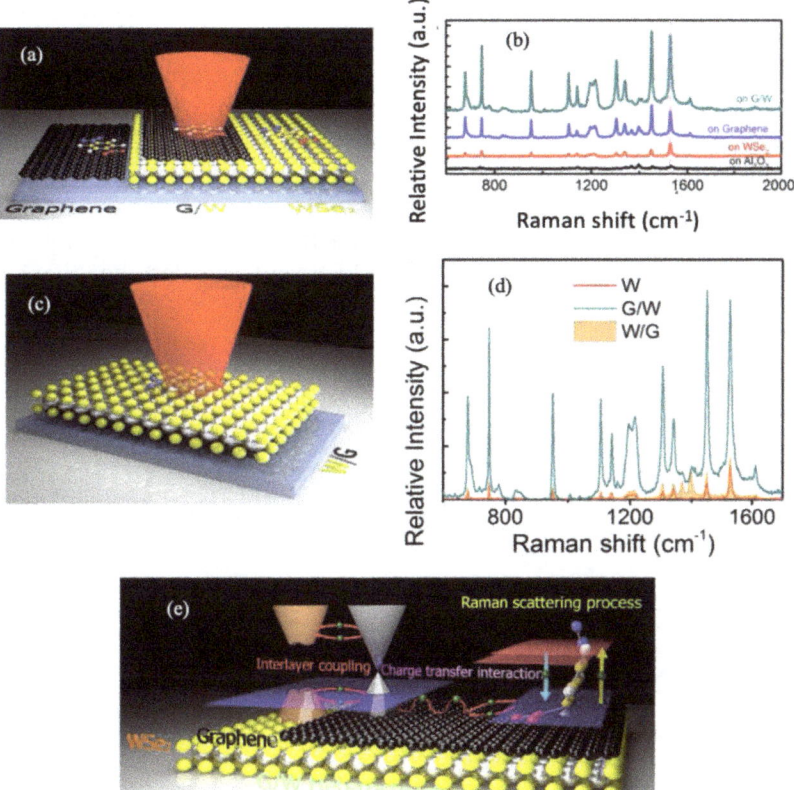

Figure 11.4. (a) Schematic of 2D heterostructures for SERS; G (graphene), G/W (WSe$_2$ monolayer) with the graphene on the top and W only. (b) CuPc molecular SERS studies based on G/W, G, W, and aluminum oxide (Al$_2$O$_3$). (c) SERS schematic of the CuPc molecular coating on W/G, with the WSe$_2$ on the top. (d) SERS studies on W, G/W, and W/G. (e) Schematic representation showing electronic transitions in the G/W heterostructure. (Reproduced with permission from [44]. Copyright 2017 American Chemical Society.)

More recently, Dandu *et al* reported that MoS$_2$/SnSe$_2$ vdW heterostructures and 1L MoS$_2$ demonstrated ten-fold enhanced SERS activity because of the nonradiative energy transfer [70]. Furthermore, SERS enhancement of 2.96×10^7 was reported on a vdW heterostructure SERS substrate consisting of a wrinkled semiconducting 2H-phase MoS$_2$ (W-MoS$_2$) platform decorated with graphene-microflowers (GMFs), using rhodamine B (RhB) as the probe molecules [71]. The high sensitivity of 5×10^{-11} M was obtained on the substrate and the enhancement is ascribed to the synergistic effects of the substantial pre-concentration of probe molecules, enhanced charge transfer, and multiple light scattering.

11.3.3 SERS substrates with both CM and EM enhancement

11.3.3.1 Hybrid metal/2D material heterostructures
It should be noted that plasmonic nanostructures could be implemented on 2D atomic materials and their vdW heterostructures to enable the superposition of EM

and CM enhancements [42, 72–74]. This is one of the unique advantages of the 2D atomic materials and their vdW heterostructures. For example, plasmonic Au nanoparticles (AuNPs) were decorated on large-sheet graphene [37, 73] using an *in situ* metal evaporation method at elevated temperatures in the range of 300 °C– 400 °C [74]. This method allows the fabrication of the SERS substrates on a commercially compatible scale with high SERS sensitivity. On the AuNPs/graphene SERS substrate (figure 11.5(a)), Lu *et al* obtained a SERS enhancement factor of R6G probe molecules four times greater than that on AuNP (without graphene) SERS substrate alone (figure 11.5(b)) [74]. This result revealed that the AuNPs can

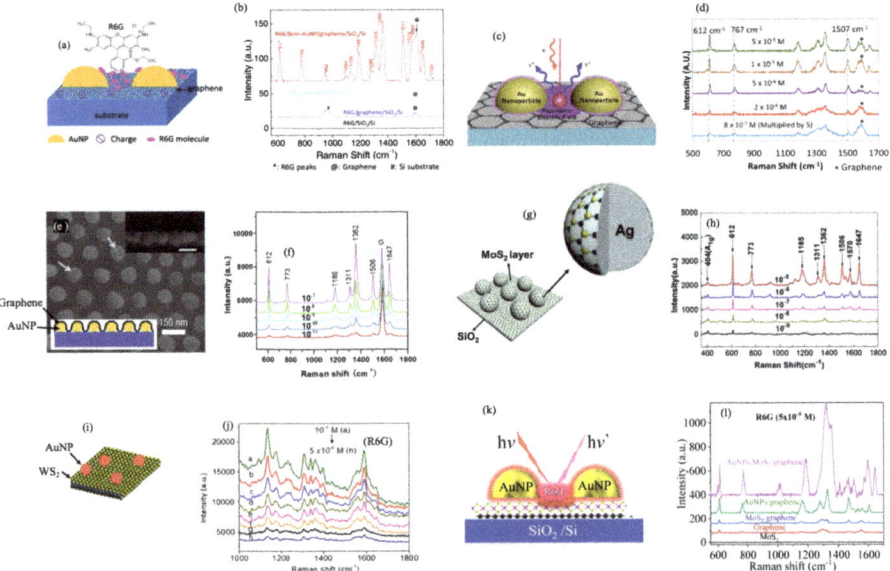

Figure 11.5. (a) Schematic description of AuNP/graphene SERS substrate with R6G probe molecules attached to and (b) comparison of Raman spectra of R6G probe molecules attached on four different substrates: AuNP/graphene/SiO$_2$/Si, AuNP/SiO$_2$/Si, graphene/SiO$_2$/Si, and bare SiO$_2$/Si, respectively. (Reproduced with permission from [73]. Copyright 2015 Elsevier.) (c) Schematic description of the enhanced electric field around plasmonic AuNPs for Raman scattering. (d) Raman spectra of R6G molecules at different concentrations in the range of 5×10^{-5} to 8×10^{-7}. (Reproduced with permission [37]. Copyright 2017 Elsevier.) (e) SEM images of top view and cross-section (top-right inset) of graphene/AuNPs. Schematic description of the graphene/AuNP SERS substrates (lower-left inset), and the Raman spectra of R6G molecules on the graphene/AuNP SERS substrates of concentrations in the range of 10^{-7} to 10^{-11}. (Reproduced with permission [75]. Copyright 2016 Elsevier.) (g) Schematic diagram of MoS$_2$/AgNPs hybrid system. (h) Raman spectra of R6G molecules of different concentrations from 5×10^{-5} to 8×10^{-9}. (Reproduced with permission [76]. Copyright 2016 Elsevier.) (i) Schematic showing the Au-WS$_2$ nanohybrid SERS platform, (j) Raman spectra of R6G molecules using concentrations from 5×10^{-4} to 8×10^{-8} on Au-WS$_2$ nanohybrid SERS. (Reproduced with permission [77]. Copyright 2018 Springer.) (k) Schematic illustration of R6G on AuNP/MoS$_2$(continuous layer)/graphene SERS substrate, (l) R6G Raman on AuNPs/MoS$_2$(continuous layer)/graphene, AuNPs/graphene, MoS$_2$/graphene, graphene and MoS$_2$. (Reproduced with permission [78]. Copyright 2019 American Chemical Society.)

form on graphene with morphology and dimensions similar to those on SiO_2/Si substrates. In addition, it confirms that the CM enhancement from graphene and the EM effect from AuNPs can be combined in the AuNPs/graphene SERS substrate for improved SERS enhancement. Despite a slightly enhanced dissipation by graphene, the LSPR effect can be induced on AuNPs as demonstrated in a finite-difference time-domain (FDTD) simulation, as shown in figure 11.5(c) [37]. Using a 633 nm laser, the detection sensitivity of 8×10^7 M has been obtained on R6G molecules (figure 11.5(d)). It should be noted that the SERS sensitivity could be affected by the excitation laser wavelength. Typically, the sensitivity of the resonance SERS (for example for R6G, the resonance wavelength is 532 nm) is several orders of magnitude higher than the cases without resonance at otherwise the same measurement conditions.

It should be noted that the stacking sequence of graphene and AuNPs could affect the SERS properties. For example, Xu *et al* covered AuNPs with graphene (figure 11.5(e)) and argued that the molecular attachment area on graphene would be increased in these graphene/AuNPs SERS substrates [75]. However, comparable SERS sensitivity of around 1.0×10^{-11} M of R6G was obtained on AuNPs/graphene/and graphene/AuNPs using the 532 nm resonant excitation as shown in figure 11.5(f), suggesting the sequence of the stacking may only generate a minor difference in SERS sensitivity. Towards a similar idea, Chen *et al* reported SERS sensitivity up to 1×10^{-9} M of R6G on MoS_2/AgNPs SERS substrate with 532 nm excitation (figure 11.5(h)) by synthesizing multilayer MoS_2 on AgNPs (figure 11.5(g)) using thermal decomposition [76]. On the other hand, Shorie *et al* reported AuNP/WS_2 flakes in SERS substrates where WS_2 flakes were obtained using liquid phase exfoliation while AuNPs were fabricated on the flasks using *in situ* deposition (figure 11.5(i)) [77]. Using R6G probe molecules, they achieved sensitivity around 1×10^{-8} M using 532 nm excitation on the AuNP/WS_2 flakes SERS substrates (figure 11.5(j)).

As we have mentioned earlier, vdW heterostructures of 2F atomic materials would allow tunable electronic structures for better CM enhancement, which has prompted many recent research works, in particular through integration with plasmonic nanostructures [78]. Figure 11.5(k) illustrates a SERS substrate based on AuNPs/MoS_2(continues layer)/graphene growth layer by layer using CVD for the bottom two layers and *in situ* evaporation for decoration of AuNPs atop [78]. In a comparative SERS study, the SERS enhancement on this AuNPs/MoS_2(continues layer)/graphene substrate and on the reference substrates of AuNPs/graphene, MoS_2/graphene, graphene only, and MoS_2 only is compared in figure 11.5(l) using R6G probe molecules (at 5×10^{-5} M). SERS enhancement is highest on the AuNPs/MoS_2(continues layer)/graphene and is ascribed to the integration of the EM enhancement from the plasmonic AuNPs and the CM enhancement from the MoS_2/graphene vdW heterostructure. In particular, the R6G probe molecules could be detected with high sensitivity up to 5×10^{-8} and 5×10^{-10} M, respectively, on the AuNPs/MoS_2/graphene SERS substrate using excitation of 633 (non-resonant) and 532 nm (resonant).

11.3.3.2 LSPR TMDC nanostructure/graphene heterostructures

It should be noted that most reported LSPR nanostructures are based on metallic materials including Au and Ag. Since Ag nanostructures tend to degrade in ambient over a time frame of 1–2 weeks, Au is the most popular material used in SERS substrates. Despite the high cost, Au LSPR nanostructures could be lossy which means that the achieved SERS EM enhancement is a compromise of the LSPR and ohmic loss on Au nanostructures. Exploration of non-metallic nanostructures for SERS is hence important. In a recent work, Ghopry *et al* reported a TMDC nanodisc (N-disc)/graphene heterostructures in which a strong EM enhancement is attributed to the LSPR effect induced in TMDC nanodisks [64]. It should be noted that the TMDC nanostructures/graphene can be fabricated using a CVD process by layer-by-layer coating of TMDC (such as MoS_2, WS_2, or a mixture of MoS_2 and WS_2) nanostructures on single-layer transferred (or directly grown [79]) on SiO_2/Si wafers as shown schematically in (figures 11.6(a)–(e)) [64, 80, 81]. The schematic presentation of the mix TMDC nanostructure/graphene SERS is shown in (figure 11.6(f)). Furthermore, different morphologies, such as nanodiscs [64, 81] and nanodonuts [80], can be obtained via control of the growth conditions.

Figure 11.7(a) shows the Raman map (using A_{1g} mode) of MoS_2 nanodiscs. The AFM images of the same sample confirm the morphology and concentration (figure 11.7(b)) as well as the lateral and vertical dimensions (figure 11.7(c)) of the MoS_2 nanodiscs [64]. This work shows that 2D TMDC nanostructure/graphene

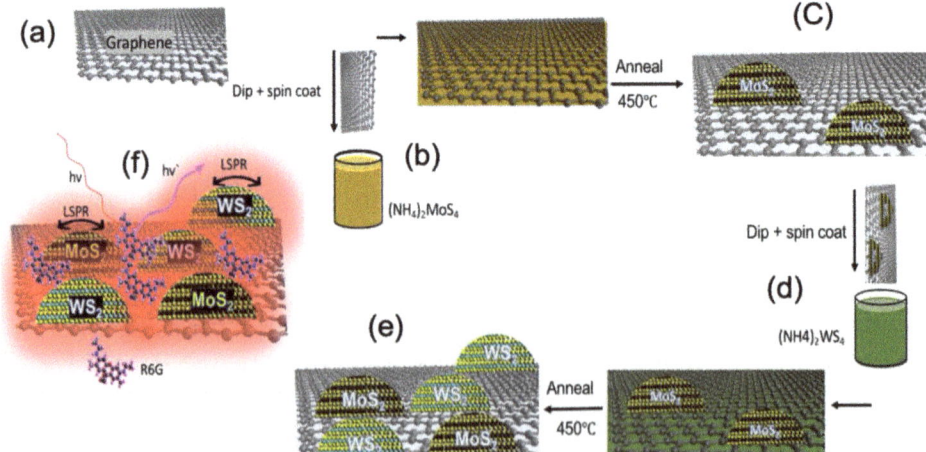

Figure 11.6. Schematic diagram of the fabrication process for SERS substrates consisting of WS_2+MoS_2 nanodiscs/graphene: (a) CVD growth followed with transfer of graphene on SiO_2/Si substrates; (b) and (c) fabrication of the MoS_2 nanodiscs on graphene using solution coating followed by a vapor transport process. (b) Graphene/SiO_2/Si samples were dip-coated with $(NH_4)_2MoS_4$ precursor solution followed by spin coating. (c) Annealing of the $(NH_4)_2MoS_4$/graphene/SiO_2/Si samples in a tube furnace filled with sulfur vapor; (d) and (e): as in (b) and (c) for the synthesis of the WS_2 nanodiscs on the MoS_2 nanodisc/graphene; and (f) the completed WS_2 nanodiscs+MoS_2 nanodiscs/graphene vdW heterostructure SERS substrate. (Reproduced with permission [81]. Copyright 2021 American Chemical Society.)

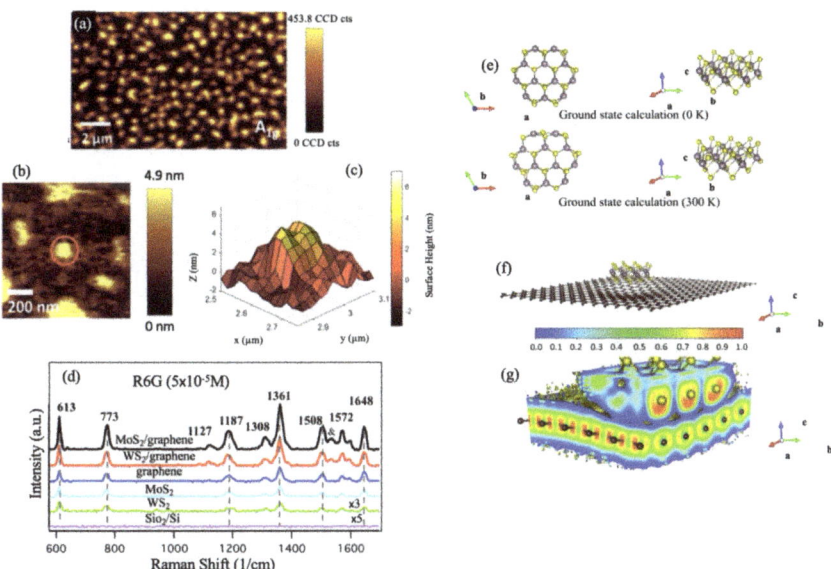

Figure 11.7. (a) Raman map (using A_{1g} mode for MoS_2) of MoS_2 nanodiscs. (b) A representative AFM image of MoS_2 nanodiscs and (c) a 3D AFM profile showing lateral and vertical dimensions of a MoS_2 nanodisc. (d) Raman spectra of R6G molecules (5×10^{-5} M) deposited on different SERS substrates including MoS_2 nanodisc/graphene and WS_2 nanodisc/graphene heterostructures, MoS_2 nanodisc only, WS_2 nanodisc only, graphene only, and bare SiO_2/Si. All spectra were taken using 532 nm excitation. (e) Monolayer MoS_2 nanodiscs after the ground state calculation at 0 K and after AIMD simulation at 300 K. Both calculations show stable configurations. (f) Vertical MoS_2/graphene bilayer heterostructure. (g) Electron localization function (ELF) of the MoS_2/graphene bilayer heterostructure shows the localized electron concentration below the sulfur atom indicating the charge transfer occurrence. (Reproduced with permission from [64]. Copyright 2019 Wiley.)

vdW heterostructures may provide a unique platform to design new SERS substrates with both EM and CM enhancements as shown in the improved SERS sensitivity of R6G probe molecules (figure 11.7(d)) [44, 66–68]. Density functional theory (DFT) (figures 11.7(e)–(g)) simulations have revealed that a weak vdW force exists between graphene and TMDC. Specifically, for MoS_2, the binding energy is estimated to be −23 meV per C atom irrespective of the adsorption arrangement [82]. Under this weak vdW force, an enhanced electric dipole moment and dipole–dipole interaction are anticipated at the TMDC/graphene interface, leading to improved charge transfer across the MoS_2/graphene interface and therefore enhanced SERS CM effect [30, 83]. While the mechanism requires further investigation, nanostructured TMDCs may enable LSPR upon photo-induced carrier doping with enhanced EM contribution to SERS in a similar way to the LSPR quantum dots and nanocrystals [84, 85].

11.3.4 Performance of the 2D materials SERS substrates

Table 11.1 highlights a set of different molecules adopted for characterization of the SERS sensitivity on various SERS substrates developed based on either 2D atomic

Table 11.1. Summary of SERS results of a list of different molecules obtained on different SERS substrates based on 2D atomic materials and vdW heterostructures.

Substrates materials	Enhancement factor	Molecule	Reference
Graphene	2–17	Pc	[41]
Graphene	63	CuPc	[50]
h-BN	13	CuPc	[50]
h-BN	10^3	Malachite green	[51]
h-BN	10^4	Methylene blue and R6G	[51]
MoS_2	16	CuPc	[50]
MoS_2	63	R6G	[52]
ReS_2	2.9	CuPc	[53]
N-doped graphene	16	RhB	[86]
Graphene/WSe_2	3.8–78.2	CuPc	[44]
GMFs/W-MoS_2	2.96×10^7	Rhodamine B (RhB)	[71]
Graphene/Ag array	$5.89 \times 1\,0^5$	Methylated DNA	[87]
Graphene/Ag	—	p-ATP	[88]

GMFs/MoS_2: wrinkled semiconducting 2H-phase MoS_2 platform decorated with graphene-microflowers.

materials or their vdW heterostructures. On some of these substrates, metallic plasmonic nanostructures, such as silver, were included. From table 11.1, it is clearly shown that the SERS substrates based on 2D materials and vdW heterostructures are suitable for a large variety of molecules with SERS enhancement factors in a broad range of a factor of few to 10^7 demonstrated.

Table 11.2 compares the SERS sensitivity of R6G probe molecules reported on series SERS substrates based on 2D atomic materials and vdW heterostructures and table 11.2 summarize a set of SERS substrates based on 2D atomic materials or their vdW heterostructures with or without plasmonic nanostructures of metallic and non-metallic materials. Considering R6G is a dye molecule with resonance absorption at around 532 nm, the Raman excitation wavelength is a critical parameter in SERS and is included in table 11.2. Typically, resonant SERS with excitation wavelength at 532 nm would lead to a much-enhanced Raman signal and hence SERS sensitivity. In addition, the inclusion of plasmonic nanostructures allows SERS enhancement via both EM and CM mechanisms as indicated in table 11.2. It should be particularly noted that non-metallic plasmonic nanostructures can provide comparable or higher SERS EM enhancement and therefore provide a low-cost approach for implementation of plasmonic EM effect for high-sensitivity SERS.

11.4 Summary and future perspectives

In summary, the progress made on nano- and atomic materials in the last decade or so has provided a promising platform in the design and fabrication of SERS substrates for the detection of molecules including pathogens. Among others, the 2D

Table 11.2. Summary of R6G SERS results obtained on selected substrates based on 2D atomic materials and vdW heterostructures.

Substrates materials	Enhancement factor	Sensitivity	Excitation wavelength	Reference
Li-MoS$_2$	1.7×10^3–3.34×10^3 (CM)	1×10^{-8} M	532 nm	[62]
T-MoS$_2$	5.6×10^2–1.7×10^3 (CM)	1×10^{-7} M	532 nm	[62]
MoS$_2$	63 (CM)	—	532 nm	[52]
WS$_2$	—	1×10^{-7} M	532 nm	[89]
1T/2H-MoS$_2$	—	10^{-8} M	532 nm	[90]
1T/2H-WS$_2$	—	10^{-8} M	532 nm	[90]
AuNPs/graphene	—	8×10^{-7} M	633 nm	[37]
G/AuNPs	4.8×10^7 (EM+CM)	10^{-11} M	532 nm	[75]
MoS$_2$/AgNPs	3.75×10^4 (EM+CM)	10^{-9} M	532 nm	[76]
AuNP/WS$_2$	6.78×10^6 (EM+CM)	1×10^{-8} M	532 nm	[77]
AuNP/graphene	4, compared to SERS on AuNP (EM+CM)	—	633 nm	[73]
AuNP/graphene	—	8×10^{-7} M	633 nm	[37]
AuNPs/ MoS$_2$(continues layer)/graphene	—	5×10^{-10} M 5×10^{-8} M	532 nm 633 nm	[78]
WS$_2$ nanodomes/ graphene	~8, compared to SERS on continuous- and single-layer WS$_2$ or single-layer graphene (EM+CM)	5×10^{-11} M	532 nm	[64]
MoS$_2$ nanodomes/ graphene	~9, compared to SERS on continuous-layer MoS$_2$ or single-layer graphene (EM+CM)	5×10^{-12} M	532 nm	[64]
MoS$_{2+}$WS$_2$ nanodiscs/graphene	14–17, compared to SERS on single-layer graphene (EM+CM)	7×10^{-13} M	532 nm	[81]
AuNP/WS$_2$ nanodiscs/graphene	12.2, compared to one on graphene	10^{-12} M	532 nm	[91]
MoS$_2$ nanodonuts/ graphene	~20, compared to one on graphene	2×10^{-12}	532 nm	[80]

atomic materials are particularly suitable for SERS applications to allow designs towards enhanced SERS sensitivity based on both EM and CM enhancements. High SERS sensitivity approaching the single molecule detection limit has been achieved on SERS substrates based on 2D atomic materials and/or their hybrids with noble metal nanostructures. These SERS substrates have additional advantages including light weight, low cost, portability, and disposability, and hence are particularly promising for on-site, noninvasive analysis of samples using portable Raman systems for detecting trace-level targets with outstanding sensitivity. It should be noted that the research into the exploration of high-sensitivity SERS substrates is only at the beginning, which can be accelerated by addressing some outstanding issues. For example, the microscopy mechanisms underlying the high-sensitivity SERS substrates based on nano- and atomic materials remains an interesting topic and systematic research is required to achieve a thorough understanding. This understanding is critical to the future design of better SERS substrates to meet the need for high sensitivity and selectivity for high-efficiency and rapid detection of pathogens relevant to specific infectious diseases.

Acknowledgments

The authors acknowledge support in part by US National Science Foundation contracts NSF-DMR-1909292 and NSF-ECCS-1809293. SG acknowledges support from Jazan University.

References

[1] Fleischmann M, Hendra P J and McQuillan A J 1974 Raman spectra of pyridine adsorbed at a silver electrode *Chem. Phys. Lett.* **26** 163–6

[2] Albrecht M G and Creighton J A 1977 Anomalously intense Raman spectra of pyridine at a silver electrode *J. Am. Chem. Soc.* **99** 5215–7

[3] Jeanmaire D L and Van Duyne R P 1977 Surface Raman spectroelectrochemistry: part I. Heterocyclic, aromatic, and aliphatic amines adsorbed on the anodized silver electrode *J. Electroanal. Chem. Interfacial Electrochem.* **84** 1–20

[4] Braun G, Lee S J, Dante M, Nguyen T Q, Moskovits M and Reich N 2007 Surface-enhanced Raman spectroscopy for DNA detection by nanoparticle assembly onto smooth metal films *J. Am. Chem. Soc.* **129** 6378–9

[5] Braun G *et al* 2007 Chemically patterned microspheres for controlled nanoparticle assembly in the construction of SERS hot spots *J. Am. Chem. Soc.* **129** 7760–1

[6] Campion A and Kambhampati P 1998 Surface-enhanced Raman scattering *Chem. Soc. Rev.* **27** 241–50

[7] Ren B, Liu G K, Lian X B, Yang Z L and Tian Z Q 2007 Raman spectroscopy on transition metals *Anal. Bioanal. Chem.* **388** 29–45

[8] Stuart D A *et al* 2005 Glucose sensing using near-infrared surface-enhanced Raman spectroscopy: gold surfaces, 10-day stability, and improved accuracy *Anal. Chem.* **77** 4013–9

[9] Vo-Dinh T, Yan F and Wabuyele M B 2006 Surface-enhanced Raman scattering for biomedical diagnostics and molecular imaging *Surface-Enhanced Raman Scattering: Physics and Applications* ed K Kneipp, M Moskovits and H Kneipp (Berlin: Springer) pp 409–26

[10] Yang D *et al* 2018 Glucose sensing using surface-enhanced Raman-mode constraining *Anal. Chem.* **90** 14269–78

[11] Moskovits M 1985 Surface-enhanced spectroscopy *Rev. Mod. Phys.* **57** 783–826

[12] Pieczonka N P W and Aroca R F 2005 Inherent complexities of trace detection by surface-enhanced Raman scattering *ChemPhysChem.* **6** 2473–84

[13] Kneipp K *et al* 1997 Single molecule detection using surface-enhanced Raman scattering (SERS) *Phys. Rev. Lett.* **78** 1667–70

[14] Nie S and Emory S R 1997 Probing single molecules and single nanoparticles by surface-enhanced Raman scattering *Science* **275** 1102–6

[15] Dick L A, McFarland A D, Haynes C L and Van Duyne R P 2002 Metal film over nanosphere (MFON) electrodes for surface-enhanced Raman spectroscopy (SERS): improvements in surface nanostructure stability and suppression of irreversible loss *J. Phys. Chem.* B **106** 853–60

[16] Jensen T R, Malinsky M D, Haynes C L and Van Duyne R P 2000 Nanosphere lithography: tunable localized surface plasmon resonance spectra of silver nanoparticles *J. Phys. Chem.* B **104** 10549–56

[17] Parihar A, Ranjan P, Sanghi S K, Srivastava A K and Khan R 2020 Point-of-care biosensor-based diagnosis of COVID-19 holds promise to combat current and future pandemics *ACS Appl. Bio Mater.* **3** 7326–43

[18] Sadique M A, Ranjan P, Yadav S and Khan R 2022 Advanced high-throughput biosensor-based diagnostic approaches for detection of severe acute respiratory syndrome-coronavirus-2 *Computational Approaches for Novel Therapeutic and Diagnostic Designing to Mitigate SARS-CoV-2 Infection* ed A Parihar, R Khan, A Kumar, A K Kaushik and H Gohel (New York: Academic) ch 8 pp 147–69

[19] Yadav S *et al* 2021 SERS based lateral flow immunoassay for point-of-care detection of SARS-CoV-2 in clinical samples *ACS Appl. Bio Mater.* **4** 2974–95

[20] Aroca R F, Alvarez-Puebla R A, Pieczonka N, Sanchez-Cortez S and Garcia-Ramos J V 2005 Surface-enhanced Raman scattering on colloidal nanostructures *Adv. Colloid Interface Sci.* **116** 45–61

[21] Baker G A and Moore D S 2005 Progress in plasmonic engineering of surface-enhanced Raman-scattering substrates toward ultra-trace analysis *Anal. Bioanal. Chem.* **382** 1751–70

[22] Gunnarsson L, Bjerneld E J, Xu H, Petronis S, Kasemo B and Käll M 2001 Interparticle coupling effects in nanofabricated substrates for surface-enhanced Raman scattering *Appl. Phys. Lett.* **78** 802–4

[23] He L *et al* 2000 Colloidal Au-enhanced surface plasmon resonance for ultrasensitive detection of DNA hybridization *J. Am. Chem. Soc.* **122** 9071–7

[24] Kneipp K, Kneipp H and Kneipp J 2006 Surface-enhanced Raman scattering in local optical fields of silver and gold nanoaggregates-from single-molecule Raman spectroscopy to ultrasensitive probing in live cells *Acc. Chem. Res.* **39** 443–50

[25] Aroca R 2006 *Surface Enhanced Vibrational Spectroscopy* (Hoboken, NJ: Wiley), p xxv 233

[26] Fang Y, Seong N H and Dlott D D 2008 Measurement of the distribution of site enhancements in surface-enhanced Raman scattering *Science* **321** 388–92

[27] Lin H X *et al* 2013 Uniform gold spherical particles for single-particle surface-enhanced Raman spectroscopy *Phys. Chem. Chem. Phys.* **15** 4130–5

[28] Potara M, Baia M, Farcau C and Astilean S 2012 Chitosan-coated anisotropic silver nanoparticles as a SERS substrate for single-molecule detection *Nanotechnology* **23** 055501–10

[29] Sivashanmugan K, Liao J D, Liu B H and Yao C K 2013 Focused-ion-beam-fabricated Au nanorods coupled with Ag nanoparticles used as surface-enhanced Raman scattering-active substrate for analyzing trace melamine constituents in solution *Anal. Chim. Acta.* **800** 56–64

[30] Li X *et al* 2015 A self-powered graphene–MoS$_2$ hybrid phototransistor with fast response rate and high on–off ratio *Carbon* **92** 126–32

[31] Huh S, Park J, Kim Y S, Kim K S, Hong B H and Nam J M 2011 UV/ozone-oxidized large-scale graphene platform with large chemical enhancement in surface-enhanced Raman scattering *ACS Nano* **5** 9799–806

[32] Guerrini L and Graham D 2012 Molecularly-mediated assemblies of plasmonic nano-particles for surface-enhanced Raman spectroscopy applications *Chem. Soc. Rev.* **41** 7085–107

[33] Mu C, Zhang J P and Xu D 2010 Au nanoparticle arrays with tunable particle gaps by template-assisted electroless deposition for high performance surface-enhanced Raman scattering *Nanotechnology* **21** 015604

[34] Willets K A and Duyne R P V 2007 Localized surface plasmon resonance spectroscopy and sensing *Annu. Rev. Phys. Chem.* **58** 267–97

[35] Atwater H A and Polman A 2010 Plasmonics for improved photovoltaic devices *Nat. Mater.* **9** 205–13

[36] Chen L, Wu M, Xiao C, Yu Y, Liu X and Qiu G 2015 Urchin-like LaVO$_4$/Au composite microspheres for surface-enhanced Raman scattering detection *J. Colloid Interface Sci.* **443** 80–7

[37] Goul R *et al* 2017 Quantitative analysis of surface enhanced Raman spectroscopy of Rhodamine 6G using a composite graphene and plasmonic Au nanoparticle substrate *Carbon* **111** 386–92

[38] Zhang C *et al* 2015 SERS detection of R6G based on a novel graphene oxide/silver nanoparticles/silicon pyramid arrays structure *Opt. Express* **23** 24811–21

[39] Seney C S, Gutzman B M and Goddard R H 2009 Correlation of size and surface-enhanced Raman scattering activity of optical and spectroscopic properties for silver nanoparticles *J. Phys. Chem.* C **113** 74–80

[40] Stamplecoskie K G, Scaiano J C, Tiwari V S and Anis H 2011 Optimal size of silver nanoparticles for surface-enhanced Raman spectroscopy *J. Phys. Chem.* C **115** 1403–9

[41] Ling X *et al* 2010 Can graphene be used as a substrate for Raman enhancement? *Nano Lett.* **10** 553–61

[42] Xu W *et al* 2012 Surface enhanced Raman spectroscopy on a flat graphene surface *Proc. Natl Acad. Sci. USA* **109** 9281–6

[43] Xu W, Mao N and Zhang J 2013 Graphene: a platform for surface-enhanced Raman spectroscopy *Small* **9** 1206–24

[44] Tan Y, Ma L, Gao Z, Chen M and Chen F 2017 Two-dimensional heterostructure as a platform for surface-enhanced Raman scattering *Nano Lett.* **17** 2621–6

[45] Ling X, Moura L G, Pimenta M A and Zhang J 2012 Charge-transfer mechanism in graphene-enhanced Raman scattering *J. Phys. Chem.* C **116** 25112–8

[46] Xie L, Ling X, Fang Y, Zhang J and Liu Z 2009 Graphene as a substrate to suppress fluorescence in resonance Raman spectroscopy *J. Am. Chem. Soc.* **131** 9890–1

[47] Xu W, Xiao J, Chen Y, Chen Y, Ling X and Zhang J 2013 Graphene-veiled gold substrate for surface-enhanced Raman spectroscopy *Adv. Mater.* **25** 928–33

[48] Hammond J L, Bhalla N, Rafiee S D and Estrela P 2014 Localized surface plasmon resonance as a biosensing platform for developing countries *Biosensors* **4** 172–88

[49] Novoselov K S *et al* 2004 Electric field effect in atomically thin carbon films *Science* **306** 666–9

[50] Ling X *et al* 2014 Raman enhancement effect on two-dimensional layered materials: graphene, h-BN and MoS$_2$ *Nano Lett.* **14** 3033–40

[51] Basu N *et al* 2021 Large area few-layer hexagonal boron nitride as a Raman enhancement material *Nanomaterials* **11** 622

[52] Zuo P *et al* 2019 Enhancing charge transfer with foreign molecules through femtosecond laser induced MoS$_2$ defect sites for photoluminescence control and SERS enhancement *Nanoscale* **11** 485–94

[53] Miao P *et al* 2018 Unraveling the Raman enhancement mechanism on 1T′-phase ReS$_2$ nanosheets *Small* **14** e1704079

[54] Coleman J N *et al* 2011 Two-dimensional nanosheets produced by liquid exfoliation of layered *Mater. Sci.* **331** 568–71

[55] Mak K F, Lee C, Hone J, Shan J and Heinz T F 2010 Atomically thin MoS$_2$: a new direct-gap semiconductor *Phys. Rev. Lett.* **105** 136805

[56] Xia F, Wang H, Xiao D, Dubey M and Ramasubramaniam A 2014 Two-dimensional material nanophotonics *Nat. Photon.* **8** 899–907

[57] Geim A K and Grigorieva I V 2013 Van der Waals heterostructures *Nature* **499** 419–25

[58] Wu J 2019 Graphene *Transparent Conductive Materials: Materials, Synthesis, Characterization, Applications* vols 1 and 2 ed D Levy and E Castellón (New York: Wiley) 165–92

[59] Qiu H *et al* 2015 Large-area MoS$_2$ thin layers directly synthesized on pyramid-Si substrate for surface-enhanced Raman scattering *RSC Adv.* **5** 83899–905

[60] Xu Y Y *et al* 2015 Layer-controlled large area MoS$_2$ layers grown on mica substrate for surface-enhanced Raman scattering *Appl. Surf. Sci.* **357** 1708–13

[61] Yin Y *et al* 2017 Significantly increased Raman enhancement on MoX$_2$ (X=S, Se) monolayers upon phase transition *Adv. Funct. Mater.* **27** 1606694–7

[62] Anbazhagan R, Vadivelmurugan A, Tsai H-C and Jeng R-J 2018 Surface-enhanced Raman scattering of alkyne-conjugated MoS$_2$: a comparative study between metallic and semiconductor phases *J. Mater. Chem.* C **6** 1071–82

[63] Song X *et al* 2019 Plasmon-free surface-enhanced Raman spectroscopy using metallic 2D materials *ACS Nano* **13** 8312–9

[64] Ghopry S A, Alamri M A, Goul R, Sakidja R and Wu J Z 2019 Extraordinary sensitivity of surface-enhanced Raman spectroscopy of molecules on MoS$_2$ (WS$_2$) nanodomes/graphene van der Waals heterostructure substrates *Adv. Opt. Mater.* **7** 1801249

[65] Nong J, Feng F, Min C, Yuan X and Somekh M 2021 Controllable hybridization between localized and delocalized anisotropic borophene plasmons in the near-infrared region *Opt. Lett.* **46** 725–8

[66] Gamucci A *et al* 2014 Anomalous low-temperature Coulomb drag in graphene–GaAs heterostructures *Nat. Commun.* **5** 5824–7

[67] Georgiou T *et al* 2013 Vertical field-effect transistor based on graphene–WS$_2$ heterostructures for flexible and transparent electronics *Nat. Nanotechnol.* **8** 100–3

[68] Levendorf M P *et al* 2012 Graphene and boron ntride lateral heterostructures for atomically thin circuitry *Nature* **488** 627–32

[69] Seo J, Lee J, Kim Y, Koo D, Lee G and Park H 2020 Ultrasensitive plasmon-free surface-enhanced Raman spectroscopy with femtomolar detection limit from 2D van der Waals heterostructure *Nano Lett.* **20** 1620–30

[70] Dandu M, Watanabe K, Taniguchi T, Sood A K and Majumdar K 2020 Spectrally tunable, large Raman enhancement from nonradiative energy transfer in the van der Waals heterostructure *ACS Photon.* **7** 519–27

[71] Qiu H *et al* 2020 Wrinkled 2H-phase MoS_2 sheet decorated with graphene-microflowers for ultrasensitive molecular sensing by plasmon-free SERS enhancement *Sens. Actuators* B **320** 128445

[72] Liu Y and Luo F 2019 Large-scale highly ordered periodic Au nano-discs/graphene and graphene/Au nanoholes plasmonic substrates for surface-enhanced Raman scattering *Nano Res.* **12** 2788–95

[73] Lu R *et al* 2015 High sensitivity surface enhanced Raman spectroscopy of R6G on *in situ* fabricated au nanoparticle/graphene plasmonic substrates *Carbon* **86** 78–85

[74] Xu G *et al* 2012 Plasmonic graphene transparent conductors *Adv. Mater.* **24** OP71–6

[75] Xu S, Jiang S, Wang J, Wei J, Yue W and Ma Y 2016 Graphene isolated Au nanoparticle arrays with high reproducibility for high-performance surface-enhanced Raman scattering *Sens. Actuators* B **222** 1175–83

[76] Chen P X *et al* 2016 A novel surface-enhanced Raman spectroscopy substrate based on a large area of MoS_2 and Ag nanoparticles hybrid system *Appl. Surf. Sci.* **375** 207–14

[77] Shorie M, Kumar V, Kaur H, Singh K, Tomer V K and Sabherwal P 2018 Plasmonic DNA hotspots made from tungsten disulfide nanosheets and gold nanoparticles for ultrasensitive aptamer-based SERS detection of myoglobin *Microchim. Acta.* **185** 158

[78] Alamri M, Sakidja R, Goul R, Ghopry S and Wu J Z 2019 Plasmonic Au nanoparticles on 2D MoS_2/graphene van der Waals heterostructures for high-sensitivity surface-enhanced Raman spectroscopy *ACS Appl. Nano Mater.* **2** 1412–20

[79] Liu Q, Gong Y, Wilt J S, Sakidja R and Wu J 2015 Synchronous growth of AB-stacked bilayer graphene on Cu by simply controlling hydrogen pressure in CVD process *Carbon* **93** 199–206

[80] Ghopry S A, Sadeghi S M, Berrie C L and Wu J Z 2021 MoS_2 nanodonuts for high-sensitivity surface-enhanced Raman spectroscopy *Biosensors* **11** 477

[81] Ghopry S A, Sadeghi S M, Farhat Y, Berrie C L, Alamri M and Wu J Z 2021 Intermixed WS_2+MoS_2 nanodisks/graphene van der Waals heterostructures for surface-enhanced Raman spectroscopy sensing *ACS Appl. Nano Mater.* **4** 2941–51

[82] Ma Y, Dai Y, Guo M, Niu C and Huang B 2011 Graphene adhesion on MoS_2 monolayer: an *ab initio* study *Nanoscale* **3** 3883–7

[83] Roy K *et al* 2013 Graphene–MoS_2 hybrid structures for multifunctional photoresponsive memory devices *Nat. Nanotechnol.* **8** 826–30

[84] Gong M *et al* 2018 Broadband photodetectors enabled by localized surface plasmonic resonance in doped iron pyrite nanocrystals *Adv. Opt. Mater.* **6** 1701241

[85] Luther J M, Jain P K, Ewers T and Alivisatos A P 2011 Localized surface plasmon resonances arising from free carriers in doped quantum dots *Nat. Mater.* **10** 361–6

[86] Feng S *et al* 2016 Ultrasensitive molecular sensor using N-doped graphene through enhanced Raman scattering *Sci. Adv.* **2** e1600322

[87] Ouyang L, Hu Y, Zhu L, Cheng G J and Irudayaraj J 2017 A reusable laser wrapped graphene-Ag array based SERS sensor for trace detection of genomic DNA methylation *Biosens. Bioelectron.* **92** 755–62

[88] Kumar S V, Huang N M, Lim H N, Zainy M, Harrison I and Chia C H 2013 Preparation of highly water dispersible functional graphene/silver nanocomposite for the detection of melamine *Sens. Actuators* B **181** 885–93

[89] Meng L, Hu S, Xu C, Wang X, Li H and Yan X 2018 Surface enhanced Raman effect on CVD growth of WS_2 film *Chem. Phys. Lett.* **707** 71–4

[90] Chen M *et al* 2020 Vertically-aligned 1T/2H-MS_2 (M=Mo, W) nanosheets for surface-enhanced Raman scattering with long-term stability and large-scale uniformity *Appl. Surf. Sci.* **527** 146769

[91] Ghopry S A *et al* 2020 Au nanoparticle/WS_2 nanodome/graphene van der Waals heterostructure substrates for surface-enhanced Raman spectroscopy *ACS Appl. Nano Mater.* **3** 2354–63

Chapter 12

Future potential of SERS-based advanced diagnosis in real-life conditions

Arpana Parihar, Vedika Khare, Ayushi Singhal, Kritika Gaur and Raju Khan

Surface-enhanced Raman scattering (SERS) has lately gained popularity for detecting residues of biomolecules due to its remarkable biochemical specificity and ultra-sensitivity, with statistical combinatorial capabilities. Several biomarkers engage together with optically active nanomaterials in highly complex contexts to create robust and unique SERS spectrum signals. SERS provides qualitative and quantitative data on the inherent physicochemical characteristics and features that could be predictive of healthy or sick conditions. Furthermore, SERS enables early prescription of focused, individualized therapy by differentiating several closely related causal agents of illnesses with comparable symptoms. This chapter discusses recent developments in the use of SERS in the diagnosis of microbiological infections and respiratory disorders. Recent technical improvements are likely to assist in realizing the full benefits of SERS in terms of acquiring deeper insights into the molecular pathogenic pathways for diverse illnesses.

12.1 Introduction

An illness diagnosis is a critical step in a disease's management, serving as a route map for the construction of a personalized medication regimen [1]. The different clinical phases of illness classification based on observed clinical signs have been explored. This critical phase necessitates extensive and impartial investigation and comprehension of the changes that the disease produces due to complicated metabolic activities and seen in biomarkers [2]. In addition to distinguishing between typically normal and aberrant cellular disease conditions, biomarkers could be useful in providing knowledge of disease severity and stage and help in designing new therapeutic and pharmaceutical medicines [3]. As a result, there is an ongoing need to develop, test, and validate assays in the future for both identified and undiscovered biomarkers for specific disorders. Diseases often include complex cellular and molecular changes, as well as complicated etiology and pathophysiology profiles. Extensive studies related to quantitative techniques are frequently employed to detect comprehensively the physiological and chemical intricacies of disease-associated biomarkers suggestive of normal or diseased states (e.g. in biofluids, tissues, etc) [4]. Researchers strive to search for and describe a range of biomarkers to boost patient outcomes to therapy, prevent diseases, and create novel treatments.

Metabolites are extracted from complex sample mixtures and the obtained metabolites are detected using mass spectrometry (MS) and gas chromatography (GC) [5]. The conventional methods, such as liquid chromatography and mass spectrometry, can indeed contribute significantly to the finding of diagnostics and pathophysiological mechanisms [6]. LC–MS is used to detect metabolomics bio-markers [7]. Multiparameter methods aid in the development of biomarkers and the discovery of intricate metabolic pathways and processes that underlie disease. Metabolites, nucleic acids, and proteins, for example, are biomarkers that can be detected straightforwardly, quickly, specifically, and sensitively [8]. For diagnosing diseases with disease-specific biomolecule alterations, GC–MS and LC–MS are not economically viable methods [9]. To improve therapeutic efficacy, patient compliance, and reduce drug toxicity, treatment drug monitoring (TDM) is necessary [10]. TDM requires non-invasive, portable equipment with affordable running costs per sample analysis. Demand has led to an upsurge in high-throughput approaches to detecting target biomarkers.

Surface-enhanced Raman scattering (SERS) has drawn a lot of attention as a powerful cutting-edge platform for disease diagnostics at the molecular level because of its improved specificity and quantitative sensitivity [11]. SERS is a form of nano-based infrared spectroscopy that amplifies Raman signals and also enables trace studies of therapeutically significant proteins at room temperature. It combines Raman spectroscopy with plasmonic nanoparticles. Currently, there is a lot of interest in the development of portable handheld Raman devices and reproducible enhancing substrates, which are guiding SERS for point-of-care (POC) biosensing. This could help with biosafety concerns about delivering contagious biological material to laboratories, particularly during an epidemic of an extremely infectious disease. Two-dimensional nanomaterial improved nano-sensors have shown promise in the detection of several disease-specific biomarkers [12]. Furthermore, because of SERS's intrinsic specificity and ultra-sensitivity, subclinical conditions such as pancreatic cancer, which does not manifest symptoms until late in the disease, could be clinically diagnosed with greater specificity [13].

SERS has now been effectively employed in a variety of domains ever since its inception, along with environmental [14], antimicrobial resistance [15], food [16], and pharmaceutical [17] setting. As an intriguing research hypothesis approach for disease characterization in biological fluids, animal cells, and tissues *in vitro* and *in vivo*, SERS, on the other hand, has only lately come to light [18]. SERS patterns provide detailed information on the molecular structures and concentration variations that distinguish different illnesses with minimal sample processing. SERS has produced encouraging findings in the determination of worldwide nucleotide patterns for sick and healthy states by combining human biofluids with bare NPs directly [19]. The plasma of blood from individuals with nasopharyngeal carcinoma and control subjects were distinguished from one another by Feng *et al* with a classification sensitivity of 90.7% and specificity of 100% [20]. Similarly, Shao *et al* employed SERS fingerprints which were discovered by combining Ag colloidal fluid and blood with a congenital Raman device equipped with a 785 nm laser intensity to distinguish between cohorts of people with liver disease and healthy individuals [21].

Further research suggests SERS's responsiveness, yet it ought to be mentioned that because SERS picks up signals from all the biomolecules in a clinical specimen, non-directional biomarker detection in chemically varied materials is difficult [22]. SERS spectral data are therefore combinations of complicated stretching vibrations, which are difficult to evaluate and adapt to targeted treatments. In varied situations, non-invasive SERS physiological indicators need not reflect the structural character of the true diagnostic biomarkers. We emphasize that chemical/molecular specificity along with the technique's ultra-sensitivity frequently serve as SERS' primary analytical strengths in clinical diagnostics. Targeting recognized biomarkers established previously using alternative methods such as GC–MS or LC–MS, polymerase chain reaction (PCR) is an important tool to maximize the benefits of SERS. For instance, Subaihi and associates separated therapeutic drugs in human urine using reversed-phase LC, then validate their accuracy by utilizing SERS [23]. Furthermore, the SERS technique, which Graham, Faulds, and others have used extensively [24], detects specific illness indicators. In this instance, SERS-active reporter molecules and recognition components adsorbed on the NP surface are used to detect SERS signals indirectly from the target analytes. Notably, Gracie *et al* extended the previously reported picomolar quantitative detection of actual meningitis pathogens [25] by using AgNPs labeled with a fluorescent reporter and biotin modification probes to detect multiple DNA sequences extracted from meningitis etiological agents in clinical samples [26]. SERS produces analyte-specific characteristic peaks with just an exceptionally limited range and a fluorescence-free baseline. SERS can provide 'yes' or 'no' answers to diagnostic questions about the presence or absence of sickness in this situation, as well as quantitative data based on specific single or multiple biomarkers. When used to its full potential SERS is, without a doubt, an excellent candidate for fast and precise qualitative and qualitative diagnostics, in addition to the analysis of unique clinical markers to disclose a variety of infection stages and severity.

The main aim of the current chapter is to provide an overview of the SERS-based advanced integrated platform. Further, its potential relevance as a sensitive and information-rich bioanalytical platform for quick disease detection using specific biomarkers has been discussed.

12.2 Surface-enhanced Raman scattering: a brief overview

Smekal theorized the Raman effect in 1923 and Sir C V Raman discovered and confirmed it empirically using simple optical components and proposed a model in 1928 [27]. Raman spectroscopy is a type of visual reading platform that employs the scattering of irradiated light after interacts with polarized molecules even when being probed by a one-color light source. Because the large bulk of scattered photons possesses the same intensity as the input light (known as Rayleigh scattering —Rayleigh scattering is the deflection of electromagnetic energy by objects with a radius smaller than one-tenth the frequency of the light), they cannot communicate important biochemical information [28]. Consequently, during traditional Raman spectroscopy only a tiny percentage of the nascent photons are inflexibly scattered (Raman scattering), the photons of reduced intensity than incoming radiation (Stokes scattering) being collected. Raman spectroscopy equipment has evolved greatly in both technical and physical terms throughout the years. Raman spectroscopy is becoming more popular and accessible in the fields of biotechnology and biochemistry because of strong and stable lasers, new monitoring systems, fiber optics, and software technology. Despite this, the Raman effect scattering remains very efficient, with an exchange of photons rate of fewer than one out of every 10^6–10^8 input photons. High energy thickness, lengthy collecting periods, and clinically implausible doses are typically necessary to obtain acceptable signal-to-noise ratios in spectral response. Fluorescence and photodegradation are typically initiated under measurement conditions, masking Raman spectral lines, which restricts the applicability of Raman spectroscopy, specifically, when it is used to identify illnesses in biofluids or cells when biomarkers could be expressed at trace levels and high specimen purity is required [29]. It is encouraging that SERS is currently receiving significant attention to circumvent the fundamental inefficiencies of standard spectroscopic techniques.

Fleischmann and colleagues at the University of Southampton (UK) discovered the SERS phenomenon accidentally in 1974. They observed that Raman emissions in a pyridine mono-layer accumulated on electrochemical process abrasive regions over Ag electrodes increased [30]. That aberrant finding was believed to be triggered by the higher surface area of rough silver electrodes and also the current enhanced local concentrations of deposited pyridine molecules. The discovery inaugurated a brand-new era of physical and surface chemistry and piqued the curiosity of quantitative engineers and scientists.

At present, there is no detailed explanation for the SERS phenomenon [32]. In principle, SERS involves the interaction of electromagnetic energy and biomolecules deposited on or around nanometer-sized rough metallic particles that have diameters less than the spectrum of stimulation radiation [33, 34] (figure 12.1). Even though no detailed definition for the SERS phenomenon has been found to date, independent experiments have been done by Van Duyne and Creighton in which the configuration of biomolecules deposited on the metallic surface revealed two simultaneously operating theories [39]. The electromagnetic (EM) theory, which is thought to be the primary method, is a physiological process that requires the visual excitation of an applied electric field and charged movements induced by collective oscillations of electrons within the conduction band of NPs (surface plasmon). This step creates 'hotspots' of localized plasmon resonance surface (LSPR) near NP surfaces [40]. As a consequence, whenever the Raman lines come into contact with LSPR, they create increased spectrum emissions having enhancement factors of 106–108 when compared to standard Raman lines. The SERS

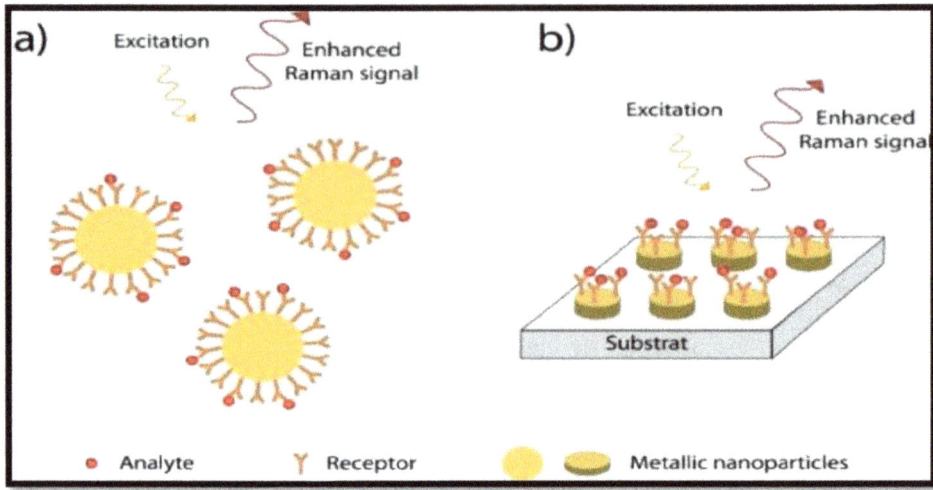

Figure 12.1. Principle of SERS sensors (a) in solution or (b) on the surface. (Reproduced with permission from [84]. CC BY 4.0.)

intensity (I) is exactly equal to the fifth degree of the local electromagnetic intensity, according to EM theory [41]. The function of E that is fE $(1/d)12$ fluctuates inversely towards the distance (d) among reactant as well as nanoparticle surfaces. As per the complex EM equation, with small variations in d and E leading to huge increases in I. An optimal SERS is achieved whenever an acceptable number of substances are inside regions with significant LSPR, inside the interlayer space of aggregate nanoparticles [42].

Charge-transfer or chemical enhancement (CM) is the second approach, and it is predicated on a resonance Raman scattering-like phenomenon. It shows that electrical stimulation of covalent bond associated conduction electrons inside chemical bonding created among solutes and the NPs surfaces is implicated. CM enhances the polarizability of physical adsorption and individual creativity by 10^3 orders magnitude for the overall SERS EF [35]. In contrast to CM, EM is a relevant process when biomolecules are covalently linked to nanoparticles, which occurs often at mono-layer coverage. It is also important to mention how to get a fluorescent dye bridge, the Raman effect may well be set to 10^{14} magnitude order [36]. This would be performed via excitation of the electrically excited state of specific chromophores near or bonded to the particle surface, which results in surface-enhanced resonance Raman scattering (SERRS). Overall, numerous experimental factors, including laser wavelength, NP shape, and dispersion medium, must be modified to obtain this ideally large SERS amplification. Importantly, appropriately aggregated NPs, excitation frequencies that coincide with the plasmonic band of the NPs, and enhancing media with a low refractive index all result in significant and repeatable EFs [37]. The consistency and reliability of SERS are greatly improved when flow injections plus microfluidics capabilities are combined [38]. Microfluidics devices are made up of microchannels that equally combine a tiny amount of material using nanoparticles moving at a steady and controlled rate [39–44]. Combined microfluidics–SERS removes the consequences of nanoparticle diffraction caused by regional warming, photodissociation, etc. Recent research has focused on building microfluidic SERS to improve *in situ* biosensors, which is critical for the use of therapeutic SERS in medical services [29].

12.3 Biochemical molecule affinity of SERS-active substrates

Rough surfaces of metal, thin steel films, and colloid NPs are among the hard and scattered surfaces currently used as SERS augmentation media. Colloids formed on metals (Au and Ag) are used extensively in biotechnological investigations because of their simplicity of fabrication and customization, and because they are relatively inexpensive, have excellent durability, and possess a large EF [29]. Furthermore, Au and Ag nanoparticles are naturally drawn to compounds containing highly electronegative or charging elements (e.g. nitrogen, oxygen, sulfur, etc). Several markers, including metabolite, nucleotides, and peptides (the reactants, intermediates, and final products of genetically predetermined processes), exhibit strong SERS activity because they include a polarizable partially positive-conjugated complex including one or more electronegative elements [30, 31]. SERS may also detect centrosymmetric molecules since the symmetric molecular properties change once biomolecules are bound to the surfaces of nanoparticles. As a result of the deadlock concept, SERS has opened up brand-new pathways for utilizing distinctive diagnostic data acquired from symmetric markers that would otherwise have been unavailable via Raman or Fourier-transform infrared (FT-IR) spectroscopy.

SERS measurements are often performed using label-based and label-free techniques. The direct interactions of the analytes with NPs are assessed using intrinsic (or label-free) SERS [34]. The resulting spectral data include a wealth of essential data regarding the structure and dynamics of the system in molecules connected directly to nanoparticles. Extrinsic (or label-based) SERS, in contrast, integrates the optical activities of plasmonic substance (Ag, Au, Cu, and so on) surface modification with SERS-active chemical messengers (so-called Raman reporters) that are resonant with a broad range of stimulation wavelengths [29, 36]. This enables assessment of the NP surface, such as an enzyme, antibody, or aptamer, attached to epitopes of particular target solutes (for example, metabolites, nucleotides, or bacterium), and it also provides the enhanced characteristics. The Raman reporters record the SERS radiation directly. When several biodegradable identification components are utilized, extrinsic SERS detects biomarkers quantitatively and multiplexed in complicated liquid samples.

12.4 SERS-based integrated devices: a step towards the future

Optical biosensors provide an innovative approach for detecting viruses because their use is risk-free and uncomplicated and their technology is efficient and affordable. Furthermore, they do not require the amplification of nucleic acids.

Fluorescence, surface plasmons, and colorimetry were all employed previously to identify viruses including HIV, Ebola, norovirus, and influenza virus, to mention only a few [45, 46]. These methods have been used in nano-biosensors, which have enabled the targeted detection of viruses as well as the imaging of individual viruses and also in COVID-19 [24]. Diagnostic instruments that may be utilized at the point of care (POC) can also be optical biosensors [24, 47]. POC diagnostics make use of gathered samples rather than requiring sample preparation, allowing minimal costs for test production, and not requiring skilled personnel or costly analysis equipment. Only a few optical biosensors for viral detection are now on the market, mainly using lab-on-a-chip (LOC) methods for nucleotide amplification for fluorescence examination [48]. Improving optical imaging, in particular single viral imaging, would help in monitoring viral replication, cell contact, and discontinuation to develop therapy alternatives more swiftly. These imaging approaches are being researched to detect COVID-19 [49], but more effort is needed to bring them to the market. Optical biosensing can integrate detection with imaging, which, in addition to identifying a pathogen in biological samples, may give better knowledge of the disease [50]. It is critical to conduct timely and systematic assessments of emerging scientific and technological advances in the field of biosensing to create new sophisticated strategies for antibiotic recognition [41]. Optical bio-imaging is a technique that utilizes sophisticated optical technologies in conjunction with tracers that are pathogen-specific. This enables the targeting and detection of anomalies in the disease pathway at the molecular level. There are several benefits to optical bio-imaging compared to other common imaging technologies such as CT, MRI, and PET. Femtomolar sensitivities, large spatial resolution, non-invasiveness, non-ionizing scanning, inexpensive technology and labor, simplicity of mobilization, quantitative information, and a fast reaction time are among the benefits [51, 52]. Another application was seen under bio-generative engineering by 3D printing [26]. Direct imaging without any prior preparation of the materials presents several obstacles, even though it is advantageous for the investigation of biological matter produced *in vivo*. Loss of light directionality is caused by the presence of thick tissues in samples, which leads to a greater degree of scattering [53]. Because the thick biological tissues have high absorption, the light intensity is diminished; as a direct consequence of this, the signal-to-noise ratio suffers. The emission and excitation frequencies in the near-infrared window (NIR 1) (700–900 nm) or a secondary NIR window (NIR 2; 1.0–1.7 m) may aid in mitigating the absorbing and scattering characteristics that all these tissue samples exhibit [54]. The science of optical imaging has evolved to the point that it may be used as a testing method for a variety of viral diseases as a consequence of current research involving fluorescence monitoring and imaging, surface plasmonics, and interface Raman spectroscopy scattering [55]. The SERS effect, discovered in the 1970s, indicated that Raman scattering efficiency may be increased by up to 10^6 when the sample is placed on or near nano-textured surfaces of plasmonic metals [56]. Given optimal conditions, this enhanced Raman spectroscopy effectiveness has immense promise as an optical bio-imaging technique, enabling deep and detailed resolution, and volumetric scanning of biological materials. Solid surfaces coated with metal nanoparticles were produced and proposed as effective and reproducible SERS-active media [57]. SERS outperforms conventional advanced optical technologies in terms of sensitivity and molecular specificity. It was used to detect viral diseases such as West Nile disease, influenza, adenoviruses, and Rift Valley disease, among many others [58].

Thanks to their versatility, microfluidic devices have been demonstrated to be an effective method in the development of chemical processing. It offers various benefits in comparison to traditional batch-mode methods, which include rapid reaction kinetics, accurate manipulation of fluids, reduced reagent usage, automation, and more [59]. The concept of a 'lab on a chip' originates from the incorporation of downstream applications into the process of nanomaterial creation in microsystems. Surface-enhanced Raman spectroscopy (SERS) is an excellent illustration of what may be accomplished in combination with microfluidic devices [60]. Raman spectroscopy is a quick and non-label detection approach for nondestructive examination. It has depth information as well as a good transmission ratio. Raman spectroscopy may be used to analyse materials without destroying them [61]. Since most materials exhibit very weak Raman spectroscopy it has limited applications in the development of more effective sensor devices. The SERS approach, which boosts Raman scattering by a factor of ten thousand with the help of localized surface plasmon resonances brought about by metallic nanoparticles, can alleviate this problem [62, 63]. To a significant extent, the enhancement factor is determined by the nanoparticle features and the length, structure, and surface finish are examples of such characteristics. Microfluidics is used in SERS microfluidic systems to ensure accurate management of the synthesis of nanomaterials and also to produce on-site SERS-based detection with reduced cross-contamination and higher amplification factors, and make the implementation easier compared to traditional techniques [64–68]. Walter *et al*, for example, successfully showed a SERS-based microfluidic system that incorporates a laser microscopy configuration mounted on top of a small aperture to enable extremely precise recognition and detection of several strains of *Escherichia coli* [69]. To detect low concentrations of bacteria, Pazosperez *et al* used AgNPs as SERS amplifying indicators, and Raman spectroscopy would boost the signal for bacterium concentration by several orders of magnitude. A Raman microscope that used a 785 nm laser was used to identify and evaluate many strains of bacteria at a 10^6 colony forming unit concentration [70]. Other investigations have been reported by Madiyar *et al* on various SERS microfluidic platforms for the detection of many foodborne pathogens (e.g. *Listeria innocua, Salmonella typhimirium, S. enteritis, L. monocytogenes, Pseudomonas aeruginosa*, and methicillin-resistant *Staphylococcus aureus* (MRSA) 35 and 86) [71]. In 2015 Chen *et al* described a label-free near-infrared SERS (NIR-SERS) method for detecting pathogens in drinking water. The process is based on the creation of AgNPs in a bacterial cell solution *in situ*. It can identify *E. coli, P. aeruginosa*, MRSA, and *Listeria* spp., and it can attain a minimum limit of detection of 10^3 CFU ml^{-1} in 5 min [72]. Furthermore, one recent study suggested a microchannel of spiral shape for SERS-based molecular detection. They studied the connection geometry's effect on manufacturing efficiency to regulate particle size and minimize shear stress in microchannels, shown in figure 12.2. This enables high-resolution on-chip SERS sensing. The viability of microfluidic systems of SERS has been investigated. Only analyser compounds with a large dispersing cross-section, including rhodamine 6G (R6G) and crystal violet (CV), are used. Their proposed SERS microfluidic technology was utilized to identify an ssDNA sequence with 43% coding regions for application in the detection of cancer [73].

Another research group developed an immune-specific assay that uses SERS nanoprobes as the testing platform. Gold shells which are isolated nanoparticles, also known as Au-SHINs, were produced by combining gold nanoparticles measuring 100 nm in diameter with a silicon substrate shell 4 nm thick and coating it with Nile Blue (Raman reporter), shown in figure 12.3. The necessary SERS components were then coated with anti-ZIKV NS1 monoclonal antibodies before

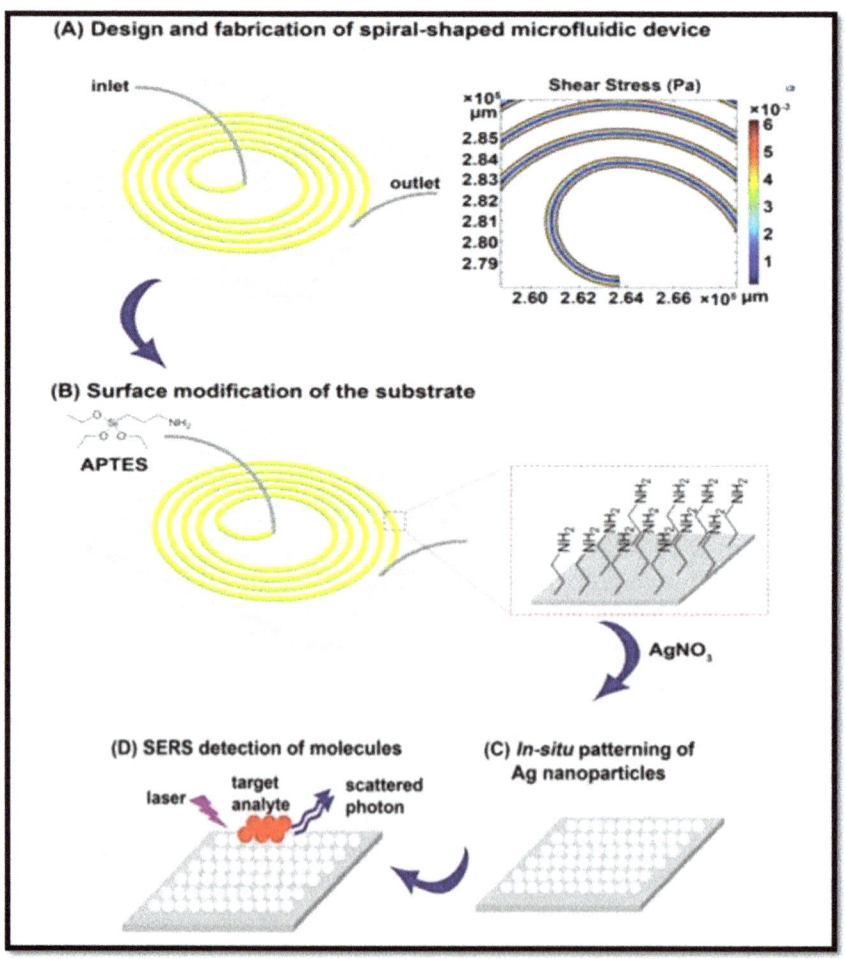

Figure 12.2. Biomolecular detection system schematic. (A) Fabrication of the microfluidic device, (B) surface modification, (C) *in situ* structuring of silver nanoparticles, and (D) on-chip SERS detection of biomolecules. (Reproduced with permission from [73]. Copyright 2021 American Chemical Society.)

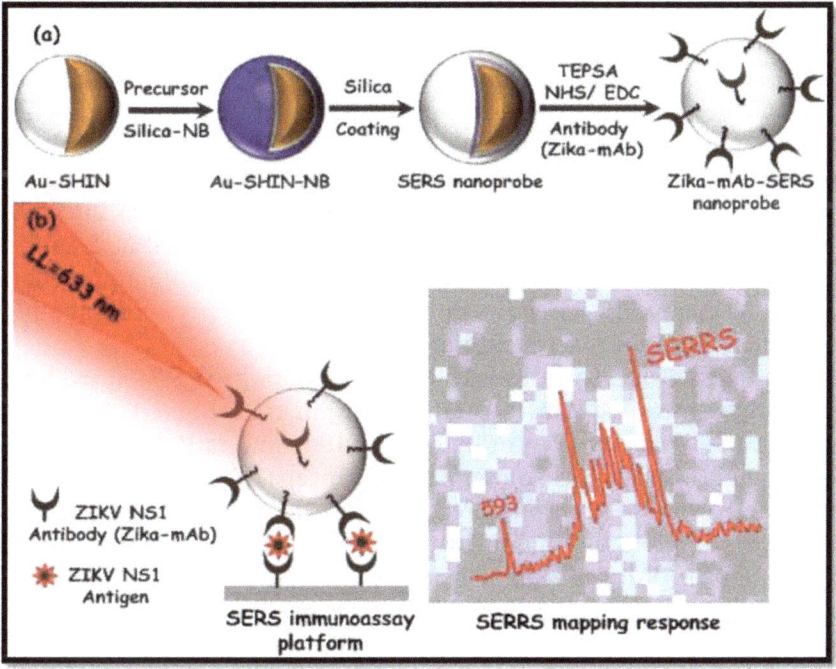

Figure 12.3. (a) Zika-mAb-SERS nanoprobe assembly diagram: Au-SHIN (100 nm Au core + 4 nm silica shell thickness); Au-SHIN + NB Raman reporter layer; Au-SHIN + NB Raman reporter layer + final 10 nm silica shell (SERS nanoprobe); conjugation onto Zika NS1 monoclonal antibodies (Zika-mAb). (b) SERS immunoassay platform for detecting various Zika NS1 concentrations. The platform is illuminated by a 633 nm laser line and the SERRS signal from NB molecules, which are situated nearby. Area mappings are used to record the proximity of gold nanoparticles (4 nm). Brighter areas imply greater NB band intensity at 593 cm^{-1}. (Reproduced with permission from [74]. Copyright 2018 American Chemical Society.)

being encapsulated in a protective silica shell. The cross-reaction between DENV NS1 and ZIKV NS1 antigens was not detected at concentrations of ZIKV NS1 as low as 10 ng ml^{-1} when it was examined [74].

He *et al* have developed a highly-sensitive, increased-efficiency, and practicable on-site UO_2^{2+} detecting SERS-based microfluidic biosensor for quick detection in actual samples. Uranyl ions (UO_2^{2+}) present substantial health and environmental concerns; hence its identification and monitoring are crucial. With the microfluidic-SERS biosensor, the lowest concentration of UO_2^{2+} that could be detected was 3.71×10^{-15} M. In the presence of 15 additional metal ions, a selectivity towards UO_2^{2+} reaction that was almost 20 000 times greater than previously was also attained. The recovery in polluted tap water and river water ranged from 95.2% to 106.3% for the high-throughput based microfluidic-SERS biosensor, which appears impressive in terms of real UO_2^{2+} identification (relative standard deviation (RSD) 6.0%, $n = 6$). Even though the SERS microfluidic biosensor that was created in this work was implemented to detect UO_2^{2+}, the high-efficiency and reusable system has the potential to be extended to detect various analytes on-site [75]. Leong *et al* designed a portable breathalyzer that identified COVID-19 patients in five minutes with >95% specificity and sensitivity across 501 individuals in a clinic case-control research study in Singapore, as illustrated in figure 12.4. The authors recorded significant changes in vibrational signatures caused by interactions between multiple molecular receptors and breath metabolites using the SERS-based breathalyzer and developed a classification algorithm for high-throughput spectrum studies based on partial least squares discriminant analysis (PLSDA), which was integrated with portable Raman instruments to provide an instant result (within 5 min, and no sample preparation was required). Through research and simulation, the authors discovered a substantial link between COVID-19 patients and breath volatile organic chemicals (BVOCs) as breath biomarkers [76].

Li *et al* designed a surface-enhanced Raman scattering (SERS)-based lateral flow assay (LFA) biosensor, aided by a catalytic hairpin assembly (CHA) amplification approach, for the dynamic monitoring of miR-106b and miR-196b, both of which have been linked to laryngeal squamous cell cancer (LSCC). Two hairpin DNAs may self-assemble into double-stranded DNA in the presence of target miRNAs, exposing the biotin molecules modified on the surface of palladium (Pd)–gold (Au) core–shell nanorods (Pd–AuNRs). This quick analytic technique was used successfully to find target miRNAs in clinical blood from healthy persons and patients with LSCC at various stages. The results agreed with the quantitative real-time PCR (qRT-PCR). As a result, the CHA-assisted SERS-LFA biosensor would emerge as a viable alternative technique for miRNA detection, with enormous practical application potential in detecting LSCC. The discussed SERS-LFA device schematic is shown in figure 12.5 [77].

Another group of researchers, Zheng *et al*, designed a microfluidic chip-based SERS immunoassay biosensor for the simultaneous detection of numerous breast cancer cell indicators in samples. An immunoassay uses tagged Ag-immune aggregates to identify breast cancer biomarkers in actual samples. Silver NPs are put on the SERS activated immune was extracted from the bottom of microfluidic chambers. To eliminate SERS signal crosstalk, they constructed a multi-channel on

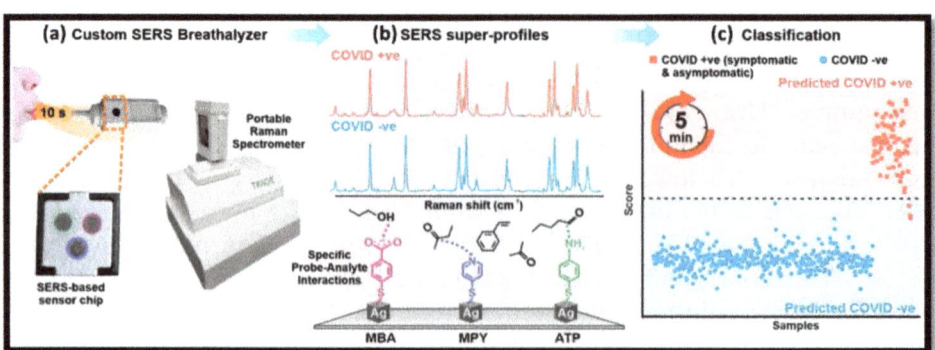

Figure 12.4. A schematic depicting the SERS-based approach for identifying COVID-positive individuals by using volatile organic compounds in their breath (BVOCs). (Reproduced with permission from [76]. Copyright 2022 American Chemical Society.)

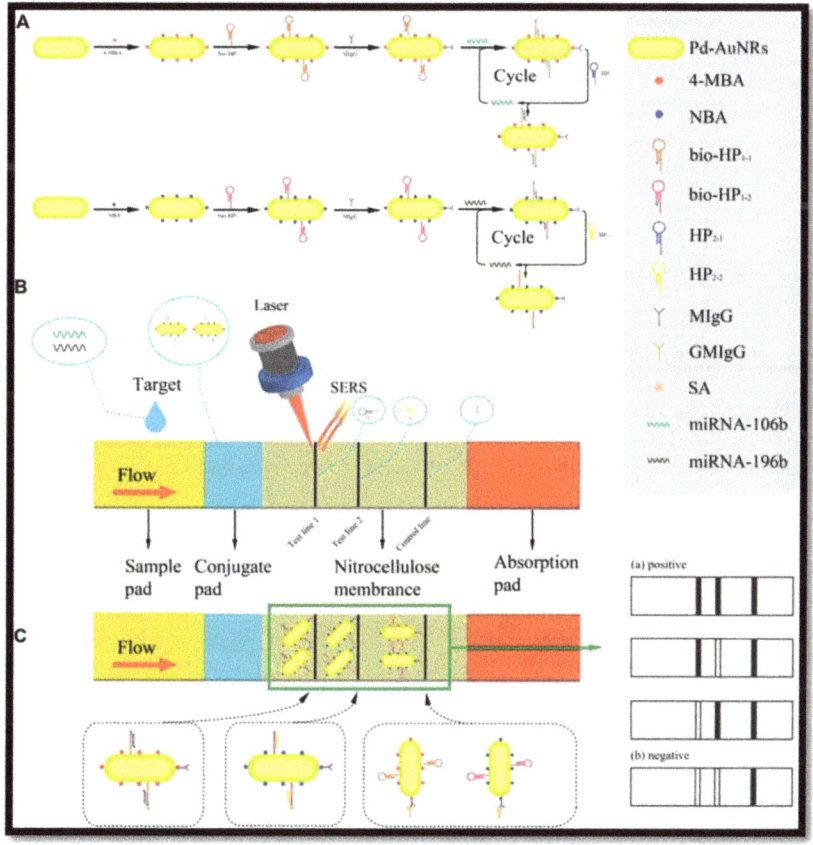

Figure 12.5. (A) Illustration of the synthesis technique for two SERS tags and the related CHA reaction concept. (B) A detailed example of how to assemble the test strips and the SERS-LFA biosensor for simultaneous detection of miR-106b and miR-196b. (C) The idea of the double-positive result, as well as schematics of additionally conceivable outcomes. (Reproduced with permission from [77]. CC BY 4.0.)

a microfluidic device. In the tests, CA153, CEA, and CA125, are used as biomarkers for breast cancer that may be identified simultaneously in human blood with good specificity and sensitivity [44]. Using linear regression, the suggested SERS micro-fluidic biosensor can identify biomarkers in actual samples [78]. Moreover, a multidisciplinary research project incorporating SERS spectroscopy, nanoparticles, and microfluidics is presented by Teixeira *et al*. By employing microfluidics to assemble NPs on paper, they created a paper-based sensing device with better efficiency and repeatability. A hybrid and modular PDMS-paper device was employed to deposit GNSs and Au@AgNRs. Using a reservoir-like PDMS device, unique anisotropy NPs self-build on a substrate surface, allowing for dynamic manipulation of hydrophilicity and evaporating. The sensitivity of Au@AgNRs and GNSs towards the Raman model molecule 1-naphthalenethiol (1-NAT) was 10–12 M for both. For example, PDMS-paper substrates have been used to lyse colorectal cancer and PBMC, as shown in figure 12.6 [79].

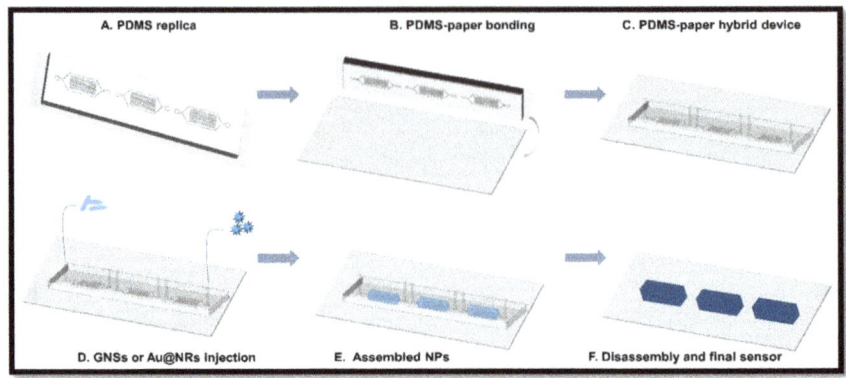

Figure 12.6. Diagram showing the manufacture of the hybrid PDMS-paper device (A)–(C), the injection and self-assembly of the NPs (D), and the injection of a Raman model molecule or lysed cells (E), before the paper sensor is finally disassembled for analysis (F). (Reproduced with permission from [79]. CC BY 4.0.)

SERS may detect an analyte's inherent fingerprint in a complex matrix. SERS sensing is one of the most promising analytical methods for on-site, label-free, nondestructive detection. However, many analytes and matrix substances have similar or overlapping spectra. Manually distinguishing them is either difficult or impossible. Hopefully, the use of machine learning (ML) will increase the efficacy of SERS considerably [85]. The uniformity of the SERS substrate's enhancement factor is critical for ML approaches, as substantial variance in the dataset raises the variance in predictions, limiting the methods to semiquantitative or quantitative analysis. With medium or large datasets, CNN consistently outperforms other ML algorithms in terms of prediction accuracy [80, 85]. Thrift and Ragan demonstrated that applying a CNN model to bundles of SERS spectra offers a robust, simple technique for concentration estimation down to 10 fM utilizing SM detection events as shown in figure 12.7. They also show that transfer learning or reusing the weights of a trained CNN model significantly decreases the quantity of data needed to train CNN models on new analyte molecules. These findings pave the way for the unambiguous interpretation of massive spectrum datasets, as well as the use of SERS in critical ultra-low concentration chemical detection applications such as metabolomic profiling, water quality monitoring, and basic research [80].

The spread of SARS-CoV-2, the pathogen causing COVID-19, is a worldwide public health problem. The key to controlling this illness is precise and timely SARS-CoV-2 antibody screening [81]. Liu *et al* described a SERS-LFIA-surface-enhanced Raman scattering-based lateral flow immunoassay for high-sensitivity anti-SARS-CoV-2 IgM/IgG detection. $SiO_2@Ag$ tags tagged with layers of Raman dye demonstrated excellent SERS signals, morphologies, and consistency (figure 12.8). Anti-human IgM and IgG were immobilized on the strip's test lines to collect anti-SARS-CoV-2 IgM/IgG immune complexes. Portable Raman instruments readily captured the SERS signal intensities of IgM and IgG test zones for high-sensitivity IgM and IgG analysis. SERS-LFIA showed a lowest detection limit for IgM and IgG 800 times greater than normal Au nanoparticle-based LFIA. The proposed

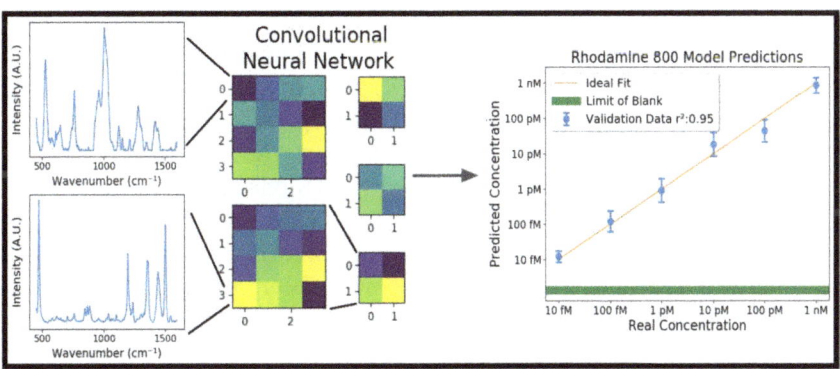

Figure 12.7. Pre-processed SERS spectrum with an R800 concentration of 1 μM. The inset depicts the 1441 cm^{-1} vibrational mode signal distribution of a 1 μM R800 dataset, an RSD of 13.1% is observed with a schematic of a CNN mode, and representative Rhodamine 800 concentration is predicted by the CNN model on a test dataset acquired during k-fold cross validation. (Reproduced with permission from [80]. Copyright 2019 American Chemical Society.)

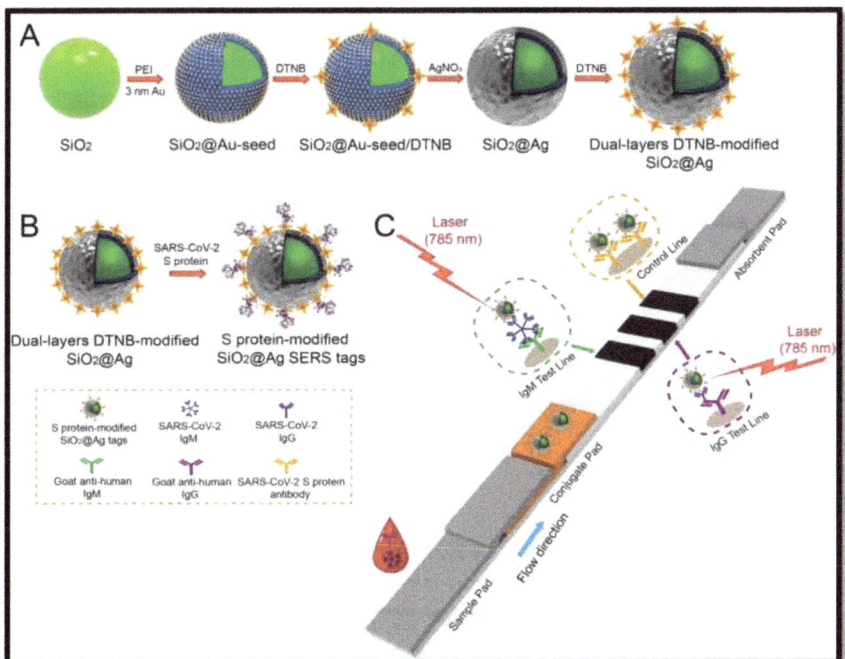

Figure 12.8. (A) Diagrammatic representation of the process used to make the dual-layer DTNB-modified SiO$_2$@AgNPs. (B) Making SiO$_2$@Ag SERS tags with SARS-CoV-2 S protein modifications. (C) The SERS-LFIA strip's great sensitivity and simultaneous analysis of anti-SARS-CoV-2 IgM/IgG [82].

assay was evaluated on 19 positive serum samples from COVID-19 patients and 49 negative serum samples from healthy persons. The approach showed good accuracy and specificity for SARS-CoV-2 patients [82].

Anti-spike antibodies are detected in multifluid cellular compartments using three different types of SERS nanotags (AuNPs functionalized employing an identical Raman sensor compound along with an IgM, IgG, or IgA, capture antibodies). The detection test accurately finds the seropositive people while employing ELISA and SPR cross-reactivity of SARS-CoV-2 sera against the P.1 and B.1.617.2 VOCs studied. Chisanga *et al* recently investigated SERS-based tool to assess numerous bridges and the longevity of three isotypes (IgG, IgM, and IgA,) guided it against existing SARS-CoV-2 spike as well as P.1 and B.1.617.2 VOCs in a single blood serum native and mutated spike allergens have been immobilized on a sensing element in four spatially distributed channels using a portable SPR device micro-fluidic cell as shown in figure 12.9 [83, 84]. Microfluidics integrated systems have been employed widely for disease diagnostics [85–87]. A summary of reported SERS biosensors is provided in table 12.1.

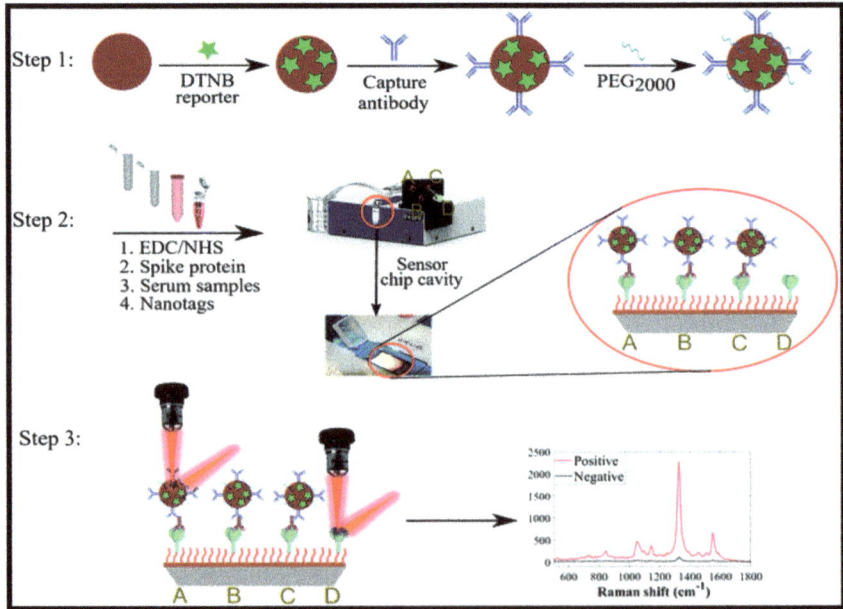

Figure 12.9. Diagram showing a multiplexed SERS detection technique. Step 1: Create nanotags (SERS-active). Step 2: Inactivation of several spike proteins onto the surface of a gold-coated biosensor using EDC/NHS chemistry in spatially separated fluidic channels: (A) native, (B) P.1, (C) B.1.617.2, and (D) followed by further anti-spike antibody detection using an evaluation and monitoring capturing antibody. To inject samples into the channels, sterile syringes were employed. Step 3: SERS was used to identify immunocomplexes; whenever the targeting antibody was abundant in patient blood serum and labeled as the A, B, and C channel, a high DTNB sign (positive, red trace) was found, however, when the targeted antibody was missing form the serum in the D channels, a weak signal (negative, black trace) was observed. It should be noted that the aforementioned approach is an exemplary IgG nanotag diagnostic methodology for anti-spike IgG. With the same synthesis pathways and detection techniques IgA and IgM antibodies were used, as well as the respective nanotags [83].

Table 12.1. Summary of the the reported SERS biosensors with targeted microorganisms, nanomaterials used, and limit of detection.

Sr. No.	Reported biosensors	Nanomaterial	Target	Limit of detection	Reference
1.	SERS in a microfluidic device for quick, high specificity, and consistent bacterial strain differentiation	Ag colloid	*E. coli*	—	[69]
2.	Immunodiagnostics depend on biosensing devices from the research lab to the point of care	AgNPs	Bacterial strains	10^6 CFU ml^{-1}	[70]
3.	Foodborne pathogen diagnosis at the point of care using SERS	—	*E. coli, Salmonella typhimurium, methicillin-resistant*	10 CFU ml^{-1}	[71]
4.	Label-free NIR-SERS differentiation and detecting of foodborne pathogens via *in situ* Ag colloidal particle biosynthesis	Ag colloid	*E. coli, P. aeruginosa,* MRSA, and *Listeria* spp.	10^3 CFU ml^{-1}	[72]
5.	Microfluidic ground silver nanoparticle structuring *in situ* structure and chemical detection using Raman spectroscopy	Ag	Single-stranded DNA	—	[73]
6.	Zika immunoassay based on surface-enhanced Raman scattering nanoprobes	Au	Zika NS1	12.5 ng ml^{-1}	[74]
7.	Ultrasensitive uranyl ion measurement using a newly built slightly elevated SERS-based microvascular device	ZnO–Ag	Uranyl ion (UO$_2^{2+}$)	3.71×10^{-15} M	[75]
8.	Non-invasive and point-of-care surface-enhanced Raman scattering (SERS)-based breathalyzer for mass screening of coronavirus disease 2019 (COVID-19) under 5 min	AgNPs	Breath volatile organic compounds (BVOCs)	—	[76]

No.	Description	Material	Target	Value	Ref.
9.	SERS-based lateral flow assay for rapid and ultrasensitive quantification of dual laryngeal squamous cell carcinoma-related miRNA biomarkers in human serum using Pd–Au core–shell nanorods and catalytic hairpin assembly	Palladium (Pd)–gold (Au) core–shell nanorods (Pd–AuNRs)	miR-106b and miR-196b, associated with laryngeal squamous cell carcinoma (LSCC)	—	[77]
10.	Identification of several breast melanoma indicators in real-time and at great sensitivity that used a SERS microfluidic chip	AgNPs	CA153, CA125, and CEA breast cancer biomarkers	CA153 and CA125 = 0.01 U ml^{-1} CEA ~ 1 pg ml^{-1}	[78]
11.	Manufacturing of a minimal cost and ultrasensitive SERS-based paper biosensing machine using a microfluidic method	Gold silver nanorods (Au@AgNRs)	PBMCs and SW480	~10^{-2} M	[79]
12.	Quantification of analyte concentration in the single molecule regime using convolutional neural networks	AuNPs	Rhodamine 800	1 fM	[78]
13.	A SERS-based horizontal stream immunoassay for the quick and impacted identification of anti-SARS-CoV-2 IgM/IgG in clinical specimens has been developed	SiO$_2$@Ag	SARS-CoV-2	—	[79]
14.	In non-hospitalized individuals, a SERS-based test for multimodal assessment of cross-reactivity and retention of antibody against the spikes of both the native, P.1, and B.1.617.2 SARS-CoV-2 was developed	AuNPs	SARS-CoV-2, P.1 and B.1.617.2 VOCs	—	[81]

12.5 Conclusions and future outlook

In this chapter we provided examples of SERS and demonstrated how adaptable this technology is as a tool for disease diagnostics. Using this the SERS frequencies of biomarkers can be calculated for malignancies, systemic diseases, and lung diseases. Both direct and indirect SERS play critical roles in the focused analyses of specific indicators in individual biological fluids or cells, and their application has been expanded to diagnose various disorders. However, to use analytical skills fully and hasten the translation of SERS to the clinic, certain technological and methodological challenges must be addressed immediately. We know that the strength or area of the SERS signal is proportional to the number of solutes in the solution allowing for reliable statistical identification of disease. Repeatability and linearity are sometimes lost because of NP surface saturation in label-free SERS, when some compounds are beyond the LSPR, or because of radiation source instabilities or uneven progressive accumulation. In data analysis, an appropriate starting plan (international standard) can be used to standardize numerous indication ranges to a specific IS optimum. Because metabolite and standard solution spectral regions are impacted comparably, this reduces spectrum signal fluctuations, particularly where isotopologues have been used. Alternatively, the conventional addition approach can be utilized, which adjusts as per surrounding data. The quantitative diagnosis and prognosis of disorder markers in a healthcare situation would become more secure and reliable. A further aspect that might require more investigation to streamline SERS analysis is the application of functional labels, i.e. nanoparticles (label-based SERS), for direct determination of specific markers across complex settings.

The use of SERS in combination with simultaneous measurement instruments yields positive results as well; it is clear that SERS has extended applicability among diagnostic approaches and recovery, as well as sensitivity when compared to spectrometry and chromatography analysis for various biomarkers. Moreover, in recent times many substantial challenges have already been addressed, which include inappropriate interaction or interactions among untargeted species, Np, and collecting components. For resolving issues, layers of protection or cornerstone, and biocompatible coating materials like polymer and silica have now been utilized efficiently.

Another critical area of emphasis for future effective interpretation of biological SERS is the allocation of wavelength bands. Metabolomics and isotopic labeling investigations have been critical in understanding the major contributions of purines (adenine, guanine) and pyrimidines (cytosine, thymine, and uracil) to typical SERS spectral bands. Nonetheless, consistent operating methods and a uniform referencing library of biomaterials for SERS are still needed to enable consistency, simplicity, and an in-depth understanding of molecular mechanics and energy metabolism. Also, it is essential to note that SERS would be proven useful and agreeable to clinicians simply if existing issues are properly resolved. The SERS community should strive to provide preliminary details such as sample processing, NP production and their properties, how NPs and solutes are placed in direct contact, the high-intensity wavelength used, sensor fusion parameters, and data management engaged as a component of the minimal level disclosure rules.

Finally, according to recent discoveries, theranostics, he simultaneous diagnosis and treatment of illness, is a new and exciting field of diagnostic techniques wherein SERS could play a key role. Because their Ag- and AuNPs have wide bandwidth performance and huge potential for putting into operation, they are appealing for illness diagnostics, photothermal treatment, and TDM. This means that nano-particles can concurrently be administered along with restorative drugs to respective designated targets, with visual intensification, and fast quantifiable disease assess-ment at detectable levels. Because of their great biocompatibility, AuNPs may move across cell components into the cytoplasm, providing a picture of internal chemical activities and metabolomic patterns. Whether paired with mechanized microfluidic devices or LOC sensors and advanced computer vision, SERS could enable a real-time in/off/online system for monitoring targeted therapy activities and patients' reactions to innovative drugs. A theranostics–SERS interface, in combination with machine variant analysis (MVA) clearly seems to have the ability to change patient safety, antimicrobial resistance (AMR) biochemistry, and drug discovery in the coming years by expanding clinicians' diagnosis and therapeutic toolkits.

Acknowledgments

The authors would like to thank the Director of CSIR-Advanced Materials and Process Research AMPRI Bhopal, India, for his attention and encouragement in this effort. AP's fellowship under the DST-WoS-B (DST/WOS-B/HN-4/2021) initiative is gratefully thanked. RK would like to thank the Science and Engineering Research Board (SERB) for funding the IPA/2020/000130udy.

References

[1] Vogenberg F R, Barash C I and Pursel M 2010 Personalized medicine: part 1: evolution and development into theranostics *P&T* **35** 560

[2] Condrat C E *et al* 2020 miRNAs as biomarkers in disease: latest findings regarding their role in diagnosis and prognosis *Cells* **9** E276

[3] Dhama K *et al* 2019 Biomarkers in stress related diseases/disorders: diagnostic, prognostic, and therapeutic values *Front. Mol. Biosci.* **6** 91

[4] Gonzalez-Covarrubias V, Martínez-Martínez E and Bosque-Plata L 2022 The potential of metabolomics in biomedical applications *Metabolites* **12** 194

[5] Shpatov A V, Tatyana S F, Popov S A, Sinitsyna O I, Salnikova O I, Zheng G, Yan L, Sinelnikova N V, Pshennikova L M and Kochetov A V 2020 Lipophilic metabolites from five-needle pines, *Pinus armandii* and *Pinus kwangtungensis*, exhibiting antibacterial activity *Chem. Biodivers.* **17** e2000201

[6] Chandramouli K and Qian P-Y 2009 Proteomics: challenges, techniques and possibilities to overcome biological sample complexity *Hum. Genomics Proteomics* **8** 239204

[7] Roca M, Alcoriza M I, Garcia-Cañaveras J C and Lahoz A 2021 Reviewing the metabolome coverage provided by LC–MS: focus on sample preparation and chromatography—a tutorial *Anal. Chim. Acta* **1147** 38–55

[8] Xu Y, Hassan M M, Sharma A S, Li H and Chen Q 2021 Recent advancement in nano-optical strategies for detection of pathogenic bacteria and their metabolites in food safety *Crit. Rev. Food Sci. Nutr.* **63** 486–504

[9] Gebara N *et al* 2022 Single extracellular vesicle analysis in human amniotic fluid shows evidence of phenotype alterations in preeclampsia *J. Extracell. Vesicles* **11** e12217

[10] Escudero-Ortiz V, Domínguez-Leñero V, Catalán-Latorre A, Rebollo-Liceaga J and Sureda M 2022 Relevance of therapeutic drug monitoring of tyrosine kinase inhibitors in routine clinical practice: a pilot study *Pharmaceutics* **14** 1216

[11] Liang X, Li N, Zhang R, Yin P, Zhang C, Yang N, Liang K and Kong B 2021 Carbon-based SERS biosensor: from substrate design to sensing and bioapplication *NPG Asia Mater.* **13** 8

[12] Parihar A, Singhal A, Kumar N, Khan R, Khan M and Srivastava A K 2022 Next-generation intelligent MXene-based electrochemical aptasensors for point-of-care cancer diagnostics *Nano-Micro Lett.* **14** 100

[13] Rawla P, Sunkara T and Gaduputi V 2019 Epidemiology of pancreatic cancer: global trends, etiology and risk factors *World J. Oncol.* **10** 10

[14] Zhao L, Zhu D, Shafik W, Mojtaba Matinkhah S, Ahmad Z, Sharif L and Craig A 2022 Artificial intelligence analysis in cyber domain: a review *Int. J. Distrib. Sens. Netw.* **18** 15501329221084882

[15] Tjandra K C, Ram-Mohan N, Abe R, Hashemi M M, Lee J-H, Mei Chin S, Roshardt M A, Liao J C, Kin Wong P and Yang S 2022 Diagnosis of bloodstream infections: an evolution of technologies towards accurate and rapid identification and antibiotic susceptibility testing *Antibiotics* **11** 511

[16] Xu M-L, Gao Y, Han X-X and Zhao B 2022 Innovative application of SERS in food quality and safety: a brief review of recent trends *Foods* **11** 2097

[17] Yilmaz H, Yilmaz D, Taskin I C and Culha M 2022 Pharmaceutical applications of a nanospectroscopic technique: surface-enhanced Raman spectroscopy *Adv. Drug Delivery Rev.* **184** 114184

[18] Liu H, Gao X, Xu C and Liu D 2022 SERS tags for biomedical detection and bioimaging *Theranostics* **12** 1870

[19] Aitekenov S, Sultangaziyev A, Abdirova P, Yussupova L, Gaipov A, Utegulov Z and Bukasov R 2022 Raman, infrared and Brillouin spectroscopies of biofluids for medical diagnostics and for detection of biomarkers *Crit. Rev. Anal. Chem.* 1–30

[20] Feng S, Chen R, Lin J, Pan J, Chen G, Li Y, Cheng M, Huang Z, Chen J and Zeng H 2010 Nasopharyngeal cancer detection based on blood plasma surface-enhanced Raman spectroscopy and multivariate analysis *Biosens. Bioelectron.* **25** 2414–9

[21] Shao Q, Zhang X, Liang P, Chen Q, Qi X and Zou M 2022 Fabrication of magnetic Au/Fe$_3$O$_4$/MIL-101 (Cr)(AF-MIL) as sensitive surface-enhanced Raman spectroscopy (SERS) platform for trace detection of antibiotics residue *Appl. Surf. Sci.* **596** 153550

[22] Sinha A, Basu M and Chandna P 2022 Paper based microfluidics: a forecast toward the most affordable and rapid point-of-care devices *Prog. Mol. Biol. Transl. Sci.* **186** 109–58

[23] Lewis M *et al* 2022 An open platform for large scale LC–MS-based metabolomics *ChemRxiv* 10.26434/chemrxiv-2022-nq9k0

[24] Sloan-Dennison S, O'Connor E, Dear J W, Graham D and Faulds K 2022 Towards quantitative point of care detection using SERS lateral flow immunoassays *Anal. Bioanal. Chem.* **414** 4541–9

[25] Gracie K, Correa E, Mabbott S, Dougan J A, Graham D, Goodacre R and Faulds K 2014 Simultaneous detection and quantification of three bacterial meningitis *Chem. Sci.* **5** 1030–40

[26] Sharma N, Gautam H, Tyagi S, Raza S, Mohapatra S, Sood S, Dhawan B, Kapil A and Das B K 2022 Clinical use of multiplex-PCR for the diagnosis of acute bacterial meningitis *J. Family Med. Prim. Care* **11** 593

[27] Kademani B S, Kalyane V L and Kademani A B 1994 Scientometric portrait of Nobel Laureate Dr CV Raman *Indian J. Inf. Libr. Soc.* **7** 215–49

[28] Young A T 1981 Rayleigh scattering *Appl. Opt.* **20** 533–5

[29] Chisanga M, Muhamadali H, Ellis D I and Goodacre R 2019 Enhancing disease diagnosis: biomedical applications of surface-enhanced Raman scattering *Appl. Sci.* **9** 1163

[30] Kumar Sur U 2013 Surface-enhanced Raman scattering (SERS) spectroscopy: a versatile spectroscopic and analytical technique used in nanoscience and nanotechnology *Adv. Nano Res.* **1** 111

[31] Eustis S and El-Sayed M A 2006 Why gold nanoparticles are more precious than pretty gold: noble metal surface plasmon resonance and its enhancement of the radiative and non-radiative properties of nanocrystals of different shapes *Chem. Soc. Rev.* **35** 209–17

[32] Polubotko A M 1990 SERS phenomenon as a manifestation of quadrupole interaction of light with molecules *Phys. Lett.* A **146** 81–4

[33] Wang C, Zhao X-P, Xu Q-Y, Nie X-G, Younis M R, Liu W-Y and Xia X-H 2018 Importance of hot spots in gold nanostructures on direct plasmon-enhanced electrochemistry *ACS Appl. Nano Mater.* **1** 5805–11

[34] Nguyen V-Q, Ai Y, Martin P and Lacroix J-C 2017 Plasmon-induced nanolocalized reduction of diazonium salts *ACS Omega* **2** 1947–55

[35] Cong S, Liu X, Jiang Y, Zhang W and Zhao Z 2020 Surface enhanced Raman scattering revealed by interfacial charge-transfer transitions *Innovation* **1** 100051

[36] Xu H, Wang X-H, Persson M P, Xu H Q, Käll M and Johansson P 2004 Unified treatment of fluorescence and Raman scattering processes near metal surfaces *Phys. Rev. Lett.* **93** 243002

[37] Ding S-Y, You E-M, Tian Z-Q and Moskovits M 2017 Electromagnetic theories of surface-enhanced Raman spectroscopy *Chem. Soc. Rev.* **46** 4042–76

[38] Yang K, Zhang S, Zhang G, Sun X, Lee S-T and Liu Z 2010 Graphene in mice: ultrahigh *in vivo* tumor uptake and efficient photothermal therapy *Nano Lett.* **10** 3318–23

[39] Sen A K, Nath A, Sudeepthi A, Jain S K and Banerjee U 2022 Microfluidics-based point-of-care diagnostic devices *Advanced Microfluidics-Based Point-of-Care Diagnostics* (Boca Raton, FL: CRC Press), pp 99–120

[40] Singhal A, Parihar A, Kumar N and Khan R 2022 High throughput molecularly imprinted polymers based electrochemical nanosensors for point-of-care diagnostics of COVID-19 *Mater. Lett.* **306** 130898

[41] Parihar A, Ranjan P, Sanghi S K, Srivastava A K and Khan R 2020 Point-of-care biosensor-based diagnosis of COVID-19 holds promise to combat current and future pandemics *ACS Appl. Bio Mater.* **3** 7326–43

[42] Singhal A, Sadique M A, Kumar N, Yadav S, Ranjan P, Parihar A, Khan R and Kaushik A K 2022 Multifunctional carbon nanomaterials decorated molecularly imprinted hybrid polymers for efficient electrochemical antibiotics sensing *J. Environ. Chem. Eng.* **10** 107703

[43] Parihar A, Pandita V, Kumar A, Parihar D S, Puranik N, Bajpai T and Khan R 2021 3D printing: advancement in biogenerative engineering to combat shortage of organs and bioapplicable materials *Regen. Eng. Transl. Med.* **8** 173–99

[44] Ranjan P *et al* 2020 Biosensor-based diagnostic approaches for various cellular biomarkers of breast cancer: a comprehensive review *Anal. Biochem.* **610** 113996

[45] Kadadou D, Tizani L, Wadi V S, Banat F, Alsafar H, Yousef A F, Barceló D and Hasan S W 2021 Recent advances in the biosensors application for the detection of bacteria and viruses in wastewater *J. Environ. Chem. Eng.* **10** 107070

[46] Saylan Y, Erdem Ö, Ünal S and Denizli A 2019 An alternative medical diagnosis method: biosensors for virus detection *Biosensors* **9** 65

[47] Pashchenko O, Shelby T, Banerjee T and Santra S 2018 A comparison of optical, electro-chemical, magnetic, and colorimetric point-of-care biosensors for infectious disease diagnosis *ACS Infect. Dis.* **4** 1162–78

[48] Zhuang J, Yin J, Lv S, Wang B and Mu Y 2020 Advanced 'lab-on-a-chip' to detect viruses–Current challenges and future perspectives *Biosens. Bioelectron.* **163** 112291

[49] Qiu G, Gai Z, Tao Y, Schmitt J, Kullak-Ublick G A and Wang J 2020 Dual-functional plasmonic photothermal biosensors for highly accurate severe acute respiratory syndrome coronavirus 2 detection *ACS Nano* **14** 5268–77

[50] Yao J, Yang M and Duan Y 2014 Chemistry, biology, and medicine of fluorescent nanomaterials and related systems: new insights into biosensing, bioimaging, genomics, diagnostics, and therapy *Chem. Rev.* **114** 6130–78

[51] Jin K-T, Yao J-Y, Ying X-J, Lin Y and Chen Y-F 2020 Nanomedicine and early cancer diagnosis: molecular imaging using fluorescence nanoparticles *Curr. Top. Med. Chem.* **20** 2737–61

[52] Faisal F, Nishat M M and Oninda M A M 2018 Spectroscopic characterization of biological tissue using quantitative acoustics technique *2018 4th Int. Conf. on Electrical Engineering and Information & Communication Technology (iCEEiCT)* (Piscataway, NJ: IEEE), pp 38–43

[53] Boas D A, Pitris C and Ramanujam N 2016 *Handbook of Biomedical Optics* (Boca Raton, FL: CRC Press)

[54] Li H, Wang X, Ohulchanskyy T Y and Chen G 2021 Lanthanide-doped near-infrared nanoparticles for biophotonics *Adv. Mater.* **33** 2000678

[55] Liu J, Jalali M, Mahshid S and Wachsmann-Hogiu S 2020 Are plasmonic optical biosensors ready for use in point-of-need applications? *Analyst* **145** 364–84

[56] Crawford B and Vo-Dinh T 2020 Plasmonic nanoparticles for cancer bioimaging, diag-nostics and therapy *21st Century Nanoscience—A Handbook* (Boca Raton, FL: CRC Press), pp 18–21

[57] Serebrennikova K V, Berlina A N, Sotnikov D V, Zherdev A V and Dzantiev B B 2021 Raman scattering-based biosensing: new prospects and opportunities *Biosensors* **11** 512

[58] Ambartsumyan O, Gribanyov D, Kukushkin V, Kopylov A and Zavyalova E 2020 SERS-based biosensors for virus determination with oligonucleotides as recognition elements *Int. J. Mol. Sci.* **21** 3373

[59] Liu Y and Jiang. X 2017 Why microfluidics? Merits and trends in chemical synthesis *Lab Chip* **17** 3960–78

[60] Garcia-Lojo D, Gomez-Grana S, Martin V F, Solis D M, Taboada J M, Perez-Juste J and Pastoriza-Santos I 2020 Integrating plasmonic supercrystals in microfluidics for

ultrasensitive, label-free, and selective surface-enhanced Raman spectroscopy detection *ACS Appl. Mater. Interfaces* **12** 46557–64

[61] Esmonde-White H J *et al* 2016 Using Raman spectroscopy to characterize biological materials *Nat. Protoc.* **11** 664–87

[62] Demirel G, Usta H, Yilmaz M, Celik M, Alidagi H A and Buyukserin F 2018 Surface-enhanced Raman spectroscopy (SERS): an adventure from plasmonic metals to organic semiconductors as SERS platforms *J. Mater. Chem.* C **6** 5314–35

[63] Pilot R, Signorini R, Durante C, Orian L, Bhamidipati M and Fabris L 2019 A review on surface-enhanced Raman scattering *Biosensors* **9** 57

[64] Fan M, Andrade G F S and Brolo A G 2020 A review on recent advances in the applications of surface-enhanced Raman scattering in analytical chemistry *Anal. Chim. Acta* **1097** 1–29

[65] Kumar S L 2021 Microfluidics technology for nanoparticles and equipment *Emerging Technologies for Nanoparticle Manufacturing* (Cham: Springer), pp 67–98

[66] Jahn I J, Žukovskaja O, Zheng X-S, Weber K, Bocklitz T W, Cialla-May D and Popp J 2017 Surface-enhanced Raman spectroscopy and microfluidic platforms: challenges, solutions and potential applications *Analyst* **142** 1022–47

[67] Wang H-L, You E-M, Panneerselvam R, Ding S-Y and Tian Z-Q 2021 Advances of surface-enhanced Raman and IR spectroscopies: from nano/microstructures to macro-optical design *Light Sci. Appl.* **10** 161

[68] Zhao Z, Chen C, Wei S, Xiong H, Hu F, Miao Y, Jin T and Min W 2021 Ultra-bright Raman dots for multiplexed optical imaging *Nat. Commun.* **12** 1305

[69] Walter A, März A, Schumacher W, Rösch P and Popp J 2011 Towards a fast, high specific and reliable discrimination of bacteria on strain level by means of SERS in a microfluidic device *Lab Chip* **11** 1013–21

[70] Poschenrieder A, Thaler M, Junker R and Luppa P B 2019 Recent advances in immuno-diagnostics based on biosensor technologies—from central laboratory to the point of care *Anal. Bioanal. Chem.* **411** 7607–21

[71] Madiyar F R, Bhana S, Swisher L Z, Culbertson C T, Huang X and Li J 2015 Integration of a nanostructured dielectrophoretic device and a surface-enhanced Raman probe for highly sensitive rapid bacteria detection *Nanoscale* **7** 3726–36

[72] Chen L, Mungroo N, Daikuara L and Neethirajan S 2015 Label-free NIR-SERS discrimination and detection of foodborne bacteria by *in situ* synthesis of Ag colloids *J. Nanobiotechnol.* **13** 45

[73] Nie Y, Jin C and Zhang J X J 2021 Microfluidic *in situ* patterning of silver nanoparticles for surface-enhanced Raman spectroscopic sensing of biomolecules *ACS Sens.* **6** 2584–92

[74] Camacho S A, Gomes Sobral-Filho R, Henrique P, Aoki B, José C, Constantino L and Brolo A G 2018 Zika immunoassay based on surface-enhanced Raman scattering nanoprobes *ACS Sens.* **3** 587–94

[75] He X, Wang S, Liu Y and Wang X 2019 Ultra-sensitive detection of uranyl ions with a specially designed high-efficiency SERS-based microfluidic device *Sci. China Chem.* **62** 1064–71

[76] Leong S X *et al* 2022 Noninvasive and point-of-care surface-enhanced Raman scattering (SERS)-based breathalyzer for mass screening of coronavirus disease 2019 (COVID-19) under 5 min *ACS Nano* **16** 2629–39

[77] Li G, Niu P, Ge S, Cao D and Sun A 2021 SERS based lateral flow assay for rapid and ultrasensitive quantification of dual laryngeal squamous cell carcinoma-related miRNA

biomarkers in human serum using Pd–Au core–shell nanorods and catalytic hairpin assembly *Front. Mol. Biosci.* **8** 813007

[78] Zheng Z, Wu L, Li L, Zong S, Wang Z and Cui Y 2018 Simultaneous and highly sensitive detection of multiple breast cancer biomarkers in real samples using a SERS microfluidic chip *Talanta* **188** 507–15

[79] Teixeira A, Hernández-Rodríguez J F, Wu L, Oliveira K, Kant K, Piairo P, Diéguez L and Abalde-Cela S 2019 Microfluidics-driven fabrication of a low cost and ultrasensitive SERS-based paper biosensor *Appl. Sci.* **9** 1387

[80] Thrift W J and Ragan R 2019 Quantification of analyte concentration in the single molecule regime using convolutional neural networks *Anal. Chem.* **91** 13337–42

[81] Coronaviridae Study Group of the International Committee on Taxonomy of Viruses 2020 The species severe acute respiratory syndrome-related coronavirus: classifying 2019-nCoV and naming it SARS-CoV-2 *Nat. Microbiol.* **5** 536–44

[82] Liu H *et al* 2021 Development of a SERS-based lateral flow immunoassay for rapid and ultra-sensitive detection of anti-SARS-CoV-2 IgM/IgG in clinical samples *Sensors Actuators* B **329** 129196

[83] Chisanga M *et al* 2022 SERS-based assay for multiplexed detection of cross-reactivity and persistence of antibodies against the spike of the native, P.1 and B.1.617.2 SARS-CoV-2 in non-hospitalised adults *Sens. Diagn.* **1** 851–66

[84] Boujday S, Chapelle M L, Srajer J and Knoll W 2015 Enhanced vibrational spectroscopies as tools for small molecule biosensing *Sensors* **15** 21239–64

[85] Cui F, Yue Y, Zhang Y, Zhang Z and Zhou H S 2020 Advancing biosensors with machine learning *ACS Sens.* **5** 3346–64

[86] Avinash K, Parihar A, Panda U and Parihar D S 2022 Microfluidics-based point-of-care testing (POCT) devices in dealing with waves of COVID-19 pandemic: the emerging solution *ACS Appl. Bio Mater.* **5** 2046–68

[87] Parihar A and Khan R 2022 3D printed human organoids for personalized medicine: high throughput system for drug screening and testing in current COVID-19 pandemic *Biotechnol. Bioeng.* **119** 2669–88

Ingram Content Group UK Ltd.
Milton Keynes UK
UKHW050736260523
422388UK00003B/46